Mental Health Dimensions of Self-Esteem and Emotional Well-Being

Joseph W. Donnelly

Montclair State University

Norm Eburne

Western Oregon University

Mark Kittleson

Southern Illinois University at Carbondale

Allyn & Bacon

Boston • London • Toronto • Sydney • Tokyo • Singapore

Vice president: Paul Smith
Series editor: Joe Burns
Series editorial assistant: Annemarie Kennedy
Composition and Prepress Buyer: Linda Cox
Cover administrator: Brian Gogolin
Photo researcher: Helane Manditch-Prottas
Editorial-production service: Shepherd, Inc.
Electronic composition: Shepherd, Inc.

Copyright © 2001 by Allyn & Bacon
A Pearson Education Company
Needham Heights, Massachusetts 02194

Internet: www.abacon.com

Library of Congress Cataloging-in-Publication Data

Donnelly, Joseph W.
    Mental health : dimensions of self-esteem and emotional well-being / by Joseph W.
  Donnelly, Norm Eburne, and Mark Kittleson.
       p. cm.
    Includes bibliographical references and index.
    ISBN 0-205-30955-0
      1. Mental health. 2. Psychology, Pathological. I. Eburne, Norm. II. Kittleson, Mark J.,
  1952- III. Ttile.

RA790 .D64 2001
616.89--dc21
                                                                        00-042093

Printed in the United States of America

10 9 8 7 6 5 4 3 2 1   05 04 03 02 01 00

CONTENTS

6 Communication and Social Well-Being   107

7 Stress   127

PREFACE

In the Fall of 1971, a young freshman enrolled in Dr. Norm Eburne's personal health class at Mankato State College (now Minnesota State University at Mankato). Eburne was a garden variety 1970's vintage young professor who had recently completed a doctoral program in which he conducted attitude assessments for the Psychiatric Research and Training Project of the Oregon Health Sciences University. With this background, he understandably infused his classes with mental health. This young student—Mark Kittleson—became very enthusiastic about health education, and he and Eburne initiated a connection that has lasted throughout these thirty years. After several classes together (as well as training runs over the roads of southern Minnesota), Norm became Mark's advisor and friend.

Mark graduated with a head full of the importance of mental health in health education and began his professional career. Norm moved to Oregon to become a Family Health Specialist with the Oregon State University Extension Service. About this time, another young man—Joseph Donnelly—was entering junior high school in the Chicago area. Mark Kittleson was now off to the University of Maine and then Youngstown State University to hone his craft as a health educator and to complete doctoral studies.

About the time Eburne moved to Western Oregon University (the Oregon College of Education) to initiate a health education major, Mark began work at Southern Illinois University–Carbondale. One of his first assignments was to the dissertation committee of a doctoral candidate named Joseph Donnelly. Donnelly's research focused on self-esteem, and Kittleson contacted his friend and old advisor Eburne, who was now doing some work with Mental Health and the American Family Project and the Center for the Study of Human Potential, to discuss some ideas. A circle of mentor–mentee (now mentor)–mentee was beginning to form.

Joseph had completed his doctorate, gone to work for Hofstra University and initiated postdoctoral training at Governor's State University in counseling by the time the three authors actually gathered together to discuss ideas about mental health and its role in the total human experience. In 1987, Dr. Kittleson published a relatively simple study regarding the status of mental health coverage in the most popular textbooks. His findings revealed that despite the perceived importance of certain topics, very little, if anything was covered in the most popular health textbooks. Most of the books then had a major focus on mental illness. In fact, the texts in use for most mental health courses are, in actuality, mental *illness* books.

Thus, the stage was set for the writing of a book that discusses mental health—a book written *by* health educators *for* health educators. Remarkably, the three authors have very similar beliefs regarding the scarcity of mental health texts and how these texts and their chapters should be structured. Despite their connection, how Norm, Mark, and Joseph obtained such beliefs is difficult to determine. Mark never recalls Dr. Eburne discussing this in any of his classes; Dr. Kittleson never formally discussed any of these issues with Joseph; and Dr. Donnelly never really discussed these issues with either Norm or Mark. It was through a continuing informal communication that each became aware of the frustration that existed and developed a burning desire to try to remedy this dearth of books.

In addition, the three felt that a mental health book should focus on mental health and on what constitutes a mentally healthy person. The consensus among the three men was that for people to be truly mentally healthy they needed to have positive self-esteem and realistic self-awareness; effective coping skills; clear communication skills; and good decision-making skills. They felt that a mentally healthy person needed to be a risk taker, a person who understood that to grow (emotionally, physically, or intellectually), risks had to be taken.

Thus, this book is based on those premises and other important components. The authors agree that mental health is vastly different from mental illness; however they also acknowledge the need for a chapter that discusses the more common mental and emotional problems that people encounter. Thus, the authors have included discussion on locating and using mental health resources. Finally, because of the incredible amount of research regarding the function of the brain, especially in the past fifteen years, the authors also include a discussion of the biomedical aspects of one's emotions.

In addition, the authors were adamant about using only the most up-to-date resources available. So, while some classic studies regarding mental health were identified, so were the latest studies. The authors also agreed on the importance of to having activities that focused on the major issues of particular chapters. The hope was to have at least one such activity per chapter, although some chapters have more.

The authors hope this book provides you with the necessary content and instructional strategies for entering the complex and ever-changing field of mental health. If you should have any questions or suggestions, please feel free to contact the authors.

Mark J. Kittleson, Ph.D.
Professor & Director of Graduate Studies
Department of Health Education and Recreation
Southern Illinois University
Home Page: http://www.kittle.siu.edu
HEDIR: http://www.hedir.siu.edu
IEJHE: http://www.iejhe.siu.ed

ACKNOWLEDGEMENTS

Many people need to be acknowledged in the completion of this book. Certainly all three of the authors' families had to deal with the incredible amount of time needed to complete such a task. Such support will be forever remembered. In addition, we are appreciative of the support provided to us by our editor, Joe Burns. Also special thanks to Tanja Eise, our assistant editor, for her continual willingness to respond to questions and provide guidance in this process. Further, we would like to recognize Danielle Castiglia for her preparation of Chapter 11, *Mental Health Resources and Helping Professions.* We offer additional thanks to Danielle Sorbello for keeping the three of us on track with countless details, guidelines, and chapter overviews. Wendy Hollenbeck deserves recognition for her contribution as chapter editor; her insightful suggestions have strengthened the transition of these twelve chapters. Carolyn Eadie's continual suggestions and support have added to the depth and scope of this project. These individuals did a great amount of the detail work, making sure that everything fit in well. Also, we would like to acknowledge our respective universities for continual support over the years: Dr. Joseph Donnelly, Montclair State University; Dr. Norm Eburne, Western Oregon University; Dr. Mark Kittleson, Southern Illinois University at Carbondale.

Finally, we—the authors—would like to acknowledge and thank each other, (not only for) our long-term friendships but also for our professional respect and expertise to help see this book through completion. It was very tough to work on something this difficult with personal friends, and, at times, each of us has had difficulty balancing such friendship with the professional demands of the project.

ABOUT THE AUTHORS

Joseph W. Donnelly, Ph.D., is a professor in the Department of Health Professions, Physical Education, Recreation, & Leisure Studies, Program of Health Professions at Montclair State University in Upper Montclair, New Jersey. He instructs courses within a variety of health-related areas, including, but not limited to, Teaching of Health Education; Bio-Medical, Psychosocial Perspectives on Drugs (graduate and undergraduate levels); and Mental Health. Additionally, courses that he has instructed at other universities include Health Counseling, Health Psychology, Mental Health, Stress Management, and Self-Esteem: Application and Theory.

He has conducted presentations on self-esteem, stress management, and motivational training for teachers, school administrators, and students. As the keynote presenter for the New York Counseling Association, he also has conducted several national, regional, and state presentations on a variety of health-related topics.

Dr. Donnelly has written numerous articles for health-related journals as well as the popular press. His expertise on topics such as mental health, self-esteem, and substance use and abuse have appeared in publications such as *Parents, Professional Counselor,* and *Self-Esteem Today,* as well as numerous health-related peer-review publications.

Before embarking on his teaching career, he obtained a Counseling and Psychology concentration at Governor State University in Chicago, Illinois. This enabled him to infuse the importance of mental well-being within a variety of health-related areas.

Norm Eburne, Ph.D., has been a professor in the area of health for over thirty years. His expertise lies in the psychosocial aspects of health behavior, in particular, the influence of values and attitudes on health-related decision making, as well as how peer groups—and society in general—influence the health behavior of individuals.

Part of Dr. Eburne's success in reaching so many different people is that he uses a variety of teaching modalities, such as training in mental balance and the marshal arts. He has worked as a family health specialist with the USDA's Extension Service, 4-H, and numerous youth health programs. His consulting programs have included *Family Mental Health Promotion* for General Mills and *Helping Rural Youth Adjust to College Life* for Farmland Industries. Additionally, he has developed programs for the Society for the Study of Human Potential and the Mandalla Society.

Dr. Eburne has taught at a number of universities and is currently professor of health education at Western Oregon State University. He teaches Health Methods, Mental Health, Drug Education, Stress Management, and School Health Education.

Mark J. Kittleson, Ph.D., has been professor in the Department of Health Education and Recreation at Southern Illinois University at Carbondale since 1989. He currently holds the position of Director of Graduate Studies in the health education program. Before this, he spent fourteen years in various work locations, including ten years at Youngstown State University, Ohio, where he completed his doctorate in 1986. He has focused on the needs assessment of teachers, public health workers, and health care workers regarding HIV transmission. In addition, he has assessed the impact of the Internet on conducting research in health education/public health.

Dr. Kittleson has also coordinated worksite health promotion activities among businesses in the southern Illinois area; served on two national committees (SABPAC and the Joint Commission to Establish Graduate Standards in Health Education); and taken national leadership in Communications Technology/Internet Development for the health education profession.

During the early 1990s, Dr. Kittleson developed the Health Education Directory (HEDIR) for the connection of over 2,500 health educators internationally, as well as the dissemination of information and expertise in this field. In 1998, he launched the *International Electronic Journal of Health Education,* for which he serves as editor.

Dr. Kittleson teaches Worksite Health Promotion, Research Foundations in Health Education, Vital Statistics, Teaching Strategies in Health Education, and Stress-Management.

CHAPTER

1 Holistic Mental Health

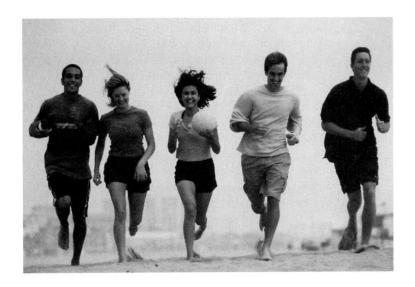

The Health of Human Beings

Most human beings place a high value on their health. Only happiness is stated as a greater prize or possession when individuals are asked what is most important to them in life. While there is no universally accepted definition; *health* has been defined in many ways by a variety of individuals and organizations. Almost half a century ago Turner (1951) cited the World Health Organization's definition of health–"a complete state of physical, mental, social, and emotional well-being and not merely the absence of disease or infirmity"—as vital to considering the health status of the total human being. The very term *health* comes from the Anglo-Saxon word "haelth" meaning, hale or whole. Very often when people consider health the issue that most comes to mind is *"physical health"* or the health of the body. However, when we consider all of the ramifications of the human experience and keeping in mind the definition of the World Health Organization, we must include all aspects of the human experience when we describe the health of human beings.

Further, the U.S. Surgeon General has recently concluded that the connection between mind and body is very important as it relates to health (National Institutes of Mental Health, 2000a). Students studying for a test are at higher risk for becoming ill closer to the time of the exam; persons who have suffered from a heart attack recover more quickly if their emotional state is stronger; and persons with terminal illnesses enjoy a higher quality of life if they are surrounded by friends and family (American Psychiatric Association, 2000).

Throughout history, there have been many and varied descriptions of the dimensions of human health. Generally, these descriptions involve some combination of body and mind; body, mood, and mind; body, mind, and spirit; or body, mind, spirit, and relationships. Regardless of the precise division, the concept of a multiple-dimensioned human being has had a place in the way health has been described for centuries. This concept considers that there is a biological or physical aspect of the person as well as a mental or thinking portion, a portion that relates or interacts with others and a portion that aspires to some sort of goodness. In the mid-twentieth century, Earl Pullias (1963) described health as the "optimum functioning of the human organism in all its complexity from the subtle processes of metabolism to the most sensitive perception of beauty or truth or love." When any significant aspect of this functioning goes awry, the quality of human life is threatened. The extent of the threat depends upon the nature and degree of the malfunctioning. Advanced illnesses whether centered in body, mind, or soul rapidly destroy the effectiveness and meaning of life. These three aspects of humans are so related and interdependent that serious malfunctioning in any one area rapidly affects the others.

Optimum health could be described as a balanced development of each of the dimensions of human well-being. The task is to identify all of these dimensions and to define what exactly constitutes a positive level of development. Someone whose arteries are smooth and uncluttered with a heart as strong as a cannon firing at a steady fifty-five beats per minute, but who is unable to establish meaningful or lasting relationships with others, would not be considered to be in optimum health. Likewise, a well-adjusted, happy and content individual with a solid network of friends and loved ones, who could not control his or her temper, self-doubts, drug use, or tendency to engage in high-risk personal behavior, could not be considered to meet the definition of *healthy*. It is understandable that when human beings think about their health the physical dimension is what most often comes to mind. From the standpoint of defining health and, perhaps more to the point, the loss of health, there are many more methods of assessing the physical human condition than there are for those problems that afflict us in other ways. It is rather easy to consider a physical illness because there are fairly well-defined measures of physical health that can be used to gauge whether or not a state of health exists. However, there are many conditions—other than those that are purely biological or physical—that suggest that we are not healthy. While the noted psychiatrist Thomas Szasz (1987) suggests that without an anatomical or biochemical defect there is no mental illness, he is definitely in the minority. When someone says, "Physically I'm doing fine but my head is a little messed up" or "Things are going pretty well for me except for my relationships with the opposite sex" or "My life is going really well right now, but I just don't feel any sense of purpose or direction" they cannot be considered to be in a state of total health. With the aforementioned examples in mind, it is easy to find fault with Dr. Szasz's concept of total health. Granted, reductionist thinking can decrease everything to the molecular level. When the behavior, thoughts, and feelings of an entire human being or between a group of human beings are considered, then the big picture rather than the smallest one should be considered. People face the world with wholeness and as complex and integrated beings, and physical and mental wellness are inseparable partners in the human state.

The Complex Nature of Human Health

Differing methods have been utilized to describe the complex nature of human health. Most attempt to describe how other parts or dimensions of the human being interact with the body or physical dimension. The notion of a body and a mind has been considered for centuries as has a body, mind, and spirit. In the early days of the holistic health movement, Mattson (1982) described a unity of the mind, body, and spirit as the fundamental principle of the holistic health philosophy. One very comprehensive view of total health or wellness includes mental, emotional, social, physical, intellectual, environmental, occupational and spiritual dimensions. That may be one of the most elaborate descriptions. A review of literature and interviews of leading professionals in the health education field (Eburne, Smith, & Graff-Haight, 1993) reveals that a majority describe human health as including the following five dimensions: physical, social, mental, emotional and spiritual. For the purpose of this book, the authors have agreed to consider health from these five dimensions. Curiously, many regard those dimensions other than the physical to comprise mental health in a broader sense, than when mental health is defined as one of the facets of human health. This is somewhat confusing, so—for purposes of clarity in this textbook—the terms *mental health* or *comprehensive mental health* are used to describe the dimensions other than physical health, that is, the mental, emotional, social, and spiritual dimensions. It is important to continually maintain the perception that human beings include all the dimensions and that each of these dimensions has a vital and contributory role in the total well-being of all. A model that illustrates these five dimensions of human health should demonstrate their interrelated and equal roles.

Physical Health

Physical well-being is both complex and multifaceted. It concerns levels of nutrition, rest, exercise, growth and development, and aging, as well as freedom from infectious, communicable, and chronic disease. Physical health involves all of the

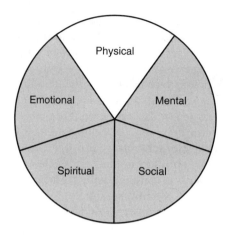

Physical health: biological or physical
Mental health: reasoning/decision making ⎤
Social health: interactions and relationships ⎬ Comprehensive
Spiritual health: beliefs and hopes   ⎪ mental
Emotional health: feelings and reactions ⎦ health

body systems—the nervous system, the skeletal system, the muscular system, the integumentary system (skin), the endocrine system (hormones), and the circulatory system. Personal behavior, environment, and genetic makeup all contribute to the status of physical health. There is a great deal of interaction between physical health and mental health. This relationship is a two-way street. A person's mental health status can have a definite bearing on that person's physical health (psychosomatic or psychophysiologic influence) and the degree to which one's physical body functions productively and effectively can factor into the various mental health dimensions. Many issues regarding self-esteem (both positive and negative) center around physical health. Further, the ability to manage stress, cope with emotional responses, and perhaps even produce the chemicals used in mental functioning involve aspects of the physical dimension of health. It is vital to remember that mental health can be both positively and negatively impacted by physical health status and, in turn, can provide a detracting or contributory effect on a person's physical well-being.

Mental Health

The mental health dimension of human health could be called the psychological dimension, the reasoning dimension or perhaps the intellectual dimension. This would certainly prevent some of the potential confusion that exists when a segment of comprehensive mental health is also referred to as mental health. However, using a term such as *intellectual health* also might be confusing and can introduce a potential for bias or prejudice. Definitions of *intellect* include: (1) the ability to perceive, reason, and understand; and (2) great mental ability or high intelligence. This second definition is what dissuades us from using the term *intellectual* health here. Although perception, reasoning, and judgment are critical to this dimension of human health, the judgment and reasoning of people with "average" or lower intelligence can be as effective in dealing with life as are those of people with superior intelligence. The notion that superior intelligence is indicative of better mental health or is in any way a major factor in any comprehensive view of mental health is not accurate, and it would not be our wish to promote such a notion. Later chapters discuss the fact that there is some indication that people with high levels of what has been traditionally labeled as *intelligence* have no immunity to departures from mental health and certainly do not seem to have any greater levels of what could be described as mental health. We certainly do not wish to give the impression that we do not value learning, intelligence, or advanced reasoning ability; these are attributes to be prized. Rather, we hope to convey that high levels of mental health are possible regardless of innate intellectual ability or advanced levels of education. Effective decision making, the capacity to form reasonable judgments, and the ability to learn and comprehend—as well as common sense and similar attributes that create the foundation for solving many of life's problems—are by no means exclusive to those with high intelligence. The term *psychological health* would likewise open the door to misinterpretation and confusion. Psychology is a complex, ever-expanding science. Since there are so many schools of thought, sub-specialties and approaches to the science and practice of psychology we wish to avoid possible confusion and mislabeling for a broad field of study by avoiding this term.

For the purposes of this textbook, *mental health* in its most specific sense implies reasoning ability. The manner in which a person accesses information and utilizes it in the decision-making process is critical here. Individuals with high levels of health in this dimension are able to assess situations accurately and make decisions that are appropriate, for everyone's best interest is concerned, in light of the available choices and resources. Realistic acceptance of life's circumstances and the utilization of choices and options available are characteristics of positive mental health. Can someone have a below-average intellectual capacity or an incomplete education and still be characterized as mentally healthy? One merely has to consider the highly successful and heroic efforts that occur regularly in special education, or consider the productive, well-adjusted, and effectively functioning individuals who have not had the opportunity to complete a formal education, to conclude that the answer is *yes*.

Social Health

Human beings are social creatures who normally seek, enjoy, and sometimes even crave the companionship of others. Most individuals thrive in the presence of a supporting, loving, and accepting social environment. On the other hand, some of the most severe forms of unhappiness result from difficulties involving human interaction. Individuals with a high degree of social well-being are able to connect with others, formulate relationships, and, if desired, maintain those relationships. This often reflects a style of interacting with others that demonstrates concern and consideration. Socially healthy people are more harmonious in their dealings with others and demonstrate helpfulness and cooperation. Skills in handling disagreements and managing conflicts are earmarks of the socially healthy. Perhaps ability or simply a willingness to attempt to understand all of the ramifications of a relationship makes the socially healthy individual better at solving problems associated with human interaction. A trusted friend with whom one can share concerns, issues, and problems in life is a tremendous buffer against negative outcomes resulting from a departure from any aspects of health. Further, such a friend (or circle of friends) can serve as a highly effective health promotion mechanism. Close interpersonal relationships can teach people to accept faults and imperfections in others and thereby perhaps lead the way to accepting such things in themselves. In their work *Healthy Pleasures,* Ornstein and Sobel (1989) suggest that the quality (intensity) of the relationships may be of more value than the quantity (number) of friends a person has. They do suggest, however, that people attempt to have more than one close relationship. Their thinking is that if human beings have multiple selves then multiple friends can more effectively connect with these selves. Further, they believe that if a single person comprises another person's sphere of intimacy then the latter person may not develop or maintain the skills necessary for establishing and maintaining friendships. In such circumstances, the loss of the single intimate friend can yield devastating results. Social health skills are needed to maintain a circle of close friends and to enable people to work and interact productively and enjoyably with other people. Further, social health allows people to work cooperatively, honestly, effectively, and fairly with those in positions of authority as well as with subordinates and peers. A combination of self-respect and respect for the welfare and rights of others is a solid foundation upon which to build social health.

Emotional Health

Emotions are both easy and difficult to understand. All people have experienced emotions and thus are familiar with them. On the other hand, many people have difficulty controlling their emotions or understanding the cause or impact of these emotions. Recent evidence offered by Goleman (1995) suggests that people may experience emotional responses to their experiences, perceptions, and environment before they deal with the same experiences intellectually. This may make it easier to understand some of the "passion-based" behaviors that often seem to be counterproductive to good mental health. Unfortunately, it also adds complexity to efforts to effect a cognitive or willful control over some emotional responses. Many regard emotion as a disturbance or agitation of normal feelings that might serve to upset normal thinking or functioning. Emotions are many and varied reactions and are so often a blend of responses that defy description. Ekman (1992) suggests that many facial expressions that reflect emotional responses—such as fear, sadness, and anger—are universally recognized regardless of culture, language, or exposure to technology. His work supports the notion that emotions and the reactions to them are common to all humans and not the product of learning or culture. There are many emotions other than those of fear, sadness, joy, and anger. A brief list of emotions experienced by humans includes shame, anxiety, terror, contentment, rage, indignation, guilt, hate, nervousness, relief, delight, surprise, fondness, and so many others that they could fill a chapter. Whether the aforementioned are merely subcategories of a smaller number or the "tip of the iceberg" regarding the range of human emotional responses is a matter for conjecture. The key issue is to recognize that humans are subjected to emotional responses and that these can be positive as well as negative. Once people recognize that they can and do have emotional responses, they are able to examine them as to their power and ability to influence their lives. An examination of their own emotional responses allows responsible people to analyze the cause of and reaction to these responses. The more they are able to recognize and dissect emotional responses the more likely they will be able to discuss their own and others' emotional reactions. The emotionally healthy person is able to recognize a feeling response in himself or herself as well as in others and then analyze whether it is a productive or non-productive reaction. Emotional health implies that an individual can utilize thoughts, judgment, and reason to moderate the impact that emotions—positive or negative—have on behavior.

Spiritual Health

Throughout history, most societies have held to some sort of belief system that involves something beyond themselves. That is, there has been and continues to be a notion that there is a power, force, or purpose that extends beyond the tangible aspects of the human experience. In some cases, these notions are highly organized and even structured into a precise pattern of belief and behavior; and, in other cases, the experience is quite free of structure and organization. In both extremes, however, there seems to be a unified notion that something either within human beings or influencing them from an external source will prompt or promote them to attempt to do "good" things. The majority of contemporary thinking includes this issue (termed the *spiritual dimension*) in descriptions of comprehensive or total human health. Whether it be through attaining membership in an organized religion, attending worship service, meditating, praying, reading sacred or inspiring books, communing with nature, or providing helping service to others, human beings tend to involve themselves in efforts that aid in a search for an understanding of the meaning of life. An unfortunate outcome of this is that at times individuals become so involved or devoted to their own method of understanding or confronting the meaning and purpose of life that they can become intolerant of the methods employed by others. Spiritually healthy individuals are able to hold firmly to a belief system, have faith in and gain strength from a belief in something beyond themselves, yet do not feel the need to belittle, demean, or interfere with the spiritual focus of others. Unfortunately, this has not always been the case.

Human history is filled with examples of people being discriminated against and at times even harmed because of their particular method of expressing or acting out their spirituality. Perhaps because of this sad aspect of human intolerance that developed out of an effort to strengthen one's own belief by demonstrating its superiority to another, many individuals, have come to regard organized belief systems as anti-intellectual and even anti-freedom. In his book, *Love, Medicine, and Miracles,* Siegel (1988) referred to some outwardly pious people who were not very spiritual. Such people, he said, can give others "spiritual ulcers." Unfortunate situations where hurt and negative outcomes result from the practice or defense of a belief system probably have much less to do with spiritual health than some other aspects of human nature. Siegel expressed the opinion that spirituality has great potential to heal and promote a very positive state if expressed openly and freely. The spiritual dimension of health can serve as a foundation for positive mental health in that it assists people in their search for understanding and meaning in life.

The Scope of Mental Health Issues

Health as a Spectrum

Since health is more than the absence of disease, it is not always easy to define or describe the healthy state. *Health* has been described as a continuum with optimal health at one extreme and absence of health at the other. One might also visualize a spectrum with deep, rich color at one end (health) and absence of color at the other end (illness). Health is seldom, if ever, constant; and, while someone may be functioning at the very well end of the spectrum or continuum one day, that same person may on another day, be at the other end for various reasons. This fluid condition of health status can be unsettling to some but a recognition of the inevitability of changes in health status can lead to acceptance and effective functioning even when alterations in health occur. Some major goals of this book are to assist in the recognition of acceptable ranges in mental health status and to promote behaving, thinking, reacting, and interacting styles that will continually encourage movement toward the positive ends of the mental, emotional, social, and spiritual spectrums. Not one of these dimensions of mental health functions in a totally independent fashion. Similarly, physical well-being is influenced by and exerts influence on mental health. The promotion of mental health involves a search for resilience, self-efficacy, coherence, harmony, balance, integrity, adaptability, and many other attributes that encourage growth, success, and joy in living.

Health Interdependence

In a fifteen-year study of the relative health status of members of a health maintenance organization (HMO), Voght, Pope, Mullooly, and Hollis (1994) discovered that those with the highest indices of mental health had the lowest risk of developing gastrointestinal illness and hyperimmune diseases. Further, they noted that those with the highest levels of worry demonstrated an increased risk of developing cancer, certain types of heart disease, and stroke. They also noted that those with the lowest indices of mental health had the highest risk for hypertension (high blood pressure).

Eisenberg (1997), in discussing world mental health, noted the interconnectedness of health problems. Examples he gave of this interconnectedness included depression, heart and lung disease, sexually transmitted diseases, and other behavior-related diseases on one hand; and the psychosocial pathologies such as violence, alcoholism, abuse of women and children, and underlying social conditions such as war, poverty, and discrimination on the other. He described this interconnectedness as a *self-perpetuating spiral.*

Knapp (1997) points out the relationship between economic status and mental health. He believes that there is a recurring and interconnected pattern of mental health problems in children and adolescents that have to do with financial considerations. He points out that there is poor coordination between agencies providing mental health care to children and youth and that mental health problems in this age group foreshadow the mental health of a future generation of adults. He believes that lack of attention to the mental health of children and adolescents has implications for a spiral of child abuse, juvenile crime, family dysfunction, and adult mental, emotional, and social problems. These problems contribute to the risk of leading to having more problems of a similar nature for future generations. The World Health Organization (1995) publication *Bridging the Gap* comments about the relationship between mental illness, stress, suicide, family disorganization, substance abuse, and poverty. The publication states that as poverty increases so does the risk of these problems; the publication follows with the somber comment that this condition creates a situation where a longer life is more of a punishment than a prize.

Balance seems to be the key to enjoyable living. When considering the many dimensions of health, it is easy to focus on those things that cause the most difficulty or perhaps those areas of life where the most success occurs. For some who might do very well socially but have difficulty with their emotional reactions, it could become easy to derive a sense of reward and satisfaction from interpersonal relationships while downplaying emotional issues. Others, however, might fail to capitalize on the strength of their social health and focus excessively on the emotional difficulties they experience. In the first case, a problem is downplayed and strength becomes the focus. There is both positive and negative to be found in this. Likewise, there are both positive and negative factors related to the second scenario. How could things be improved in both cases without diminishing the positive attributes involved? One notion is to work on the things that need the most work. This would mean that focus on the weakness would become a matter for self-improvement. Another thought is to attempt to maximize the positive attributes. This thinking is based on the notion that people are better off if they maintain and seek to improve those things that are the most successful and productive. A descriptive analogy to a set of elevators or a child's seesaw is the basis of this thinking—when one goes up, the other must descend. Ideally, people should maintain their positive attributes and seek to improve upon their weaknesses or difficulties. How much time and effort should be devoted to each? How is an effective ratio established between the focus on strengths and the focus on weaknesses? College students face such a dilemma every term: *Do I diminish my efforts in my best subjects in order to improve my weaker ones? What if I work so hard on my weak courses that I drop to average in my better subjects?* Later chapters discuss possible methods of establishing balance in mental health, utilizing each of the dimensions of mental health to strengthen the other dimensions.

The Influence of Mental Health on Human Life

The Extent of Mental Health Problems

An Institute of Medicine report (1996) suggests that the general public grossly underestimates the impact of poor mental health. The overall effect of mental disorders on families, industry, and society in general is often hidden. Even health care workers tend to underidentify mental health issues in their patients. Many aspects of physical health have a connection to mental health status. McGinnis and Foege (1993) suggest that while many of the leading causes of death in the United States are from chronic illness brought on by personal choices in health-related behavior, the causes of these health-detracting and life-shortening behaviors have their origins in mental, emotional, and social health factors. Further, Schoenborn and Horn (1993) believe that two of the behaviors most directly associated with poor physical health and a reduction in longevity—tobacco use and heavy alcohol use—are often associated with negative mood and emotion.

According to information presented in the U.S. Department of Health and Human Services Public Health Service's (1996) document, *Healthy People 2000 Midcourse Review,* suicide is the ninth leading cause of death in the country and the third leading cause of death among adolescents and young adults. The actual number of suicide deaths exceeds 30,000 each year in the United States.

Depression, a mental health problem that is unfortunately downplayed in importance by many, is considered to be one of the primary risk factors in both suicide and attempted suicide. The statement that depression is downplayed by many is evidenced by the fact that fewer than 40 percent of depressed individuals seek or obtain professional care for this condition. In spite of the fact that major depression accounts for more days in bed than any other health-related condition except for heart disease, it is still ignored. Murray and Lopez (1996) suggest that depression is the fourth leading cause of disability-adjusted life years (DALYs) worldwide, headed only by lower respiratory infections, diarrheal diseases, and conditions associated with childbirth. The DALY is a statistic utilized to present the impact of suffering, disability, and premature death as a result of a specific condition or disease. When the impact of these conditions is considered on a worldwide basis, it is easier to grasp the extent of depression on human disability. The World Bank (1993) utilized the DALY in preparing a report outlining the *global burden of disease (GBD).* This report concluded that 8.1 percent of the GBD resulted from mental health problems. The report further suggests that 34 percent of the

GBD is due to disorders that are related to such behavioral issues as violence and alcohol and tobacco use. They estimate that between 5 percent and 10 percent of all people on earth are negatively affected by alcohol-related disease. The report further predicts that depression alone will account for 5.7 percent of the GBD by the early part of the twenty-first century and that this condition will become second only to heart disease as a cause of long-term disability. The World Health Organization (1996) suggests that a combination of neurotic (a term currently being replaced by *personality disorder* in the United States), stress-related, and somatoform disorders is the third most important cause of morbidity (illness) on a worldwide basis. Further, when chronic disability is the consideration, mood disorders are the most important single cause with dementia ranked seventh and schizophrenia ninth. Bourdon, Rae, Locke, Narrow, and Regier (1992) estimate that over forty-one million U.S. adults have had a mental disorder at some time during their lives. This translates to more than one in seven adults who have had their lives and health disturbed by a departure from well-being of a psychosocial nature. Norden (1995), in his book *Beyond Prozac*, points out that mental illness strikes nearly all people but that it does so in many different forms and to varied degrees. His work cites a report that reveals that almost one-half of people between the ages of eighteen and fifty-four met the formal diagnostic criteria for at least one of fourteen serious psychiatric illnesses. Since the aged population was not considered (and this age group is at extremely high risk), it might be safe to assume that well over 50 percent of the population will experience some form of mental illness sometime during their lives. Norden also cites a study of three hundred biographies of some of history's most accomplished artists, politicians, philosophers, and scientists that reveals that 75 percent of these talented individuals suffered from some form of serious mental illness.

Cost of Mental Health Problems

Evidence of the extent of health problems might be best represented by the cost in both money and human suffering that occurs when the quality of mental health is diminished. While advocating for increased attention to mental health care, former first lady Mrs. Rosalynn Carter (1996) stated that there is an incalculable cost to humans in lost and decreased opportunity to participate in the activities of daily life due to mental illness. She suggests that the *indirect* costs to society due to such factors as premature death from suicide, loss of productivity in the workplace, support of the mentally ill homeless, added burden to the criminal justice system, and the cost of medical care necessary due to physical illness precipitated via mental and emotional problems all exceed the cost of direct treatment of mental illness. When such factors as family disruption, worker turnover, loss of productivity on the job, and excess worker absenteeism are taken into account, it is easy to accept that her estimates could be accurate.

Due to the very complex and interconnected nature of the various dimensions of human health, it is difficult to assess a precise financial cost that can be directly attributed to mental health. Perhaps due to this interconnectedness, the federal government has established an agency called the Substance Abuse and Mental Health Services Administration (SAMHSA). This government agency focuses on mental health and alcohol and other drug (MHAOD) abuse services. When this government agency calculates the costs associated with services in this area, they often factor drug, alcohol, and mental health issues together. One SAMHSA (1998) report states that MHAOD expenditures were 8.8 percent of the $942.7 billion in national health expenditures. This calculates to be $79.3 billion with estimates of $66.7 billion for the treatment of mental illness. As stated previously, accuracy is difficult in such estimates due to complex interconnections such as dual diagnosis (referring to someone who is at the same time mentally ill and chemically dependent). SAMSHA utilizes a method whereby whichever is diagnosed first—chemical dependency or mental illness—is considered to be the primary cause when determining the cost to the country for the treatment in situations where both conditions occur. Further, the estimated expenditures do not include such costs as treatment of Alzheimer's disease, mental retardation, age-related dementia or treatment of medical conditions resulting from MHAOD disorders. A National Institutes of Health (1997) report states that the total spending for MHAOD disorders is close to that expended for either heart disease or injuries and trauma. The report further states that the expenditures for MHAOD disorders exceeds the amount spent on both diabetes and cancer.

The consulting firm of Harris, Rothenberg International (1999) suggests that dependency and mental illness combined cost U.S. corporations over one hundred billion dollars each year. They further estimate that during any given week an excess of one hundred million work hours are lost due to these conditions.

The U.S. Surgeon General suggests that the cost to the nation for mental health is $178 billion per year (NIMH, 2000b). This includes mental disorders, senile dementia (including Alzheimer's disease), and substance use treatment cost. The direct costs—in the amount of $79 billion—are for treatment from various health care providers including psychiatrists, psychologists, counselors, nurses, hospitals, mental health centers, and residential treatment centers. The federal government covers a larger percentage of this cost than that of physical health care costs, since most private insurers offer less-generous coverage for mental health care. Indirect costs—in the amount of $99 billion—are for lost productivity in morbidity costs and mortality costs for workers who experience premature death.

The Stigma of Mental Health Problems

Les Campbell (1996), a worker with the Alliance for the Mentally Ill, suggests that one out of every one hundred high school graduates in the United States will eventually suffer from schizophrenia. He further states that due to our fear of the unknown the mentally ill are reduced in our minds from potentially valuable citizens to tainted eccentrics at best and fearsome maniacs at worst. This stigma associated with mental illness is taught by omission in our schools since neither the elementary or secondary schools include much accurate or clear information concerning mental illness in their curriculums. Wartik (1997), in reviewing the possible reasons why proper diagnosis of mental problems does not always occur, discusses the fact that many people go untreated for mental disorders due to the stigma associated with such disorders. There seems to be a notion held by many people that mental and emotional disorders are not beyond personal control and that psychiatric illness is somehow—at least partly if not totally—the fault of the person who is ill. The National Mental Health Association (1996) conducted a survey and found that more than 50 percent of the respondents viewed depression as a sign of weakness.

Frances and First (1998) believe that while most psychiatric disorders have existed as long as there have been human beings on earth they have only recently been understood in a manner that approaches scientific levels. While they contend that one in five people have a psychiatric disorder at any given time and one in two will have one sometime during their lifetime, many will not receive adequate treatment due to fear or misunderstanding. They make a plea for a level of compassion that would enable those with mental health problems to be given the "care, consolation, and time to heal" that is afforded those with physical ailments. Gorman (1996) believes that ignorance and the notion that seeking help regarding mental health problems represents a personal failure are responsible for the stigma associated with mental illness. The American Psychiatric Association's publication, *The Diagnostic and Statistical Manual of Mental Disorders, Fourth Edition* (1994), was expanded significantly over the third edition. This publication, which is often referred to as the psychiatrist's bible, currently categorizes a variety of "less-severe" conditions as mental disorders. Critics have suggested that this only encourages people to avoid responsibility for certain aspects of personal behavior. However, the thinking behind the expansion of characteristics could help to diminish the stigma associated with mental health problems by revealing just how often such illness occurs. If society could come to recognize that those mental health problems can occur as frequently as physical health problems, some of the prejudice, fear, and discrimination that surround mental health problems could be eased.

Summary

The body is interconnected. Each joint, limb, muscle, nerve, reaction, and function is connected to some other system. The whole human experience affects not just one small part of who a person is but the entire body. Emotionally, spiritually, mentally, and physically, actions taken and decisions made affect the human spirit.

Mental health is a complex blend of human dimensions. Further, while mental health problems are quite common, many can be prevented and most are better managed if there is early recognition and treatment. Though it is an old and tired adage, an ounce of prevention is easily worth a pound of cure where comprehensive mental health is concerned. Personal goals in the varied dimensions of mental health may vary greatly among individuals, and that is understandable. Chapter 2 considers some of the varied notions about what makes a person mentally healthy and discusses what to consider and work toward in this complex and interesting aspect of human life.

DISCUSSION QUESTIONS

1. Which of the five areas of comprehensive health do you feel is most in need of attention in your life?

2. When considering health as a spectrum of states, where on the spectrum do you fall? Where did you fall at other times in your life?

3. Can you think of a time when the interconnectedness of health became important in your life? For example, have you ever been sick during finals week? How did it affect your performance?

4. What experiences do you have with mental illness? Has it touched your life in any way?

5. Considering the financial cost of mental health problems, what do you think could be done to reduce this? What is the best strategy—increased awareness, increased treatment, or something else?

RELATED WEBSITES

http://www.hrsa.dhhs.gov/ Health Resources and Services Administration. Includes newsroom, job opportunities, and upcoming events.

http://www.health.gov Accessible health information from the U.S. government.

http://www.befitnet.com The BeFitNet Alliance. Provides information on health and fitness, sports strategies, and nutrition.

http://www.jstor.org/journals/00959006.html This site allows you to search the journal *Health and Human Behavior.*

http://www.plgrm.com/health/mental_health.html Health Topics: Mental Health. This site offers information on a variety of mental health topics.

http://www.mentalhealth.org.uk/ Mental Health Foundation. This site offers support services, advice, news, and conference information.

http://www.cdc.gov Centers for Disease Control and Prevention. This site offers current health news and resources.

http://mentalhelp.net Mental Health Net. Provides over 9,000 mental health resources.

http://www.phy.mtu.edu/apod/mind Dialectical Behavior Therapy. Includes mindfulness, interpersonal effectiveness, emotion regulation, and distress tolerance. A great focus of this site is on borderline personality disorder.

http://www.counseling.com/Ccom/reference.html This site addresses reference and resource information regarding alcohol problems, chemical dependency, emotional/mental health, and family problems and provides crisis hotlines from the American Counseling Association.

REFERENCES

American Psychiatric Association. (1994). *Diagnostic and Statistical Manual of Mental Disorders* (4th edition) Washington, D.C.: APHA

American Psychiatric Association. (2000). *Mind Body Connection: Get the Facts* [On-line]. Available: http://helping.apa.org/mind_body/index.html

Bourdon, K. H., Rae, D. S., Locke, B. Z., Narrow, W. E., & Regier, D. A. (1992). Estimating the Prevalence of Mental Disorder in U.S. Adults from the Epidemiologic Catchment Area and Survey. *Public Health Reports,* 107 (6), 663–668.

Campbell, L. (1996, Aug. 8). Outside the Cage Looking In: A Disturbing Look at How Society Defines the Mentally Ill, *San Diego Tribune,* p. B11.

Carter, R. (1996, May 7). A Positive Link of Mind and Body [Editorial]. *Los Angeles Times.*

Eburne, N., Smith, M., & Graff-Haight, D. (1993). *Comprehensive Health Education: Basic Thinking Among Leaders in the Profession.* Research presented at the National AAHPERD Convention, Indianapolis, IN.

Eisenberg, L. (1997). Psychiatry and Health in Low-Income Populations. *Comprehensive Psychiatry, 38* (March/April). 336–380

Ekman, P. (1992). An Argument for the Basic Emotions. *Cognition and Emotions, 6,* 175.

Frances, A., & First, M. (1998). *Your Mental Health.* New York: Scribner.

Goleman, D. (1995). *Emotional Intelligence,* (pp. 17–21). New York: Bantam Books.

Gorman, J. M. (1996). *The Essential Guide to Mental Health.* New York: St. Martin's Griffen.

Harris, Rothenberg International. (1999). *Value to Companies: What Research Says* [On-line]. Available: http://info@harrisrothenberg.com

Institute of Medicine. (1996). *American Psychologist, 51* (11), 116.

Knapp, M. (1997). Economic Evaluations and Interventions for Children and Adolescents with Mental Health Problems. *Journal of Child Psychology and Psychiatry, 38* (1), 3–25. Cambridge University Press.

Mattson, P. H. (1982). *Holistic Health in Perspective.* Palo Alto, CA: Mayfield.

McGinnis, J. M., & Foege, W. H. (1993). Actual Causes of Death in the United States. *Journal of the American Medical Association, 270,* 2207–2212.

Murray, C., & Lopez, A. (1996). *The Global Burden of Disease and Injuries* (Vol. 1). Cambridge, MA: Harvard University Press.

National Institutes of Health. (1997). *Disease-Specific Estimates of Direct and Indirect Costs of Illness and NIH Update.* Washington: U.S. Department of Health and Human Services.

National Institutes of Mental Health. (2000a). *Mental Health: A Report of the Surgeon General,* Chapter One [On-line]. Available: http://www.nimh.nih.gov/mhsgrpt/chapter1/sec1.html#mind_body

National Institutes of Mental Health. (2000b). *Mental Health: A Report of the Surgeon General,* Chapter Six [On-line]. Available: http://www.nimh.nih.gov/mhsgrpt/chapter6/sec2.html

National Mental Health Association. (1996). Alexandria, VA.

Norden, M. (1995). *Beyond Prozac.* New York: HarperCollins.

Ornstein, R., & Sobel, D. (1989). *Healthy Pleasures* (pp. 229–234). Reading, MA: Addison Wesley.

Pullias, E. V. (1963). The Education of the Whole Man [Monograph I]. *Quest* (Winter, p. 41).

Schoenborn, C. A., & Horn, J. (1993). *Negative Moods as Correlates of Smoking and Heavier Drinking: Implications for Health Promotion.* Bethesda, MD: National Center for Health Statistics.

Siegel, B. S. (1986). *Love, Medicine, and Miracles.* New York: Harper and Row.

Substance Abuse and Mental Health Services Administration (2000): Costs of Mental Health and Substance Abuse. Available Online: http://www.samsha.gov/media.htm#MH&SACosts

Szasz, T. (1987). *Insanity, the Idea and Its Consequences* (pp. 47–98). New York: Wiley.

Turner, C. E. (1951). *Community Health Educator's Compendium of Knowledge.* Englewood Cliffs, NJ: Prentice-Hall.

U.S. Department of Health and Human Services Public Health Service. (1996). *Healthy People 2000 Midcourse Review and 1995 Revisions SPECTRUM* (pp. 54–56). Sudbury, MA: Jones and Bartlett.

Voght, T., Pope, C., Mullooly, J., & Hollis, J. (1994). Mental Health Status as a Predictor of Morbidity and Mortality: A 15-Year Follow-Up of Members of a Health Maintenance Organization. *American Journal of Public Health, 84* (2), p. 311.

Wartik, N. (1997). Missed Diagnosis: Why Depression Goes Untreated in Women. *American Health* (June), 47–49.

World Bank. (1993). *World Development Report—Investing in Health (World Development Indicators).* Oxford, United Kingdom: Oxford University Press.

World Health Organization. (1995). *Bridging the Gap.* Geneva, Switzerland: Author.

World Health Organization. (1996). *The World Health Report 1996: Fighting Disease, Fostering Development.* Geneva, Switzerland: Author.

2 Characteristics of People Who Are Mentally Healthy

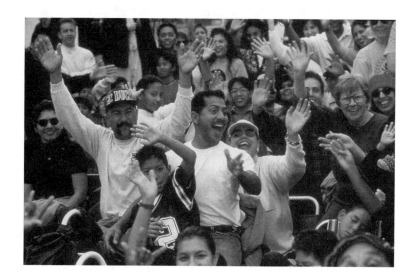

Experiences with People Who Are Mentally Healthy

There are many and varied descriptions of mental health and perhaps even more attributes posed as characteristic of those with positive mental health. Consider whether or not it is realistic to assume that any one person can possess all or most of the characteristics attributed to mental health. Much of this chapter is devoted to exploring this question.

Richie

One of the authors describes an individual whom he considers to be the most mentally healthy person he has ever known—Richie. Richie had an extremely positive outlook on life; he always attempted to see the good or potential for good in any situation. This positive outlook was often contagious; and his friends, family, and co-workers usually were infected with his upbeat approach to life. Richie did not fool himself concerning the importance of his responsibilities or the serious nature of many of the world's problems; it was just that he continually attempted to convince himself that things were good or potentially good. His attitude toward life seemed to solicit both love and support from others. He usually had the sort of support that would enable him to confront a negative situation and plan and execute a solution. But even when he was on his own, he was not afraid to stand firm including his beliefs. Richie had a very good sense of himself and neither overestimated his abilities nor employed any false modesty. He was frank and honest about issues confronting him. He managed criticism well, sometimes with a sense of humor and other times with blunt assertiveness. One of the most interesting of Richie's characteristics was his ability to see the "big picture" and thus focus on the "important" things in life. He did not allow insignificant irritations or side issues to distract him from his efforts to live life to the fullest. Richie's diverse interests always kept his mind active, and he seemed to find enjoyment in almost anything he contacted.

Richie felt good about himself, but did not fool himself into believing his talents or abilities exceeded what they actually were. In his dealings with others, he was honest and straightforward and exhibited understanding, concern, and caring. When things did not go his way, he faced his challenges in a straightforward and honest fashion. He was reluctant to blame others for any unwanted demands and generally attempted to devise a strategy to solve problems that took all dimensions into consideration. Although everyone does not have a close friend like Richie, most have met or known someone possessing characteristics in common with him. Further, they may have recognized additional or different attributes that have contributed to a positive mental health status in other friends or acquaintances.

A Person Who Is Mentally Healthy

Think of a person you know who seems to have a high degree of mental health. Think about all of this person's attributes. In your opinion, what is it that sets this person apart from your other friends and associates? Make a list of all of the adjectives that could be used to describe this person who is mentally healthy. For the sake of convenience, some possible adjectives follow; do not feel limited to these. Try to come up with some additional adjectives that would help to paint an accurate picture of the person you are remembering.

Accepting	Loving
Understanding	Optimistic
Honest	Self-controlled
Frank	Self-aware
Hopeful	Caring
Sensitive	Realistic

Diverse	Open-minded
Helpful	Assertive
Forgiving	Straightforward
Tolerant	Strong
Positive	Cooperative

Are all of these attributes essential to mental health? Probably not. Could someone who was not very mentally healthy have a good number of these attributes? Conceivably, yes. This list applies to Richie, and perhaps many of them have as much to do with his being an extremely nice person as they do with his being mentally healthy.

National Mental Health Association

The National Mental Health Association (NMHA) (1996) suggests that mental health involves

- Feelings about self
- Feelings about others
- Ability to meet and handle the demands of life

This is a very interesting *cluster* of behaviors; that is, this general list of three things encompasses a variety of other attributes and is open to a little personal interpretation. The clustering technique offers an effective method of grouping similar characteristics together to allow for a more brief and general perspective concerning mental health.

Feelings about Self

People who are mentally healthy appreciate and even take joy in their emotions rather than being troubled or subdued by them. They willingly adopt a realistic view of themselves, their talents, and their abilities and can cope effectively with both success and disappointment. Accurate assessment of abilities, honest acceptance of limitations, and reasonable pride in accomplishments promote a high degree of self-understanding. Knowledge of oneself can establish a pattern of thinking and planning that enables an approach to life that will provide satisfaction and enjoyment.

Feelings about Others

Those who are mentally healthy are able to focus on the needs and interests of others, establish and maintain productive and fulfilling relationships, and give and receive love. By respecting the differences found in others, people who are mentally healthy develop a sense of caring and understanding regarding other people.

This can help in the development of personal relationships that are both enduring and rewarding. Trusting and caring associations with others provide a significant source of power in fostering mental health.

Ability to Meet and Handle the Demands of Life

People who are mentally healthy accept responsibility in a reasonable manner, plan effective strategies to meet impending and future responsibilities, and do not fear the future or the unknown. They accept their responsibilities and attempt to make the best use of their talents and abilities. This is done to meet life's demands in the best way possible. They plan for the future by setting reasonable goals for themselves and are generally able to manage the unexpected. By changing what they can and adjusting to what they cannot change, they are able to meet life's demands when they arise.

Describing Mental Health

Much of the preceding section applies to Richie and likely applies to the individuals you know who are mentally healthy. Do the characteristics described by the adjectives listed in the earlier section or the attributes described in the NMHA's cluster of three help a person attain or, in times of trouble, retain mental health? Think again about people you knew who appear mentally healthy. Do they meet the three criteria of the NMHA? If so, how do their personal characteristics help them to continue meeting the criteria?

That no two people are exactly alike is a well-accepted principle. Further, most people appreciate and even savor the differences in others, which is one reason for referring to them as *individuals.* How then can mental health be described? After all, there are certain dimensions of human health that would suggest a condition described as *healthy* and others that would be indicative of *illness.* Body temperature, blood pressure, and blood sugar are a few of the more noteworthy examples of a fairly consistent standard for measuring physical health. However, mental health tends to have a wider range of measures that differentiate between *well* and *not well.*

So then, describing the person who is mentally healthy must involve the notion that huge ranges of behavior and characteristics not only are in existence but also are acceptable and desirable. A review of the literature in the mental health field reveals numerous definitions and lists of characteristics that are considered to indicate a positive mental health status.

In *Beyond Health and Normalcy,* Shapiro (1983) suggests that those with high degrees of mental health generally do not see themselves as being the center of the universe. They tend to have compassion for others, be flexible and adaptable, derive satisfaction from intimate relationships, and have sufficient control over their bodies and minds to make health-enhancing decisions and choices. Goleman (1997) suggests five components of what he terms *emotional intelligence.* These components, which seem to be a critical factor in the development and maintenance of mental health, are self-awareness, understanding of personal motivation, empathy, altruism, and the ability to be loved and to love. There is much to consider in each of these points. Initially, self-awareness indicates more than self-esteem. Rather, this implies a knowledge of self. Self-knowledge is one of the great tasks of human beings, and it is something that few ever master completely. By becoming aware of personal motivation and its underlying reasons, a person is more likely to be able to work toward a prudent and rational pattern of behavior. A high degree of self-awareness can make the motivation behind certain behaviors more apparent. Having mastered this awareness, an individual may be able to control self-serving or potentially harmful sources of motivation and be able to consider the needs of others in decision making. To understand the needs and motives of others and consider them in decision making is certainly a factor involved in empathy. Empathic thinking and feeling certainly are positives when trying to develop an altruistic nature. Altruism—making decisions based on needs of others rather than self—is an excellent basis for unconditional love. Offer and Sabschin (1984) suggest that a person with positive mental health

1. Perceives reality as it is
2. Feels a sense of fulfillment in daily life
3. Establishes and maintains close relationships
4. Accepts his/her limitations and potentials
5. Pursues work that suits her/his talent and training
6. Values self
7. Carries out responsibilities
8. Establishes and maintains close relationships

Most of what Offer and Sabschin include in their list could be included in one of the three general attributes offered by the NMHA. Other observers of effective mental health include additional factors or present them in an alternative manner. Some feel that the list of attributes should be shorter and more manageable, allowing for a more general interpretation as well as for more individual variation. Sheehy and Cournos (1992) suggest that mental health involves three domains of human functioning. These include

1. The way people experience and express their feelings
2. How people think, reason, and learn
3. The way people behave

The first domain on the Sheehy and Cuornos (1992) list involves feelings or emotions. Emotions can cover a wide range and yield quite a spectrum of responses and, as a result, promote a rich experience in living. However, when emotional responses yield extremes in feelings and become inappropriate to the circumstances or begin to dominate one's thoughts, they are not indicators of positive mental health. While *normalcy,*—a statistical measure meaning to tend toward the middle—is never an ideal means to identify a healthy behavior, emotions that are not extreme are indicative of better mental health.

The second domain presented by Sheehy and Cournos (1992) includes a great deal of range as well as variety. Granted that a person's ability to think in a manner that reflects mental health follows logical and reasonable lines, there remain the varied thinking and reasoning styles that reflect different intelligence, language, prior experiences, and culture. A key factor here is that mentally healthy thinking implies realistic expectations of one's self and others and the ability to discern between what is going on in one's mind and what may be happening in reality. Though noted earlier that the concept of *normalcy* is not a good barometer of health status, the exception may be when it comes to the third domain, the way people behave. Fortunately infrequent, the "normal" behavior of a "society gone mad" would be an obvious exception. Bear in mind that eccentric and alternative behaviors can be compatible with mental health if they do not cause problems or discomfort for others. Generally, positive mental health includes sufficient management of personal behavior to prevent any deviance from societal norms or conventions from becoming a major interpersonal, social, or legal problem. Individuals who are mentally healthy do not engage in self-defeating behavior patterns. Karl Menninger suggests that mental health involves the effective adjustment of human beings to the world and to each other with a maximum of effectiveness and happiness.

While it is never an adequate method to describe *health* as the absence of illness, some insight into characteristics of people who are mentally healthy might be gained by considering freedom from things that might be indicative of requiring psychiatric care. Gorman (1996) provides a list of thirteen reasons to see a psychiatrist. Considering not only an absence of these reasons but also a strength in the opposite direction may lead to further insight into positive mental health. People who are mentally healthy should not feel excessively sad without reason. On the contrary, they should have a normal appetite, they should feel that life holds something positive to look forward to, and they definitely should not feel that life is not worth living. Further, individuals who are mentally healthy do not need alcohol or nonprescribed medications to aid in sleep or cheerfulness. Gorman further suggests that people who are mentally healthy should feel comfortable going out in public without unreasonable fear of other people or concern for their safety and that friends and associates would agree that their ideas are generally reasonable.

Carl Rogers (1961), a man who did much to promote the notion that mental health should be approached from a positive perspective and who was fundamentally involved in the beginning of the human potential movement, described what he termed the *fully functioning human being*. Dr. Rogers believed that the fully functioning individual

1. *Was open to life's experiences.* He believed that fully functioning individuals sought and welcomed new experiences. They could regard both sides of an issue and enjoy perspectives other than their own without becoming confrontational or defensive.

2. *Experienced life in a full and complete manner.* Rogers believed that to be fully functioning, a person should be spontaneous, adaptable, and not bound to living life in accordance to a script.

3. *Had freedom in making choices.* He felt that a fully functioning individual should be able to make choices based on the best thing to do rather than the limiting factor of prior experiences. This made for a person free of the constraints of the past.

4. *Was self-trusting.* Dr. Rogers believed that it was crucial to trust inner feelings and impressions. This inner wisdom was something that he felt humans could nurture and utilize for effective and rewarding decision making and that it could develop as it was utilized.

5. *Was creative.* Dr. Rogers believed that new ways of living and regarding life's experiences could be formulated and that these would contribute to a higher level of joy and effectiveness.

The myriad of lists, classifications, and groupings of mental health characteristics include the ability to

- Be self-accepting
- Enjoy life
- Establish and maintain relationships
- Develop intimacy
- Have a realistic view of life
- Make allowances for inadequacies in others
- Manage stress
- Find joy in life
- Live solidly in the present while remembering the past and preparing for the future

The descriptions go on and on. Most of the lists are presenting essentially the same thing in a different manner or from a different perspective or background.

Ten Characteristics of People Who Are Mentally Healthy

For the purpose of this textbook, the authors have attempted to select the prime characteristics offered by a variety of thinkers in the mental health field as those exhibiting what is generally described as mental health. Keep the following points in mind:

- No two people are alike.
- Issues associated with human behavior have a greater potential for variance than those associated with physical health.
- As in all conditions associated with human health, mental health is never a rigid or constant thing.

It is unlikely that any one person would demonstrate all of the qualities at any given time. If perhaps someone did display each of these characteristics, it is unlikely that he/she would exhibit them all of the time. If mental well-being is a fluid state with continual variations, then it is unrealistic to expect each of these characteristics to be evident at all times. However, over any given period of time, it is reasonable to expect that a person who is mentally healthy would exhibit a pattern of behavior that includes a majority of these characteristics:

1. A positive outlook on life
2. A realistic set of expectations and approaches to life
3. Effective management of emotions
4. The ability to function well with others
5. The ability to draw strength from others without being overly dependent upon them
6. Reasonable appetites
7. A spiritual nature
8. Effective coping skills
9. An honest self-regard and self-esteem
10. The ability to view the world honestly, accurately, and realistically

A Positive Outlook

If things are not going as well as expected the person who is mentally healthy believes things will improve. Having the ability to see the potential for improvement, being able to visualize the means to bring about resolution of a problem, or maintaining a realistic belief that improvement is possible is typical of a person who is mentally healthy. On the other hand, avoiding the steps needed to solve a problem or improve an undesirable situation or hoping and dreaming about a better situation when no plan or potential exists is not indicative of mental health. A realistic assessment of how things are is also important. Borysenko (1987) suggests avoiding the use of a system of thinking that can put mental processes in a restrictive and negative mode. She feels that becoming too analytical and negative limits the potential to consider—much less implement—positive reactions and responses. Perhaps El Phonse De Chateaubrilliant stated it best when he said, "We become what we consider." A desire to improve a situation where application of effort will yield a reasonably good chance of success is a positive thing; however, pining for something unrealistic is not mentally healthy behavior.

Realistic Expectations

Some feel that reality varies based on individual perspective. However, people who are mentally healthy perceive a reality that fits reasonably well with the "mainstream" and are not continually or seriously out of synch with most of society. Attempts to create a new reality or to deny the existence of what is real departs from mental health.

Facing up to reality enables the individual who is mentally healthy to live and act in harmony with the world and its people. If someone's view of the world is unreal or overly narrow, such an individual is less likely to function effectively or productively in the world.

Sociologist and philosopher Walt Schaefer (1992) believes that negative thoughts and self-talk run contrary to positive mental health. Schaefer classifies six varieties of negative thinking that can distract from positive mental well-being. These are pessimism, "catastrophizing," polarized thinking, "should-ing," blaming, and magnifying. Negative thinking is discussed more fully in a later chapter. The real issue here is to note that when people focus on issues or factors surrounding issues that are not realistic, they are not functioning at their best. The contemporary admonition to "get real" has great potential to allow individuals to cope, interact, decide, and think productively and honestly.

Management of Emotions

Located somewhere between ice-cold logic and the outright self-interest of survival are emotions. Survival is easy to comprehend, for without it there would likely be many fewer humans on the planet and perhaps none at all. Likewise, logical thinking utilizing rational, reasonable judgments based on the best available evidence allows for decision making that "makes sense." Emotions, however, often defy logic and move people toward destruction and away from survival. But without emotions, people would certainly be "less than human" and life would be much less interesting. Very few would suggest that people would be better off without love, fear, anger, remorse, and so on. The question is, how do these emotions influence people's lives? People who are mentally healthy are able to react to emotional responses in a productive fashion. They use emotional responses as a trigger for action or as barometers to provide information concerning the potential effect of an experience on them. Ekman (1992) notes that emotional reaction is very rapid. He cites evidence that people actually react emotionally before they can have any cognitive input into the process. In a sense, they may sacrifice accuracy or reason for speed.

This can produce a situation whereby immediate impressions outweigh careful analysis of factual information. While this speedy response may have been a matter of survival in prior times and perhaps can still be a factor important to survival in contemporary times, snap reactions can lead to potential harm. Perhaps the basis of the old adage, count to ten before reacting, was to enable the thinking to catch up with emotional responses. People who are mentally healthy try not to allow their emotions to govern their intellect or endanger their survival. They are able to recognize and manage the effects of emotional responses and "enjoy the ride" that emotions can provide without being adversely effected.

Functions Well with Others

Given the choice, would you rather get along well with yourself or with others? This may be a more realistic choice than first imagined. If getting along with others requires that a person surrender on a point, belief, or value, then the resulting discomfort may yield difficulties in living effectively in that relationship. So, getting along with others while still respecting the personal decisions made is extremely important. But what if the compromise is constant and causes you to feel out of tune with yourself? How would it feel to believe that you are failing to live up to your own code or belief system in order to maintain satisfactory relationships with others? In such circumstances, functioning with others is less the case in point and dysfunctioning may be a more accurate description. Methods of interacting such as always taking control on one extreme or constantly giving in to others' wishes on the other hand offer very mixed rewards. Establishing, maintaining, and in some cases terminating relationships is a skill natural to some and difficult for others. Arkoff (1995) suggests categorizing friends and associates into one of four groups. Group 1 is those with whom there is a completely positive and effective relationship. Group 2 is those with whom there is a mostly positive or productive relationship. Group 3 is those with whom the relationship is mostly negative or unproductive. Group 4 is those with whom the relationship is totally unproductive or negative. Arkoff does not have a neutral category because he feels that relationships that are not negative are in some way positive. He suggests that you ask yourself the question, Is your life rich in people? How well you interact with others and how you feel about it can be critical to positive mental health.

Draws Strength from Others without Being Overly Dependent

Having a network of friends can help ease life's burdens. Having a close trusted friend with whom to share concerns, troubles, doubts, dreams, and accomplishments can perhaps ease them even more. Having a wide pattern of casual friendships differs from having one intimate friend with whom talking and sharing is conducted under the protective shelter of trust and confidence. Research suggests that on the average men tend to have a much different pattern of friendship development and utilization than do women. Some have even suggested that the more effective utilization of friendship support for women is a critical factor in their longevity exceeding that of men. An interesting question is, Are people mentally healthy because of the support of their friendships or are those with high degrees of mental health better able to develop productive friendships? Whatever the case, using the strength and support of friends to get through difficult times in life or to help make important decisions is not the same as being unable to function without the constant support or continual input from friends. People who are mentally healthy are able to differentiate between the support of friends and the need for continued input or direction from friends.

Reasonable Appetites

Most individuals have tastes or appetites for something. Preferences allow for great individuality and variety. Food and drink are what usually come to mind when considering appetite, but there can also be tastes or preferences for risk, control, adventure, sex, drugs, and so on. To have an appetite under control allows for desire, achievement, and enjoyment. However, when control is lost, appetites can be overpowering. In such cases, appetites can control individuals rather than the other way around. Lickey and Gordon (1991) suggest that a loss of desire for food, sex, entertainment, recreation, or any other normally rewarding or pleasurable activity should be considered as indicative of a reduction in mental health status. People who are mentally healthy can and often do have healthy appetites for and derive enjoyment from things that do themselves and others no harm.

A Spiritual Nature

People who are spiritual have a sense of purpose in being and have a notion that they belong somewhere in their own big picture of the universe. A spiritual nature does not necessarily imply a formal belief system or membership in an organized religion. Spirituality does not even necessarily imply an overwhelming reverence for life or some sense of a universal oneness with humankind. It might, but such characteristics would be optional extras in people who are spiritual. Remen (1988) suggests that the spiritual dimension provides a deep sense of belonging and participation in life. So many people seek some aspect of the spirit that it can be considered to be essential to the well-being of humans. Individuals who are mentally healthy believe that there is a purpose to life and feel that they have a part to play in that purpose. They realize that there are many issues in the world that are larger than themselves and their needs.

Effective Coping Skills

Stress results when any number of things cause a reaction in people that requires extraordinary measures to maintain or return the body to equilibrium. Some sources of stress (stressors) are psychological in nature, while others are physical. While recognizing sources of stress and taking steps to eliminate stressors can be very effective, most people still experience periodic and even regular episodes of stress. Coping with stress by management of the stressor or intervention in the stress response allows the individual to maintain a life that is functional and enjoyable. Lazarus (1991) considers coping to predict how well a person can manage the demands of an encounter. He believes that there are both cognitive (changing the way of thinking about things) and behavioral (actually do something to change the relationship with the demand or threat) aspects to coping. People who are mentally healthy can accept the nature of stress and its frequency in life. They are able to use it as a motivation for behavior or to employ intervention or prevention strategies in order to continue living in a positive fashion.

Honest Self-Regard and Self-Esteem

People who are mentally healthy are not fooled by themselves. They are very much aware of who they are as well as who they are not. Most people occasionally experience being a little overconfident or perhaps unaware of their strengths at some time during their lives, but on the average they are aware of the scope of their abilities. A high degree of self-esteem without honest self-awareness can set the stage for very inaccurate opinions of oneself. People who are mentally healthy are able to assess their strengths as well as their deficiencies. This honest self-appraisal allows them to make sense of who they are and how they feel about themselves. They consider themselves as good or worthwhile due to their self-esteem. Honest self-awareness allows for constant appraisal of what is acceptable and what needs work; it can act as a means to motivate self-improvement while offering a buffer against self-doubt.

As already noted, it is rare for a person who is mentally healthy to have all of the preceding characteristics at one time. If that does occur, it is not for a prolonged period of time. A person who is mentally healthy may have many more characteristics than those described in this chapter, but this is certainly a good starting place. Subsequent chapters provide an examination of these characteristics in more depth and offer some tools for self-assessment with regard to these characteristics.

An Accurate and Realistic View of the World

Mentally healthy individuals generally perceive reality and the world around them in a manner similar to the majority of people. While there are obvious and important exceptions, concurrence as to what is and is not real is something that the mentally healthy would share. Individuals who continually view the world differently than the majority of people may simply be responding to different prior experiences that form a foundation for their interpretation. Such individuals may also have a greater or lesser capacity for the intake and utilization of information. However, when someone consistently and forcefully disagrees with the predominate views of society there is a potential for problems. These problems can occur even if the individual with the alternate perceptions is more intelligent, sensitive, or possesses keener powers of observation. While alternate views and opinions are often prized as the basis of new thinking and intellectual progress they have often created problems for some individuals. For the mentally healthy individual an accurate and realistic view of the world includes the ability to determine when and when not to focus on these different perspectives.

A realistic view of the world enables individuals to accurately perceive who and what they are. It also allows them to develop a sense of just where they fit in the grand scheme of things. Mentally healthy people honestly consider their importance, significance and role in contemporary life. Misinterpretations can produce inaccurate assumptions that may devalue or inflate individuals' consideration of the importance of themselves as well as other issues in life. The relative importance of such things may be altered to the extent that individuals take offense when none was intended or become oblivious to criticism or failure. Important questions to consider when fine tuning an accurate and realistic view of the world include:

"Are contemporary perceptions being influenced by past experiences?"
"Is this really important beyond the present moment?"
"How important is this in the grand scheme of things?"
"What impact will this have one month, one year or five years from now?"

Mentally healthy people are able to enjoy the present while preparing for the future utilizing lessons from the past. In a sense each individual is three individuals, the individual they are, the individual they once were and the individual they will become. Too much focus on any one of these can distort the accuracy of one's view of the world and become counter-productive to mental health. It is important to value, honor and respect the influence of the past. However failure to let go of past glory, success, failure, or relationships can create the type of burden sometimes termed excess baggage. A realistic view of the world includes accepting and coming to grips with the residual impact of prior life experiences. Failure to recognize and address these earlier occurrences can have a negative impact on present and future living. While nothing can be done to change the past, much can be done concerning how the past is regarded and utilized. Perhaps the most important aspect of prior life experiences is their influence on the accuracy of a contemporary view of the world and as a factor in influencing hope for the future.

To live only for or in the moment is risky because it can promote denial of the two other eras (the past and future) of the self. Focus on the here and now without concern for anything beyond the present distorts a realistic view of the world. While the future in inevitable and unavoidable, the nature of the future can be, in part at least, molded by our management of the past as well as our present actions, thoughts and plans. An accurate and realistic view of the world includes preparation for the future. While the slogan "good things come to those who wait" has merit, it might be more productive to consider that better things come to those who prepare. However, to only live for and dream about the future, denying the needs and realities of the present is not indicative of positive mental health. An accurate and realistic view of the world is promoted via an extended view. This extended view considers such things as what has happened in the past, how this impacts the present, what is happening in the present and how contemporary occurrences will influence the future.

Recognition of Mental Health Characteristics

A Comparison of Characteristics

Think again of the person you described at the beginning of the chapter. How does he or she compare to the characteristics described in the chapter? Please write your answers in the following spaces:

Characteristic	Does Compare	Does Not Compare
1. A positive outlook		
2. Realistic expectations		
3. Management of emotions		
4. Functions well with others		
5. Draws strength from others without being overly dependent		
6. Reasonable appetites		
7. A spiritual nature		
8. Effective coping skills		
9. Honest self-regard and self-esteem		
10. Accurate and realistic view of the world		

Reasons for Mental Health Characteristics

What enabled the person being described to develop these positive characteristics? Since most people would agree that it is not simply luck that allows them to be the way they are, what factors in their backgrounds contribute to a positive mental health status?

Consider the person used in the preceding comparison. Look at such factors as childhood experiences, the conditions of this person's home life, the types of early life experiences, and recent challenges, successes, and failures he/she has experienced. What types of friends does he/she have? Do this person's friends approach his/her level of mental health? Since the person described is an acquaintance, mutual experiences may be common. Ask yourself how much your personal mental health is like that of the person you have described. Are you very close or quite dissimilar in characteristics?

_____

_____

_____

_____

Developing Mental Health Characteristics

List any of the characteristics discussed in the chapter that you feel you would like to develop.

_____   _____

_____   _____

List any reasons that might be responsible for you not having the desired characteristic(s).

_____   _____

_____   _____

Keep this list in mind as you progress through the textbook, and refer back to this activity as more information is presented and you have the opportunity to react to this information.

Self-Assessment

Take a moment to examine how you measure up to the NMHA's indicators of mental health. Consider the extreme as well as the average feelings you experience regarding each of the three criteria.

Feelings about Self

1. Most positive _____

2. Typically positive _____

3. Least Positive _____

How positive do you feel about yourself most of the time?

5 ------------------ 4 ------------------ 3 ------------------ 2 ------------------ 1
Very positive   Fairly positive   Not very positive

How positive do you feel about yourself on the average?

5 ------------------ 4 ------------------ 3 ------------------ 2 ------------------ 1
Very positive   Fairly positive   Not very positive

Feelings about Others

1. Most positive feelings about others _____

_____

2. Typical (average) feelings about others _____

_____

3. Least positive feelings about others _____

_____

How do you feel about (most) other people most of the time?

5 ------------------ 4 ----------------- 3 ------------------ 2------------------ 1

Very positive   Fairly positive   Not very positive

Ability to Meet and Handle the Demands of Life

1. Everyday demands _____

_____

2. Serious demands _____

_____

How well do you cope with everyday demands?

5 ------------------ 4----------------- 3 ------------------ 2------------------ 1

Very well   Fairly well   Not too well

How well do you cope with the serious demands of life?

5 ------------------ 4----------------- 3 ------------------ 2------------------ 1

Very well   Fairly well   Not too well

Remember: It is not the purpose of this book to have people self-diagnose, and this exercise is far from sophisticated enough to enable anyone to do so. This is to simply awaken awareness for you on a personal level. With that in mind, write a few comments to assess how well you are functioning mentally in terms of

1. Interacting with others: _____

_____

_____

2. Life's demands: _____

_____

_____

Summary

People who are mentally healthy have a variety of personal characteristics in common. Some exhibit all of the attributes discussed in the chapter, while others may have a varying mix of the attributes. Individual patterns of behavior are one of the critical factors in creating individual differences. No one could, or even should be expected to, demonstrate all of these attributes all of the time. However, people who are mentally healthy exhibit many or most of these much of the time. In fact, the number of these characteristics they display (and the frequency with which they display them) may be critical to defining an individual's mental health status.

DISCUSSION QUESTIONS

1. Rank the characteristics discussed in this chapter in order of importance to mental health. Arrange them with *a* being the most important.

   a. _____   f. _____
   b. _____   g. _____
   c. _____   h. _____
   d. _____   i. _____
   e. _____   j. _____

   Can you justify your ranking? If your answer is no, discuss why it would not be possible to make such a ranking.

2. Another approach would be to assign a numerical value to each of the characteristics. Using a scale from 1 to 4, assign a value of 1 to those attributes with the highest value to healthy mental functioning and a 4 to those of less value.

3. Which of the following makes the greatest contribution to the development of the characteristics of people who are mentally healthy? Be prepared to defend your answer.

   a. Family
   b. Friends
   c. Culture
   d. Religion
   e. Education
   f. Life experiences such as travel
   g. Popular media

4. Would you consider mental health to be an inborn trait that is stronger in some than in others or something that is nurtured as a result of life's experiences?

REFERENCES

Arkoff, A., 1995 *Illuminated Life*. Boston: Allyn & Bacon. pg 77.
Borysenko, J. (1987). *Minding the Body, Mending the Mind*. New York: Bantam Books.
Ekman, P. (1992). An Argument for the Basic Emotions. *Cognition and Emotions*. 2, 98–102.
Goleman, D. (1997). *Emotional Intelligence*. New York: Bantam Books.
Gorman, J. M. (1996). *The Essential Guide to Mental Health*. New York: St. Martin's Griffen.
Lazarus, R. (1991). *Emotion and Adaptation*. Oxford: Oxford Press.
Lickey, M. & Gordon B. (1991). *Medicine and Mental Illness*. New York: W. H. Freeman & Co.
National Mental Health Association. (1996). *Characteristics of Mentally Healthy People*. Alexandria, VA: Author.
Offer, D. & Sabschin, M. (1984). *Normality and the Life Cycle*. New York: Basic Books.
Remen, R. (1988). On Defining Spirit. *Noetic Sciences Review*, Autumn.
Rogers, C. (1961). *On Becoming a Person*. Boston: Houghton Mifflin.
Schaefer, W. (1992). *Stress Management for Wellness* (2nd Ed.) Dallas: Harcourt, Brace & Jovanovich.
Shapiro, D. (1983). *Beyond Health and Normalcy*. New York: Van Nostrand Reinhold.
Sheehy, M. & Cournos, F. (1992). *What Is Mental Illness,* New York: Simon and Schuster.

CHAPTER

3

Emotional Well-Being

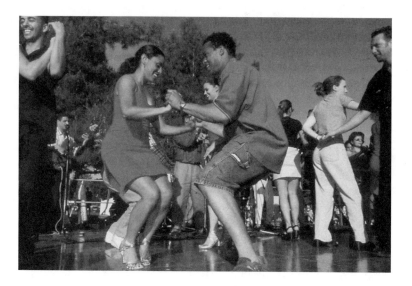

During the twentieth century, people devoted extensive time to studying the underlying factors of emotions. Psychologists, psychiatrists, and neurologists have all been interested in unlocking the secrets of the mind. Why do people feel happy or sad? What makes them feel angry? These may seem like simple questions. However, years of research have gone into finding an answer. Emotions are an essential part of life. In fact, many people will argue that it is emotions that drive behavior. If this is true, then emotions are a very powerful phenomenon. They affect the ability to make decisions and work toward goals, set up boundaries and internal guidance systems, communicate and guide interactions with others, and create a source of unity among human beings. Ultimately, they are at the core of overall psychological well-being. With this in mind, it is important to understand and accept the world of emotions. To achieve true emotional well-being, people need to become aware of how emotions affect their lives and develop the ability to understand and accept how they feel.

What Is Emotion?

First and foremost, a working definition of emotions is needed. What exactly is an emotion? This question has long been under debate, and often the answer depends on a person's philosophical and theoretical orientations. In everyday language, emotions are synonymous with feelings. Most psychologists agree that feelings, or subjective experiences, are a large part of emotions. They do, however, contend that there are several other components that make up emotions.

Emotions can be characterized by expressive reactions, including smiles or frowns; physiological reactions, including increases in heart rate and the production of tears; coping behavior, such as seeking comfort from one's mother or running away; and by the specific cognition or thoughts a person has (Cornelius, 1996). Together, these four areas give way to a more specific definition of emotions. Each part is essential to the definition. It is still under debate, however, which parts are the most important in describing emotions. Based on this information, *emotions* can be defined as a complex set of organized psychophysiological reactions that consist of cognition, actions, and somatic reactions (Folkman & Lazarus, 1988).

There is one more defining characteristic to emotions that needs to be discussed. Emotions are individualized and differ among people. Words such as *happy, sad, fear,* and *jealousy* are used to describe feelings. The degree to which these feelings are experienced and how people react to them are what separate one individual from another. There is a wide continuum of emotions. When people experience an event, they have certain feelings that fit somewhere on this continuum. What triggers one person to feel slightly upset can trigger another person to feel severely distraught and depressed. At times, people have a degree of emotion that is characterized by a psychological disorder or mental illness. It is not the emotion itself that causes a psychological problem; rather, it is the degree to which a person experiences that emotion and how that person copes and reacts to it.

Emotional well-being is dependent upon the understanding and processing of and coping with emotions. This chapter explores both the physiology and psychology of emotions. Hopefully, the reader will gain a better understanding of where emotions come from, how people process emotions, and the ways in which emotions affect lives. In addition, strategies for achieving emotional well-being are introduced and discussed.

The Physiology of Emotions

The Brain

To understand fully the concept of emotions, a basic understanding of the brain and the role it plays is needed. The brain is the most important part of the human nervous system. It is the focal point of organizing nerve impulses that carry information throughout the body. The brain controls all automatic vital functions such

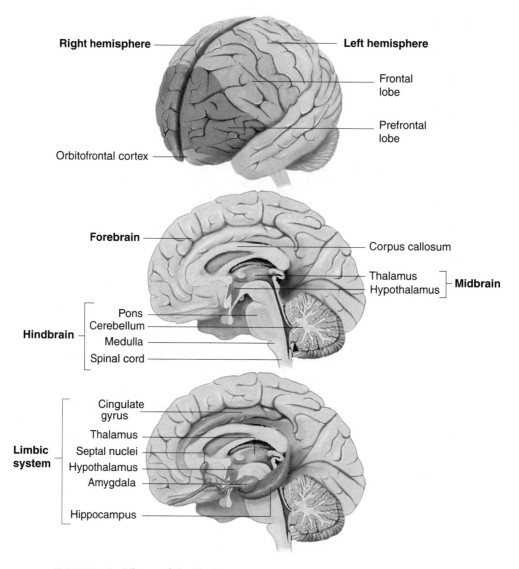

FIGURE 3.1   Views of the Brain

as breathing, digestion, and hormone release, along with processes such as smell, touch, muscle movement, and strength. In addition, the brain is the cognitive center of the body. It is the place where ideas are generated, memory is stored, and emotions are experienced (Hafen, Karren, Frandsen, & Smith, 1996). The very emotions that powerfully affect people's lives are originated in the brain, thus giving the brain a strong influence over the body. In fact, some see the main function of emotions as coordinating the mind and body. An emotion organizes areas such as perception, thought, memory, behavior, physiology, and social interaction to provide a person with the best means for coping with a situation that generates the specific emotion (Pally, 1998). The emotions produced by the brain are essentially a combination of feelings and physical responses. Over the years, there have been several areas of the brain identified as being important in the generation and processing of emotions.

There are three main divisions of the brain: the forebrain, the midbrain, and the hindbrain. Each division has several structures that contribute to various types of physiological and psychological processing. The *forebrain* has been shown to host the major structures involved in the perception and processing of emotions. The two primary structures of the forebrain involved in emotions are the cerebral cortex and the limbic system. The *cerebral cortex* is the folded, twisted tissue that comes to mind when imagining what a brain looks like. It controls higher order abstract functioning and is divided into two hemispheres, the right and left, that are connected by the corpus callosum. Each hemisphere specializes in specific areas. Generally speaking, the right hemisphere is associated with unconscious awareness, perception of faces and patterns, comprehension of body language and social cues, creativity, intuitive reasoning, visual-spatial processing, and overall comprehension. The left hemisphere controls language, speech communication, verbal intelligence and memories, and information processing in the areas of math, typing, grammar, logic, analytic reasoning, and perception of details (Bancroft, 1999).

The idea that the right and left hemispheres are specialized for different types of thinking has been backed by research over the years. Originally, researchers thought the right hemisphere was superior in the processing of all emotional expressions. However, new research suggests that the two hemispheres play distinct emotional roles. More recently, it has also been proposed that the two hemispheres are specialized for different emotional experiences. This type of division of labor may be more efficient. Research from people with neurological problems such as epilepsy supports this notion. For example, one documented case involved a woman who experienced seizure attacks to both the right and left hemispheres. A team of clinicians found that when the seizure attacks were to the left hemisphere she would become depressed and agitated, whereas with attacks to the right hemisphere she would become manic and careless (Miller, 1988). Other researchers have found that when people experienced positive emotions the left hemisphere was more active and when they experienced negative emotions the right hemisphere was more active (Miller, 1988; Moretti, Charlton, & Taylor, 1996). This is further supported by studies showing that people who are under distress and who are pessimistic have increased activity in the right hemisphere. In addition, people who have at some point in their lives been clinically depressed show decreased left hemisphere activity when compared to people who have never been clinically depressed (Goode, Schrof, & Burke, 1991). Although findings over the years have varied in this area, there is strong support for the belief that emotional processing is done in both hemispheres.

The *limbic system* is another area of the brain that is important in studying emotions. The limbic system is a collection of brain structures that are involved with emotion, motivation, behavior, memory storage, and recall. The major structures that make up this system are the hippocampus, amygdala, parts of the thalamus and hypothalamus, and the septal nuclei. The hippocampus helps convert short-term memories into long-term memories. It stores memories that are of emotional and motivational significance to a person. The amygdala's job is to sense the emotional significance of all experiences. This is the structure that is responsible for the ability to feel complex emotions like love and anxiety. It causes an emotional influence on perception and thought. As a result, damage to this area can create misperceptions in societal cues. In addition, violent tendencies have been linked to this structure. The thalamus is the relay station for incoming sensory signals and outgoing motor signals that pass to and from the cerebral cortex. The hypothalamus is the structure in the brain that controls and monitors the ability to feel extreme pain or pleasure. It is the most primitive part of the limbic system and is where all emotions originate as raw, undirected feelings. In a sense, the hypothalamus is the emotional core of being. The septal nucleus is involved with the ability to form emotional and social bonds with others. It also can exert discouraging effects on mood. Stimulation of this structure is known to generate strong feelings of pleasure. It taps into the emotional pool of the hypothalamus and, because of this, is able to exert emotional influence upon the entire brain. It is also interconnected with the hippocampus and can counteract the amygdala. The limbic system is primarily concerned with emotions and their behavioral expression. It is thought to produce such emotions as fear, anxiety, and joy in response to physical and psychological signals (Bancroft, 1999).

Nerve Cells and Communication

In studying emotions, it is also necessary to have a basic understanding of how messages are communicated throughout the brain and body. There is a multitude of research that supports the notion that psychological disorders are caused in part by some defect in the transmission of messages in the brain. In fact, this is the basis for prescribing medications for clinical disorders such as depression or anxiety. In some way, these medications have an effect on the ways in which nerve cells communicate in the brain.

There are three major parts of nerve cells: the cell body, the dendrites, and the axon. The *cell body* is the large part of the nerve cell that contains the nucleus. *Dendrites* are hairlike projections from the cell body that receive information. The *axon* is somewhat like an extremely long dendrite with branches at the end. At the end of these branches are structures called *synaptic knobs*. The space between the synaptic knob of one nerve cell and the dendrite of the next cell is called the *synapse* (Levinthal, 1999).

Synaptic knobs have structures called *synaptic vesicles* that produce and store chemicals called *neurotransmitters*. Nerve impulses cause the release of neurotransmitters, which then flood the synapse and bond to special receptors on the dendrite. The receptors and neurotransmitters have similar shapes, and the neurotransmitter fits the receptor like a key in a lock. The bonding of the neurotransmitter to the receptor causes a change in electric potential in the nerve cell. These changes in electric potential are called *nerve impulses,* and they allow nerve cells to communicate with each other (Levinthal, 1999).

This communication comes in two basic forms: one type, called *excitation,* tells cells to work harder, to fire more impulses. The second type, called *inhibition,* tells cells to relax, to fire fewer impulses. Because impulses occur at a very rapid rate (many times per second) and each impulse requires the presence of a neurotransmitter, the body "recycles" these chemicals. After a neurotransmitter bonds to a receptor and transmits the impulse, it is released from the receptor and returns to the synaptic knob. This process is called *reuptake.* Reuptake is a process that allows neurons to have a constant supply of neurotransmitters available. If reuptake does not function correctly, the healthy nerve cell replaces the neurotransmitter.

Neurotransmitters. Following are brief descriptions of five neurotransmitters: acetylcholine, norepinephrine, dopamine, serotonin, and endorphins.

Acetylcholine was the first neurotransmitter discovered. There are two types of receptors for acetylcholine: muscarinic and nicotinic. *Muscarinic receptors* are named after the drug muscarine; and, when acetylcholine binds to them, it stimulates the parasympathetic nervous system. This part of the nervous system functions to generally relax the body. If a drug is antimuscarinic, it interferes with acetylcholine's ability to stimulate the parasympathetic nervous system. Atropine, for example, is a drug used to dilate the eyes during eye examinations, and it works by preventing the parasympathetic response of pupil contraction.

There is a class of hallucinogens that are able to block the effects of acetylcholine on the parasympathetic nervous system. Called *anticholinergic drugs,* the effects they produce include reduced production of mucus and saliva and the elevation of body temperature, heart rate, and blood pressure. Psychoactive effects include delirium, confusion, and loss of memory of events during the drugged state. These drugs come from natural sources such as the mandrake plant, henbane, jimsonweed, and deadly nightshade. These plants—which create a feeling of flying, as well as other hallucinogenic effects—were major components of witches' potions during medieval times.

Nicotinic receptors are responsive to nicotine. They are found on motor neurons and throughout the cerebral cortex of the brain. Acetylcholine (as well as nicotine) stimulates these receptors to relax muscle tightness; and, at extreme doses, antinicotinic drugs can create severe and rapid paralysis. The poisons curare and botulinus toxin (botulism) either block acetylcholine from entering nicotinic receptor sites or from being released from the synaptic knobs (Levinthal, 1999).

Norepinephrine is concentrated in the hypothalamus and limbic system, as well as in parts of the peripheral nervous system. In the brain, norepinephrine is related to regulation of mood states and is also believed to be involved in the control of seizures. Recent research has shown that genetically engineered rats lacking norepinephrine are more susceptible to induced seizures than rats with normal levels of this neurotransmitter (Palmiter, 1999). Monoamine oxidase (MAO) inhibitors, which inhibit MAO enzymes (which function to inactivate a number of neurotransmitters including norepinephrine, serotonin, and dopamine), increase the levels of norepinephrine in the brain and are for this reason often used to treat depression, which is characterized by decreased levels of these neurotransmitters.

In the peripheral nervous system, norepinephrine stimulates the sympathetic nervous responses, creating what some have called a "flight or fight" situation. Examples demonstrating changes in levels of neurotransmitters with a drug-induced state follow. Related to this function of norepinephrine are the amphetamines and cocaine. Amphetamines work by either mimicking norepinephrine at the receptor sites or by inducing the release of the neurotransmitter from the synaptic knob. This explains the highly stimulating effects of amphetamines: faster breathing and heart rate, higher blood pressure and body temperature, decreased appetite, and a boost in alertness and energy. Cocaine works by blocking the reuptake of norepinephrine and dopamine from the receptors, causing the neurotransmitters to have a more pronounced effect (Levinthal, 1999). Recent research into the mechanisms of ketamine's ("Special K") effect have shown that it selectively inhibits norepinephrine and serotonin receptors (Nishimura & Sato, 1999).

It is important to realize that each individual person has a natural level of energy. Some people simply have more energy than others do. This is particularly important in U.S. society, which is characterized by high energy and constant motion. Some people choose to augment their energy level by consuming drugs such as caffeine, cocaine, crack, or amphetamines. When this happens, the body may heighten its energy level for a period of time; however, it will eventually return to the "normal" level of the person. In fact, the energy level may return to a level that is lower than the "normal" level. This process is called *rebalancing* or a *rebound effect*. The body can only retain a high level of energy for so long, then exhaustion sets in, and the body must rebalance. For example, on a continuum of one to ten, if an individual's natural level of energy is a five, consuming a substance may energize him or her to an eight. It is only natural that the body will rebalance at a level lower than five in order to recuperate and maintain homeostasis.

Dopamine, another transmitter, is important for two aspects of behavior: motor control and emotionality. Parkinson's disease, characterized in its early stages by a marked deficiency in motor control, is caused by degeneration in the dopamine-releasing neurons of the midbrain. The second function of dopamine is in controlling emotionality. Defects in dopamine-producing neurons in the cortex and limbic system that cause the brain to produce too much dopamine are believed to play a major role in the development of schizophrenia. Overdose of L-dopa, a drug used to treat Parkinson's disease by increasing dopamine production, produces schizophrenic-like symptoms. Drugs used to treat schizophrenia work by blocking dopamine from entering receptor sites, thereby causing elevated levels of serum dopamine to exist (Levinthal, 1999). Recent research into the roots of these disorders has shown associations between dopamine D4 receptors and other neuropsychiatric disorders, including attention-deficit/hyperactivity disorder, mood disorders, and Parkinson's disease, as well as specific personality traits such as novelty seeking (Tarazi & Baldessarini, 1999).

Serotonin is concentrated in a number of places. In the pons and medulla of the hindbrain, it regulates sleep patterns. In the limbic system, it regulates mood, like norepinephrine. Increased levels of serotonin have been correlated with an increase in aggression, confidence, and leadership abilities. In the midbrain, decreased levels of serotonin have been correlated with increased irritability and extreme emotion, such as depression, or mood swings. It is also believed that sex hormones like estrogens and androgens have an effect on serotonin regulation (Fink, Sumner, Rosie, Wilson, & McQueen, 1999). MAO inhibitors have been shown to increase the production of serotonin, and tricyclic antidepressants have been shown to slow down the reuptake of serotonin and norepinephrine. For these reasons, the preceding two classifications of drugs are used in the treatment of clinical depression. There is an increase in emotions and a higher state of happiness evident when individuals consume these drugs.

There are, however, a number of people who will try to *self-medicate.* This means that some people elect to consume drugs—such as cocaine, crack, and amphetamines—that will produce a similar effect. These drugs produce an increased state of happiness that cannot be sustained. This is an unnatural way of increasing happiness. If an individual continues to use these aforementioned drugs, he or she may experience a state known as *anhedonia.* This is a state when an individual ceases to experience emotions at the higher or lower level. Essentially, one may say that this person is catatonic or possesses a placid personality. This person may reacquire their emotions in time, but there are no guarantees.

Endorphins are actually a group of neurotransmitters that chemically resemble morphine. Three groups exist: enkephalins, beta-endorphins, and dynorphines. They are known as *endogenous opioid peptides,* or endorphins. Increased levels of endorphins are produced in response to pain and have an anesthetic effect. This effect is so intense that scientists must control for it when studying response to pain (Lautenbacher, Roscher, Kohl, Vedder, & Krieg, 1999). Endorphin levels measured in the placental bloodstream of pregnant women peak during labor. Morphine and other opiate drugs such as heroin do not change levels of endorphins or reuptake of these chemicals; instead, they directly stimulate endorphin receptors (Levinthal, 1999). In this way, they are unlike other illicit drugs in that they act directly on the existing neurotransmitter receptors to produce effects.

Each of these neurotransmitters is produced naturally in our bodies. It is important to realize, however, that when people choose to self-medicate or act as their own biochemist, the amount of neurotransmitters and balance within our bodies becomes irregular. This type of substance abuse is not beneficial to achieving emotional well-being.

Emotional Processing

Having the preceding basic knowledge of the brain, it is easier to examine a model of emotional processing. As mentioned earlier, emotions connect the mind with the body as well as create unity between individuals. How exactly is this done? Well, the first step includes the appraisal of stimuli. During this stage, the brain focuses on evaluating incoming stimuli in order to assess its significance to the organism. In its most simplistic form, stimuli can be either rewarding or aversive. Stimuli appraised as rewarding lead to positive emotions such as happiness, whereas stimuli appraised as aversive lead to negative emotions such as fear. Two appraisal centers in the brain are the amygdala and the orbitofrontal cortex (Pally, 1998). Remember, the amygdala is responsible for sensing the emotional significance of all experiences. It makes more simple kinds of appraisals such as good/bad or safe/dangerous. The orbitofrontal cortex is an area of the prefrontal cortex that receives inputs from parts of the thalamus and hypothalamus, among other areas (Pally). It is involved in the adjustment of previously formed stimulus-reinforcement associations. Because these stimulus-reinforcement associations are strong and are considered to be the basis of various emotional states, it is easy to see how this area is involved in the appraisal of more complex stimuli that build from personal experience over the course of one's life.

The second stage in emotional processing includes the brain and body changes that result from the appraisals. The amygdala and orbitofrontal cortex appraisal centers send messages to the hypothalamus and the brainstem. This in turn activates the brain and body changes of emotion through endocrine production, the autonomic nervous system, and musculoskeletal behaviors (Pally, 1998). The hypothalamus regulates a number of hormones—such as cortisol, which facilitates the metabolic reactions of emotional arousal. In addition, the hypothalamus signals to the pituitary gland when to release endorphins that decrease pain sensations and promote attachment. One final function of the hypothalamus is that it helps control the skeletal muscles through the cranial nerves to produce various *emotional* behaviors such as a smile or a frown. The autonomic, or *automatic,* responses of the body are essential to the experience of emotions and stress and are discussed in more detail later on.

The third stage of emotional processing is the feedback of brain and body changes. It is thought that during this stage the body and brain changes are *fed* back to the brain and as a result are represented as part of the whole experience. Most of the time this occurs without conscious awareness; however, when it is processed consciously it contributes to our subjective experiences (Pally, 1998).

The Autonomic Nervous System

It has been shown that emotional processing is rooted in the physiology of the brain. It is essential for people to realize that their experiences produce certain physiological reactions due to such a complex system. The autonomic nervous system plays a crucial role in the way the body reacts to various stimuli. The autonomic nervous system is involved in the automatic regulation of smooth muscles, cardiac muscles, and the glands. In other words, it controls all the involuntary functions of the body. It regulates these parts by sending impulses to them that are controlled by nerve centers in the lower part of the brain (Bancroft, 1999). The system is divided into two opposing systems that have different effects on the body: the sympathetic nervous system (SNS) and the parasympathetic nervous system (PNS).

The SNS serves to prepare the body for "flight or fight." It helps to ensure survival in the face of an environmental threat through the accumulation of energy reserves that can be utilized when needed. When a person encounters an emotional situation, particularly fear, the SNS is activated by the hypothalamus and causes physiological reactions such as increased heart rate, dilated pupils, increased strength of skeletal muscles, and increased mental activity (Bancroft, 1999; Greenberg, 1996). The PNS functions as the opposite of the SNS. It serves primarily to prepare the body for feeding, digestion, and rest. It also aids in increasing the body's supply of energy. Once the body has been energized by the SNS and the stressor has passed, the PNS helps restore calmness and helps the body rest (Bancroft, 1999).

It is apparent in the preceding discussion that emotions lead to actual physical changes that have the potential to contribute to psychosomatic disorders. Historically, individuals who presented with physical symptoms as a result of emotions were told, "It's all in your head." This is clearly not true. The body can develop chronic physical symptoms from severe anxiety, for example, that can ultimately damage the body. In fact, the body and mind are interconnected in such a way that emotions and illnesses have a close relationship.

Emotions and Physical Illness

In recent years, there has been more emphasis on the study of psychoneuroimmunology (PNI). The science of PNI focuses on the connection between the mind, the brain, and the immune system. Physicians and psychologists are beginning to realize that emotions play an extremely important role in both sickness and health. It appears to have an astounding effect on the immune system in that positive emotions help improve immune responses and negative emotions can damage immune responses (Hafen et al., 1996).

The immune system is in charge of policing the body against internal and external attackers. It is made up of lymphocytes (T cells and B cells) and antibodies that the system stores. When an antigen enters the body, certain cells help turn on cells that multiply to form an "army" to fight while other cells suppress the "army" when all is clear. Research has found support that emotions can have a profound impact on how this system operates. For example, there is a line of research that indicates guided imagery can control the immune responses (Hafen et al., 1996). In addition, other studies have shown a connection between the central nervous system and the immune system that suggests that the mind can influence sensitivity or resistance to disease. In other words, people have the ability to consciously control how their immune system functions by altering how they think.

Physicians are beginning to believe that a patient with a good attitude or "fighting spirit" has a much greater chance of recovering from life-threatening diseases such as cancer (Robinson, 1988). In addition, the ways in which a person expresses emotions also play a part in this phenomenon. For example, researchers have found that the "nonexpression" of emotions is a hallmark of the cancer personality. Keeping emotions bottled up inside, thus creating unresolved tension, has been shown to be a common personality characteristic of people diagnosed with cancer (Hafen et al., 1996). Thus, it is important to realize that it is not emotional arousal in and of itself that is harmful. In fact, emotional arousal is a normal part of living and serves many adaptive purposes. Rather, it is the inability to properly regulate emotions, resulting in either too much or not enough and how the individual copes with these situations, that is crucial.

This section has provided a brief overview of the physiology of emotions. It is clear that the brain, along with the various physiological processes it produces, has an astounding effect on our emotions. Over the years, researchers have pinpointed several brain structures that are essential to the production and processing of emotions. More recently, it has also been found that emotions are connected to illness and the immune system. This has several implications for people who are *at risk* for developing certain diseases or who already have developed a disease. In addition, it begins to bridge the gap between the body and the mind.

The Psychology of Emotions

Theories of Emotions

As has been shown, physiology plays an important part in the *science* of emotions. There is, however, another major area to examine. The study of emotions has long been linked to psychology, and the field of psychology contributes greatly to the study of emotions. In fact, the very core of psychology involves how people feel and think about selves, others, and the world. With this in mind, it is logical to think that emotions play a crucial part in both psychological theory and mental illness.

In studying emotions from the standpoint of psychology, there are several psychological theories that can be discussed. Certainly, each theoretical orientation in psychology—including psychodynamics, behaviorism, and existentialism—can offer insight into the concept of emotions. There is one orientation, however, that is the most linked to the study of emotions and is included in many emotional theories. This is the area of *cognitive psychology*. Since the 1950s, psychologists have focused on cognitive processes and their impact on behavior. This involves the study of basic information processing, including attention and memory, as well as higher mental processes such as thinking, planning, and decision making. As with many other behaviors, psychologists have analyzed emotions from this viewpoint. Cognitive or cognitive-behavioral psychologists focus on how thoughts and information processing can become distorted and lead to maladaptive emotions and behavior.

One of the most influential theorists in the modern cognitive approach to emotion is Magda Arnold (1960). Her theory identifies and explains the major components of emotion. Arnold was one of the first people to look at emotions as being a distinct type of perception. The perception of emotions is not the same as the perception of simple objects. Rather, emotions are perceived based on a judgment of how the object or event maybe harmful or beneficial (Cornelius, 1996). For example, if a person were to encounter a bear while walking in the woods, a judgment would be made as to whether or not the person thought the bear would be harmful. This judgment would result in a particular emotion. For example, the bear could be perceived as dangerous or life threatening, which would evoke the emotion of fear. The person, in turn, would respond according to this emotion, possibly trying to flee or escape the situation. This is an emotional perception. This is very different from seeing a picture in a book and perceiving it as a bear.

This notion of emotional perception is synonymous with the cognitive process of appraisal. Arnold (1960) states that at the heart of every emotion is a special kind of judgment or appraisal. As mentioned in the beginning of this chapter, there is a continuum of emotions that a person can fall into. Why can two people in the same situation experience different emotions? According to cognitive psychology, this difference in emotion is explained by the fact that people think about or appraise situations differently. This cognitive process of appraisal, therefore, is very important to the study of emotions.

Appraisal refers to the process by which individuals judge the personal relevance of their situation for good or bad. It is the evaluation they make about the significance of knowledge in relation to their personal well-being (Cornelius, 1996; Lazarus, 1991). In this context, knowledge refers to the beliefs a person has about the way the world works in general and in a specific context. This knowledge can be seen as *nonemotional* until the point that appraisals are made (Lazarus). In other words, the essence of the cognitive approach in emotions is to understand how people make judgments about events in their environments. This view holds that emotions are the result of these appraisals. They are responses to cognitive activity that generates meaning. Without this appraisal, there can be no emotions. "To arouse an emotion, the object must be appraised as affecting me in some way, affecting me personally as an individual with my particular experience and my particular aims" (Arnold, 1960, p. 171).

The cognitive view does not dismiss the fact that physiology plays a part in emotions. In fact, Arnold (1960) holds that appraising one's situation in a particular way sets a certain set of physiological responses in motion that are experienced as a type of unpleasant tension. When the action implied by the appraisal takes place, there is a relief of this tension. In addition, different emotions drive people to different actions. Thus, Arnold argued that because different emotions appear to motivate people differently, there is a distinct pattern of physiological activity for each one (Cornelius, 1996).

There is one more aspect of appraisals that needs to be discussed. Arnold referred to these cognitive appraisals as *sense judgments* in order to recognize their immediate, nonreflective nature. These appraisals are not intellectual judgments that involve an in-depth cognitive processing. Instead, they are automatic. People judge their relationships to certain objects and events with a great degree of speed that would not allow for more in-depth processing. Arnold used the example of baseball to explain this concept. A baseball player uses judgments much like appraisals to coordinate movements, speed, and direction when trying to catch a fly ball. If a player actually stopped to think about the situation and analyze the best reaction, he or she would not stay in the game long. Thus, a baseball player reacts to the game according to the appraisals the player makes (Cornelius, 1996).

Taken together, the preceding discussion of emotions leads to a more precise definition of emotions that is offered by Arnold (1960). *Emotions* are "the felt tendency toward anything intuitively appraised as good (beneficial) or away from anything intuitively appraised as bad (harmful). This attraction or aversion is accompanied by a pattern of physiological changes organized toward approach or withdrawal. The patterns differ for different emotions" (p. 182).

One outgrowth of the cognitive view of emotion is the *relational theory* of emotion. In the relational theory, emotions are viewed as the process of establishing, maintaining, or disrupting the relation between the organism and the internal and external environment on matters of significance to the person (Campos, Campos, & Barrett, 1989). The relation can be with another individual or an object. Focusing on emotions as a relational process shifts the interest to include transactions between the person and his or her environment. In addition, it creates a new purpose for emotions being communicative. For example, the emotion of joy functions to signal to the person and to others to keep up the interaction. Thus, joy monitors the success of a goal and organizes expressive signals that will help continue the interaction. Sadness, on the other hand, occurs when an action is seen as being unlikely to be successful in attaining a goal. Social signals accompany sadness, and serve to gather help in a situation in which the person believes nothing more can be done (Campos et al.).

In this relational view, the appraisal process includes *relational meanings* that a person sees when confronted with a situation. The relational meanings are specific implications for personal well-being and are a function of what the person brings to the situation and what the situation has to offer the person (Cornelius, 1996). There have been two levels of appraisal identified by relational theorists. The first is the *molecular level of appraisal*. This level comprises the specific judgments made by a person to assess the costs and benefits in the person's environment. They are individual appraisal components and are essential to the concept of appraisal discussed up to this point. The second is the *molar level of appraisal* in which these individual appraisal components are combined to create *core relational themes*. These core relational themes serve as a summary of the emotional meaning of an event. They are the central relational harm or benefit in situations that underlie each emotion.

Core relational themes are disclosed by the combination of several individual appraisals such as whether the event is relevant to a person's goals, whether it will bring a person closer to or farther away from attainment of those goals, and whether or not the person can do anything about the event. Each emotion, therefore, is associated with a specific pattern of individual appraisal components and a particular core relational theme (Cornelius, 1996; Lazarus, 1991). Lazarus (1991) offers one example of a core relational theme for the emotion of anger. Suppose you are at a party and overhear a friend making a sarcastic comment about you behind your back. This situation is relevant to your goal of maintaining a friendship in that it compromises the goal. Furthermore, it is a situation in which the other person is to blame. According to Lazarus (1991), these individual appraisal components come together to form the theme "a demeaning offense against me" that generates the emotion of anger. If the situation was reversed and you were making a sarcastic comment about one of your friends, then the core relational theme would be different and the resulting emotion of guilt would follow instead of anger.

The relational approach to studying emotions has several implications for emotion theory that Campos and his colleagues (1989) discuss. First, there are certain factors that have been previously neglected in studying emotions. One important process is that of motivation. Motivation, including striving to attain goals, helps explain how the same situation can extract different affective reactions. In a sense, the emotional outcome of a situation depends on the motivational context. In addition, because of the expressive nature of emotions, social referencing can occur by the emotional signals of a person being used by others to interpret environmental events and regulate the course of action. This repetitive process can create the basis for the value system of a culture.

A second implication of this theory is an emphasis on the importance of action. One major function of emotion is to change the relation between the organism and the environment. To accomplish this, emotional regulation is needed. Part of this process includes regulating the action tendencies of the other organism in the relation. *Action tendencies* refer to preparing to use any one of a number of behaviors that can serve the same function for the environment. For example, the action tendencies can be facilitated, redirected, or prevented depending on how the person appraises the situation. This theory implies that the emotions of other people can directly affect the self.

There are two more implications that need to be mentioned. The third is the necessity of viewing human beings as living in a complex interrelationship with social and physical objects. This implies that there is some sort of shared meaning and emotional sharing among people. This breaks the trend of the traditional view that psychological well-being is dependent solely on the individual. The individual is part of a larger social system, and the relationship a person has with the environment is important in achieving good mental health. This has several implications for achieving good mental health that are discussed later in this chapter.

Finally, the fourth implication of the relational theory is the incorporation of autonomic responses. Here again is the link between psychology and physiology. Physiological autonomic responses have powerful social regulatory consequences and fit into this theory quite nicely. Take blushing, for example. Blushing is a physiological response that expresses or communicates to other people the emotion of embarrassment or shame. Similar autonomic responses can be seen in anger (flushed face) and sadness (production of tears).

Sex Differences in Emotions

The differences in how males and females perceive and interpret life events are easily seen with respect to emotional expressions. People often discuss how males and females differ in their emotional expression. In fact, the differences that exist are often a main point of tension and conflict in male/female relationships. What exactly are the differences, and why do they exist? This question has been explored for many years.

First, women are generally more emotionally expressive than men. For example, compared to men, women disclose their feelings to a greater extent. Women tend to report their negative feelings, cry, and display more nonverbal expressions than their counterparts. This is not written in stone, however, because men have been shown to express certain emotions such as anger more often and with greater intensity (Timmers, Fischer, & Manstead, 1998).

One way researchers explore this phenomenon is by looking at physiology. Is there something genetically different in males and females that leads to this difference in emotional expression? Emotional perception is a task that is completed mostly in the right hemisphere of the brain. This suggests that emotional processing may differ in males and females due to a difference in cerebral capacity within the right hemisphere. Another possibility is that it may be related to differences in the development of the temporal cortex of the brain. Researchers also leave room for the idea that social experiences may promote sex differences. Girls, for example, are encouraged more than boys in the expression and perception of emotion and nonverbal communication (Crucian & Berenbaum, 1998).

Another way to look at the gender differences in emotions is from a psychological perspective. One specific area that has been examined is regulating emotions. Emotion regulation serves to channel emotional responses in a way that is appropriate within a particular emotion culture. Emotions serve to signal social needs and communicate social intentions and interpersonal goals. What are the motives males and females have for regulating emotions? Well, some researchers have suggested there are four main types of motives: (1) the expected cathartic effects of emotion expression, (2) avoidance of gender-inappropriate impressions, (3) power-based motives, and (4) relationship-oriented motives (Timmers et al., 1998). The first two motives deal with the specific regulation of emotional expression. The expected cathartic effect deals with the nature of the emotion expression involved and is concerned with the effects for self. For example, crying may be experienced as a relief, and slamming a door in anger may be experienced as intrinsically satisfying. The second type, the avoidance of gender-inappropriate emotional impressions, concerns the emotional expression in relation to others. For example, there is a presumable norm governing the emotional expression of men and women in that men should suppress most of their emotions, whereas women are permitted to be more expressive. More recently, it has been proposed that the emotions men should suppress are those that signal powerlessness (Timmers et al. 1998).

The two remaining motives relate to interpersonal goals people want to achieve in specific situations. Generally speaking, men seem to be less concerned with the negative consequences of failing to express positive emotions toward another person. On the contrary, they expect more positive consequences from expressing more powerful emotions such as anger and pride. As a result of this, men are expected to be more concerned than women with power-based motives in which they try to regain control over themselves, over situations, and over others. Women, on the other hand, are more focused on the relational consequences of emotion expression. Generally, they are more motivated to keep others happy and to maintain close relationships with others. Therefore, this motive for women is considered to be relationship oriented (Timmers et al., 1998).

Research results do indicate that women tend to display more powerlessness when expressing their emotions, whereas men tend to display more power. Why is this? It could be because femininity has traditionally been associated with emotionality. In addition, there may be a self-fulfilling prophecy. It can be argued that because others expect women to display their emotions spontaneously, women act accordingly (Timmers et al., 1998).

The College Years

Many researchers believe that the college years are the most stressful years in a person's life. Studies have found that college students experience significant life change. During these years, students experience a wide array of emotions, including love, shyness, jealousy, anxiety, and frustration. Some of the more pertinent factors in the experience of stress during the college years are lifestyle change, friendships, and jealousy (Greenberg, 1996).

For the first time in many students' lives, they must assume responsibilities they never had to assume before. They leave the comforts of home and are suddenly expected to lead a responsible and functional life. In addition to this, the younger college student is faced with several other tasks. Greenberg (1996) lists the following tasks that need to be addressed during the college years:

1. The development of competence
2. The management of emotions
3. The freeing of interpersonal relationships
4. The development of purpose
5. The development of integrity
6. The development of identity
7. The development of autonomy

This list contains tasks that are very complex and ones that many people struggle with throughout their lives. It is certainly a lot for a traditional eighteen-year-old student to be faced with when beginning college.

The friendship factor is of particular importance to college students. They have to give up or change old friendships and develop new ones once they go on to college. This is a very challenging process. College students often have concerns about whether people will like them, whether they will find people with similar interests, and whether or not they will find friends and companionship. This leads to many stressful emotions for college students. Along with this comes a feeling of jealousy for some. Making new friends can be ego threatening. Jealousy is the fear of losing property, whether it is friends, status, or power. This is a stressor many college students experience (Greenberg, 1996).

The college years are a very exciting time of life, with many different emotions arising, often at the same time. Most college students feel happy and energetic about their newfound freedoms and new lives. There are also, however, many stressors that lead to feelings of anxiousness, frustration, and insecurity. It is important that college students become aware of their feelings and be able to process them. *Processing* simply means to think about why feelings are a particular way and how to deal with them. Developing a good social support system, using effective time management, and utilizing relaxation techniques are all good ways to maintain healthy emotional functioning during the college years.

Integrated Analysis of Three Emotions

The study of emotions has gone hand in hand with the study of poor mental health over the years. This is mostly because it is difficult to separate the two concepts. It is difficult to study what is *abnormal* without a conceptualization and a way of measuring what is *normal.* Remember that emotions in and of themselves are not bad. It is the degree and expression of emotions that can lead to poor mental health and psychological disorders. To achieve emotional well-being, an understanding is needed of the main emotions that all people experience and the effect they have on mental health. The discussion to this point has examined the physiological and psychological components of emotions. Now consider three common emotions: anger, anxiety, and depression. Each of these emotions will be explored with respect to their psychological and physiological aspects and to discuss the healthy and unhealthy expression of each.

Anger

Everyone has experienced anger—whether as a brief annoyance or as full-force rage. Anger is a completely "normal" and healthy human emotion. It can be caused by external events—for example, being angry at a specific person for taking a parking space or being angry over a traffic jam that is making a person late for class. Anger can also be caused internally—by worrying or stewing over personal problems or by memories that trigger angry feelings. Two clarifying statements can facilitate the understanding of anger. First, anger is not aggression. Anger is an emotion, whereas aggression is a behavior. Aggression is one expression of anger. Second, anger is not the same as hostility, although people tend to use these emotions interchangeably. Anger is a temporary emotion that may or may not be expressed outwardly. Hostility, on the other hand, is more of an attitude. It includes anger that is expressed in aggressive behavior motivated by hatefulness (Hafen et al., 1996).

As with other emotions, anger is accompanied by physiological changes. When a person gets angry, there are increases in heart rate, blood pressure, and muscle tension. Often, people clench their fists, become flushed, sweat, feel hot or cold, and lose self-control. In addition, during the experience of anger, adrenaline and noradrenaline are released. These two hormones cause the arousal, excitement, and energy of an emotion. They act on organs served by the sympathetic nervous system by stimulating the heart, dilating coronary vessels, constricting blood vessels in the intestines, and shutting off digestion (Hafen et al., 1996).

Throughout human evolution, anger has been important for survival. It serves as an adaptive response to threats and inspires powerful behaviors that allow people to fight and defend themselves. In the present day, however, the culture has evolved beyond people's bodies. In other words, people are now expected to deal calmly with each other despite the fact that they are still programmed to experience this fight or flight response (Hafen et al., 1996). Anger still has a beneficial purpose, however, and does help motivate people to tackle problems, correct injustices, and focus attention on important tasks. So, to some extent, a certain amount of anger is necessary for survival.

The way a person expresses and copes with anger is essential to achieving emotional well-being. As already mentioned, anger can have some productive and adaptive functions. The key is to have a healthy expression of anger. Typically, people are not taught how to express anger. They are taught early on that anger is bad and they should not express it. Being able to express anger in an appropriate way is essential for anger to be beneficial. Generally speaking, this means facing situations early on before anger is allowed to build up and using self-talk to relieve the anger (Hafen et al., 1996). It is essential to be assertive in a way that facilitates communication. People need to learn how to make clear what their needs are and how to get them met without hurting others. Being assertive does not mean being pushy or demanding; it means being respectful of self and others. The main goal in experiencing anger, therefore, is to process it and to be able to move past it.

Of course, not all people are able to express their anger in an appropriate way. When this happens, the anger is not properly worked through and has the potential to affect a person's emotional well-being. If anger remains uncontrolled and habitual, then it can damage personal and working relationships. A buildup of rage or development of hostility can lead a person to hurt others both emotionally and physically. Aggression is not an effective way of dealing with anger and, in fact, can actually escalate anger further. Further, people often use misdirected anger in which they take out their anger on a person or object; that is not the real problem. These techniques for dealing with anger are unhealthy, yet the opposite reactions are just as unhealthy. This includes holding in feelings of anger. Keeping things bottled up inside is just as dangerous and can lead to physical problems, such as a heart attack or hypertension, or psychological problems, such as depression. Physically, chronic anger is associated with fatigue, pain in the neck or jaw, hives, acne, migraines, frequent colds, and lowered skin temperature. It is also associated with other conditions, including cancer and heart problems (Hafen et al., 1996). Psychologically, anger can lead to poor relationships, aggression problems, and depression. Some of the strategies used to help control and process anger are relaxation techniques, cognitive restructuring, problem-solving strategies, and increasing communication skills.

Anxiety

A second common emotion is anxiety. Almost everyone feels anxious from time to time. It is that feeling of uneasiness, apprehension, or tension that is felt in response to a situation that is perceived as a threat. Situations that cause some sort of distress or threaten a loss can create feelings of anxiety.

For example, most people have felt anxiety at some point by the anticipation of a tough exam or a job interview. Anxiety is often associated with worry. Most people are familiar with this concept and spend a great deal of their day worrying about various aspects of their lives including family, relationships, job, finances, or school. This worry is the thinking part of anxiety.

When a threat or loss is perceived, anxiety is a normal human reaction. It provides a way for the body to prepare to deal with potential danger. At times, it helps a person to take steps that will keep something negative from happening.

The physiological response to anxiety is a complicated one. Adrenaline and cortisone are released in the bloodstream, the heart rate speeds up, breathing becomes shallow and rapid, muscles tense, sugar is released from the liver, and the mind goes on full alert. In addition, there are other physical symptoms of anxiety, including dry mouth, nausea, faintness, hyperventilation, frequent urination, sweating, hyperactivity, and sexual difficulties. Once again, there is the fight or flight response of the sympathetic nervous system. Psychologically, a person who feels apprehensive, restless, and irritable will have difficulty concentrating, relaxing, and sleeping. These various physiological and psychological reactions to anxiety can be either mild or intense depending on the person and the situation (Talley, 1999).

Normally, anxiety is temporary and dissipates when the perceived threat or loss goes away or is dealt with in some way. When it lasts a long time, however, it becomes a serious problem. When the symptoms are extremely intense, a person's ability to cope mentally with concerns and fears is diminished. In addition, anxiety can cause a feeling of panic that may require psychiatric or psychological intervention. At times, people experience anxiety that is not tied to an identifiable threat or is so severe that it is classified as a clinical disorder. In general, anxiety disorders are debilitating and disruptive to life. There are several types of anxiety disorders recognized in the *Diagnostic and Statistical Manual of Mental Disorders* (*DSM-IV*) (American Psychiatric Association, 1994), including obsessive-compulsive disorder, panic disorder, post-traumatic stress disorder, and generalized anxiety disorder. Each one is slightly different regarding where the anxiety comes from and how the person deals with it.

So what is the key to keeping anxiety within the normal limits? This question is a key to emotional well-being. The client must become aware of how anxiety and stress affects the body and how to deal with it. Adequate rest, a balanced diet, and exercise are three factors that contribute to well-being. These are extremely important and should be practiced in day-to-day life. In addition, relaxation techniques, behavioral techniques, and supportive relationships are useful in working through and preventing anxiety (Talley, 1999).

Depression

Sadness, discouragement, and hopelessness about certain situations are familiar feelings to most people. As with anger and anxiety, most people experience some form of depression at certain times in their lives. In general, depression can be viewed as a normal response that is caused by some disruption of normal life balance (Hafen et al., 1996). This disruption could be, for example, losing a job or the death of a loved one. Almost always, normal depression is the result of a recent stress. It is an unpleasant feeling; however, it is usually temporary. Further, the experience of depression is not necessarily bad. Like with other emotions, depression is a normal part of life that can play an adaptive role. For example, it can help a person face an issue and move on without becoming stuck. Feeling depressed helps individuals face thoughts and other feelings that they may not otherwise recognize or deal with. Normal depression is also self-limiting in that it has the potential to turn off after a period that has reached a certain intensity level. In these ways, it is suggested that it is normal, and even desirable, for people to have depressive feelings as long as they are brief and mild. Similarly, anyone who undergoes a painful life event would experience depression (Carson, Butcher, & Mineka, 1996).

As already mentioned, depression is normal when it is temporary. Prolonged feelings of depression, however, are unhealthy and have the potential to severely impact a person's life. For example, a person who has feelings of hopelessness and depression over a romantic breakup for longer than six months has gone beyond the scope of normal depression. This person may be stuck in the process, and the presence of depressive symptoms may be increasing in severity. Depression as an illness is much more than occasional feelings of sadness. Rather, it is a condition in which the present conditions and future possibilities are intolerable. It involves the body, mood, and thoughts. It affects the way humans eat, sleep, and feel. This also affects thought processes, often creating distortions (Carson et al., 1996; Hafen et al., 1996).

There are many symptoms that are associated with a depressive disorder including insomnia or oversleeping, weight gain or loss, restlessness, irritability, difficulty concentrating, physical symptoms such as headaches, decreased energy, lack of interest in sex or other pleasurable activities, and a feeling of hopelessness and pessimism. These are unhealthy expressions of depression. Many of these symptoms originate from physiological upset. Specifically, depression is linked to dysfunction in the midbrain. The midbrain contains both pleasure and punishment centers. When this system does not function normally, depression is thought to result. As mentioned earlier, one of the neurotransmitters that influences the midbrain functioning is serotonin. This chemical has been found to be deficient in people who suffer from depression (Hafen et al., 1996). This suggests that the illness of depression reflects a disturbance of mood that occurs when the pleasure centers of the brain are not working or when the punishment centers are working overtime. Still, there is the psychological component that holds for the idea that depression is caused by a repetition of negative life events, low self-esteem, stress, or viewing the world with pessimism. Often, the combination of physiological, psychological, and environmental factors is involved with the presence of a depressive disorder.

The important thing to remember with depressive emotions is to keep a positive attitude. Often, it is the negative thinking that leads to distortions and clinical depression. Being optimistic and talking through feelings can change this. Social supports are particularly important with depression. Family and friends are very helpful in working through problems. In addition, setting realistic goals and exercising can help keep a healthy attitude and prevent depressive feelings. People who have prolonged depression and suffer from a disorder are able to get help through psychotherapy (Hafen et al., 1996). Usually, cognitive/behavioral and interpersonal techniques are used with depressed patients. These are helpful in allowing the patient to obtain more satisfaction and rewards through actions, to change negative styles of thinking, and to recognize disturbed personal relationships that may intensify the depression. Additionally, antidepressant medications are helpful in some cases of depression.

Achieving Emotional Well-Being

The human mind experiences a wide variety of emotions on both a physiological and a psychological level. The key to achieving emotional well-being is to have effective ways of processing and dealing with feelings. Everybody is going to feel depressed, angry, or anxious at times. A person who is healthy will be able to understand why these feelings exist and move on with life.

One emotion that is often overlooked in the study of psychology is that of happiness. What exactly is happiness? Different people experience happiness in different ways. Generally, it is an overall good feeling. People who are happy perceive the world as a safer place, are able to make decisions more easily, and report greater satisfaction with their whole lives. Just as a "bad mood" can make life seem depressing, a "good mood" can create hope for the future and a content feeling with relationships and self-image (Myers, 1999). Thus, being able to experience and maintain happiness is essential to achieving emotional well-being. People need to lead their lives in a way that will promote overall healthiness. This section outlines some of the major components needed to work toward and maintain emotional well-being.

Social Support

The amount of social support a person experiences is crucial in mental health. Studies have found that one of the main factors that most often leads to good health and long life is the amount of social support a person enjoys. *Social support* can be defined as the degree to which a person's basic social needs are met through interaction with other people. It includes all the resources other people can offer. The people who make up a person's social support system are the people that the person associates with and could turn to in a time of need. They can include family members, community members, neighbors, and close friends (Hafen et al., 1996).

Many people lack social support. Especially in U.S. society, people are taught early on to be independent and successful on their own. It is often viewed as a sign of weakness when a person needs to ask others for help. This is a damaging value to instill in people. People are social beings and need to feel the support and caring of others. In today's society, people are more often likely to live alone, less likely to marry, and less likely to belong to social organizations (Hafen et al., 1996). To increase emotional well-being, this needs to change.

Having a secure social support system enhances health. In recent years, it has become apparent that amount of social support affects physical health with regard to onset and progression of disease. It influences certain behaviors that impact our health such as diet and exercise. It has a positive influence on such biological processes as immune responses and blood flow. Finally, developing and maintaining social supports satisfies a basic human need to belong and connect to other people (Hafen et al., 1996).

Take a moment to think about your social support system. Who are the key people in your life? Who can you turn to for help if you have a problem? How can you develop new social supports? These questions are essential for you to examine. Having a strong support system will help you feel happy and get through the tough times.

Optimism

People with *optimism* are those who are hopeful about the future. They generally believe good things will happen to them and approach the world in an active, productive way. Hafen and his colleagues (1996) offer the following characteristics of people who are optimistic:

1. They see the good in situations and truly expect things to go their way.

2. They see events in their lives as controllable. If something bad does happen, they can create a plan of action, follow it, and work quickly before the situation gets out of control.

3. They do not give up and are known for their perseverance.

4. They tend to see the future as a positive opportunity. They believe they will have a happy life filled with good health.

5. They are able to express acceptance or resignation when needed. They have the instinct to know when to charge forward and when to back off.

These characteristics are very different from those of people who are pessimistic. People who are pessimistic expect to fail and prepare for the worst. Research supports that people who have a pessimistic explanatory style are at risk for poor health. They tend to be poor problem solvers, allow problems to escalate, are more socially withdrawn, and are less likely to take steps to combat illness and promote health (Peterson, Seligman, & Vaillant, 1988). In general, people with a pessimistic attitude experience more stress and less pleasure.

Creating an optimistic attitude and the characteristics that go along with it is important for achieving emotional well-being. There has been support for the notion that optimism promotes health. Having an optimistic attitude can actually protect a person from getting sick in the first place. In addition, it can boost the body's healing process (Hafen et al., 1996). Mentally, people who are optimistic feel happier, have higher self-esteem, and have more productive ways of dealing with problems.

Humor

For centuries, the idea that humor may play a role in stress reduction and increased well-being has been noted. *Humor* has been defined as the ability of a person to feel inner joy (in self and surroundings) and a point of view that sees the comical in things (Hafen et al., 1996). Researchers have begun to find support that humor in fact has many physiological and psychological benefits. As a result, many hospitals and counselors are adopting humor as one type of intervention. Humor has had its impact on the psychological field for many years. According to Martin and Lefcourt (1983), Freud considered humor as being one of the highest defensive processes humans possess. According to him, humor provides a saving of emotional energy. Psychologists who came after Freud also tend to agree that a person who can learn to laugh at himself may be on the way to self-management, which leads to a healthier existence (Martin & Lefcourt, 1983).

Physically, humor can actually promote good health by boosting the immune system. It has been demonstrated in research that people who have a humorous outlook on life have greater immunity against a variety of diseases. In addition, laughter has the added benefit of decreasing pain through the release of endorphins. Physiologically, laughter increases the breathing rate, relaxes muscles, and temporarily increases heart rate and circulation. This helps increase the amount of oxygen that circulates through the blood. Through laughter, stress can be reduced and the body can feel relaxed (Hafen et al., 1996).

There are also many psychological benefits to humor and laughter. Humor serves as an adaptive coping mechanism that gives pleasure and relief to people who are distressed. This effect is produced by means of the cognitive shifts that occur and the various changes in affective quality that accompany it. Research indicates that humor has a moderating effect on stress, particularly between recent negative life events and current levels of mood disturbance (Martin & Lefcourt, 1983). A person needs to place a high value on humor and be able to produce humor in stressful situations encountered in daily life to reap the benefits.

In addition to moderating stress, humor serves other psychological benefits. Having a humorous outlook on life can have benefits on self-esteem, creativity, decision-making skills, performance, sense of power, and coping abilities. Being able to laugh at personal shortcomings and the shortcomings of others is an effective way of achieving emotional well-being. Having this attitude helps people see the world in a new perspective that is sometimes needed to overcome obstacles and move on (Hafen et al., 1996).

So, how does a person create a humorous attitude that will offer benefits? One article offers the following tips for adding and maintaining humor in life (Gallo, 1989):

1. Look for humor. Try to see the amusing side of every situation.

2. Keep a humor first-aid kit and stock it with things that always make you laugh. This can include funny cartoons, jokes, or comedy tapes.

3. Brighten up your surroundings with cheerful posters, silly bumper stickers, and humorous signs.

4. Make time for fun. Schedule a ten-minute "humor break" every day.

5. Be playful and do not be afraid to be silly.

6. Laugh when you are low. Many psychologists believe that people do not laugh because they are happy; they are happy because they laugh.

7. Encourage laughter in others. Try to make humor a contagious attitude.

8. Avoid self-degrading or put-down humor. There is such a thing as bad humor that hurts. Remember to laugh with people and not at them. Above all, always be prepared to laugh at yourself!

Cognitive Restructuring

It has already been mentioned that the appraisals a person makes about life situations are crucial in understanding that person's emotions. Psychologists have long known that how a person perceives a stressful event is more predictive of the person's response to that stress than the actual event itself. Thus, if people think about the world in unreasonable or irrational ways, they become stressed (Wallace, 1998; Hafen et al., 1996). Nowhere is this seen better than in cognitive-behavioral theories. Consider Albert Ellis and his rational-emotive behavior therapy. Ellis believes that the emotions people experience are a direct result of the thoughts and beliefs they have. He defines this human characteristic in terms of the ABCs. The *A* stands for the activating event that occurs in a person's life. Next comes the *B*, the belief that the person holds about the event. Finally, there is *C*, consequences to those beliefs typically involving feelings and emotions. According to Ellis, it is the belief that is crucial to understanding feelings. Beliefs can be either rational or irrational. If beliefs are irrational, then the individual will experience inappropriate emotions such as anxiety, depression, or anger. The key for Ellis, therefore, is to identify what the irrational belief is that is causing that emotion and then change it to a rational belief. As a result, the person will feel more appropriate emotions such as sadness instead of depression. In rational-emotive therapy, this is accomplished by the therapist disputing and challenging the irrational beliefs of the client until the point at which the client can recognize the belief as irrational. Then the therapist works with the client to note the effect of this belief, replacing irrational statements with rational ones (Carson et al., 1996).

This notion has strong implications for working toward emotional well-being. Further, it is something everyone can use, not just people who have severe psychological issues. *Reframing* a situation does not change what the actual problem is but rather the outlook toward that problem. Reframing is looking at a situation from a different point of view. It may be that you are looking at the situation with an irrational belief. Suppose you are feeling depressed because your grades for the past couple of semesters in college have been Bs and Cs. Where do these depressed feelings come from? Most likely, you hold the idea that you should be getting all As. Why should you be? Is there an underlying reason that helps to explain your grades? Are your expectations realistic reflecting the student you actually are? This is a typical irrational belief among college students. What is wrong with getting some Bs and Cs? Yes, grades are important. It is not healthy, however, to hold an unrealistic or irrational belief.

So what exactly is cognitive restructuring? First, of it is realizing that stressful situations do not cause feelings and physiological responses as much as the way a person chooses to think about those situations. The word *choose* here is crucial. This implies that in order to achieve emotional well-being a person needs to reexamine his or her way of thinking, discover a more rational way of perceiving the situation, and help develop strategies to use this new rational thought. When this is achieved, a person has a sense of control and harmony with his or her values and attitudes (Hafen et al., 1996). Following are some tips for becoming a more rational person (Wallace, 1998):

- Realize that your thoughts influence your actions. Thoughts are very powerful; make notes of irrational thoughts that may be contributing to your feelings.

- Avoid some of the common unreasonable thoughts. Irrational statements usually include the use of absolute words such as *should, must,* and *have to*—for example, "I have to be perfect at everything I do" or "I can't cope."

- Actively challenge your beliefs to manage your emotions. Take into account both positive and negative information. Balancing your thinking can lead to interpreting an event in a different way.

- Try positive thinking. This is helpful in that it offers good coping statements to help you through tough times—for example, "I will take this one step at a time" or "I've survived worse than this before."

This section has provided an overview of some of the key components in achieving emotional well-being. Of course, there are many other factors that could be discussed, including issues of hope, faith, and spirituality. Be aware that there are many factors that contribute to emotional well-being. Stress is a central component of emotional well-being. A thorough explanation of stress and stress management can be found in Chapters 8 and 9.

Self-Assessment

Consider the following emotions:

- Happiness
- Sadness
- Anger
- Anxiety

For each of these emotions, spend some time thinking about what types of things make you feel that particular emotion. Self-reflection is an important key in gaining insight about yourself. Answer the following questions about each emotion:

1. In what situations do I feel this emotion?
2. How do I express this emotion?
3. How often do I feel this emotion?
4. To what degree do I feel this emotion?
5. What are the beliefs I have that may contribute to this emotion?
6. Are my beliefs realistic and rational?
7. What can I do to improve the way in which I experience and express this emotion?

Summary

Throughout this chapter, the importance of learning to understand and accept feelings has been emphasized. This is a fundamental criterion for becoming a person who is emotionally healthy. People experience similar emotions at different levels. Not everyone has the same reaction to a particular situation. It is important to identify what causes certain emotions to develop effective coping strategies. Emotions can be viewed as being physiological and psychological in nature.

There are specific structures in the brain such as the limbic system and nerve cells, along with neurotransmitters, that allow events to be processed and expressed emotionally. The stimulation or inhibition of certain sites in the brain causes many physiological effects of emotions such as difficulty breathing, increased energy, and increased mental activity. Some of these effects are used by humans as social indicators of emotional expression such as the production of tears and a smile.

The way people process and interpret life events cognitively is another important concept in studying emotions. Cognitive psychologists have found that people's appraisals of situations have an effect on the resulting emotions they experience. Psychologically, emotions can be viewed as the process of establishing, maintaining, or disrupting the relation between the organism and the internal and external environment. In many ways, this process determines the emotions that are experienced. There are also many gender differences evident in research. In general, females tend to be more willing to express powerful emotions, whereas males are more motivated to stay in control.

All of this information can provide insight into the inner world of emotions. There are many implications in this information for learning to deal with emotions and to prevent psychological problems. It is healthy for people to experience all of the emotions, even negative emotions such as anger and anxiety. The key is in the degree. Each emotion has a healthy and an unhealthy expression. Not only are emotions important for psychological well-being, but they are also important for physical well-being. There is evidence that having a healthy attitude and appropriate expressions of emotion boosts the immune system's ability to prevent or fight off disease. This connection between emotions and sickness validates a connection of the body and the mind.

DISCUSSION QUESTIONS

1. Name and describe the major parts of the limbic system. How are they important in the study of emotions?

2. Describe the difference between the right and left hemisphere of the brain.

3. List and describe the three phases of emotional processing.

4. Give a definition of cognitive appraisal. What is the significance of the appraisals people make?

5. Using the relational view of emotions, give an explanation as to why people feel anger.

6. What are some of the main gender differences supported in the research regarding emotions?

7. What are some of the typical emotions college students experience? According to the information presented, how can you account for these emotions?

8. Pick one specific emotion and provide an explanation of a healthy and an unhealthy expression of that emotion.

9. What are the main characteristics of a person who is optimistic? Why is this healthier than being pessimistic?

10. What are some ways in which humor can serve as a coping mechanism?

11. What is cognitive restructuring? How can it be used to help a person achieve emotional well-being?

RELATED WEBSITES

http://www.nmha.org/fund/index.cfm National Mental Health Association provides information on anxiety disorders, depression, state and government affairs, education, and health care reform.

http://www.plgrm.com/health/mental_health.html Health Topics: Mental Health; provides information on a variety of subjects including addiction, behavior modification therapy, personality disorders, depression, eating disorders, stress, substance abuse, and more.

http://anxiety.mentalhelp.net/ Mental Health Net for disorders and treatment; this site outlines disorders by providing information on symptoms, treatment, on-line resources for specific disorders, organizations, on-line support, and research.

http://www.counseling.org/ American Counseling Association; includes leadership, foundations, and a search for additional specific articles and sites to find more information on various disorders and/or problems.

http://www.sis.net/onschools/february.wellness.html Strategic Information Systems; wellness issues in families and schools. Covers current legislation as well as technology and community services.

http://h-devil-www.mc.duke.edu/h-devil/emotion/emotion.htm Helping a friend with a personal concern. Anorexia nervosa, bulimia, depression, perfectionism, stress, and suicide.

http://www.wmich.edu/healthquest/index.html Health Quest Main Menu: emotional health, nutrition, fitness, sexual health, tobacco, and so on.

http://www.KatKing.com/wisdom/body-M.html Wisdom of Ancient Healing Manual; your body is *not* the enemy! The chemistry of physical, mental, emotional, and spiritual health.

http://www,phy.mtu.edu/apod/mind/ Dialectical Behavior Therapy: includes mindfulness, interpersonal effectiveness, emotion regulation, and distress tolerance. A great focus of this site is borderline personality disorder.

http://www.counseling.com/Ccom/reference.html This site addresses reference and resource information regarding alcohol problems, chemical dependency, emotional/mental health, and family problems. It also provides crisis hotlines from the American Counseling Association.

REFERENCES

American Psychiatric Association. (1994). *Diagnostic and Statistical Manual of Mental Disorders* (4th ed.). Washington, DC.: Author.

Arnold, M. B. (1960). *Emotion and Personality: Vol. 1. Psychological Aspects.* New York: Columbia University Press.

Bancroft, M. (1999, April 14). *Brain Physiology* [On-line]. Available: http://www.enspire.com./html/brain_physiology.html.

Campos, J. J., Campos, R. G., & Barrett, K. C. (1989). Emergent Themes in the study of Emotional Development and Emotion Regulation. *Developmental Psychology, 25*(3), 394–402.

Carson, R. C., Butcher, J. N., & Mineka, S. (1996). *Abnormal Psychology and Modern Life* (10th ed.). New York: HarperCollins College Publishers.

Cornelius, R. R. (1996). *The Science of Emotion Research and Tradition in the Psychology of Emotion.* Englewood Cliffs, NJ: Prentice-Hall.

Crucian, G. P., & Berenbaum, S. A. (1998). Sex Differences in Right-Hemisphere Tasks. *Brain and Cognition, 36,* 377–389.

Ellis, A. (1975). A New Guide to Rational Living. Prentice-Hall

Fink, G., Sumner, B., Rosie, R., Wilson, H., & McQueen, J. (1999). Androgen Actions on Central Serotonin Neurotransmission: Relevance for Mood, Mental State, and Memory. *Behavioral Brain Research, 105,* 53–68.

Folkman, S., & Lazarus, R. S. (1988). The Relationship between Coping and Emotion: Implications for Theory and Research. *Social Science Medicine, 26*(3), 309–317.

Gallo, N. (1989, August). Lighten Up, Laugh Your Way to Good Health. *Better Homes and Gardens*, 31.

Goode, E. E., Schrof, J. M., & Burke, S. (1991, June). Where Emotions Come From. *U.S. News & World Report*, 54–62.

Greenberg, J. S. (1996). *Comprehensive Stress Management*. Guilford, CT: Brown & Benchmark.

Hafen, B. Q., Karren, K. J., Frandsen, K. J., & Smith, N. L. (1996). *Mind/Body Health, the Effects of Attitudes, Emotions, and Relationships*. Boston: Allyn & Bacon.

Lautenbacher, S., Roscher, S., Kohl, G., Vedder, H., & Krieg, J. (1999). Corticotropin-Releasing Hormone Lacks Analgesic Properties: An Experimental Study in Humans, Using Non Inflammatory Pain. *Pain, 83*, 1–7.

Lazarus, R. S. (1991). Cognition and Motivation in Emotion. *American Psychologist, 46*(44), 352–367.

Levinthal, C. F. (1999). *Drugs, Behavior, and Modern Society* (2nd Ed.). Boston: Allyn & Bacon.

Martin, R. A., & Lefcourt, H. M. (1983). Sense of Humor as a Moderator of the Relation between Stressors and Moods. *Journal of Personality and Social Psychology, 45*(6), 1313–1324.

Miller, L. (1988, February). The Emotional Brain. *Psychology Today, 22*(2), 34–42.

Moretti, M. M., Charlton, S., & Taylor, S. (1996). The Effects of Hemispheric Asymmetries and Depression on the Perception of Emotion. *Brain and Cognition, 32*, 67–82.

Myers, D. G. (1999, April 14). *Happiness* [On-line]. Available: http://www.hope.edu

Nishimura, N., & Sato, K. (1999). Ketamine Stereoselectively Inhibits Rat Dopamine Transporter. *Neuroscience Letters, 274*, 131–134.

Pally, R. (1998). Emotional Processing: The Mind-Body Connection. *The Journal of Psycho-Analysis, 79*, 349–361.

Palmiter, R. (1999). Norepinephrine-Deficient Mice Have Increased Susceptibility to Seizure-Inducing Stimuli. *Journal of Neuroscience, 19*, 10985–10992.

Peterson, C., Seligman, M. E. P., & Vaillant, G. E. (1988). Pessimistic Explanatory Style Is a Risk Factor for Physical Illness: A Thirty-Five Year Longitudinal Study. *Journal of Personality and Social Psychology, 55*(1), 23–27.

Robinson, D. (1988, January). Medical Report: Can a Fighting Spirit Defeat Disease? *50 Plus*, 23–25.

Tarazi, F., & Baldessarini, R. (1999) Dopamine D4 Receptors: Significance for Molecular Psychiatry at the Millennium. *Molecular Psychiatry, 4*, 529–538.

Talley, J. E. (1999, April 14). *Emotional Health, Anxiety* [On-line]. Available: http://h-devil-www.mc.duke.edu/h-devil/maps/emotion.map?400,170

Timmers, M., Fischer, A. H., & Manstead, A. S. R. (1998). Gender Differences in Motives for Regulating Emotions. *Personality and Social Psychology Bulletin, 24*(9), 974–985.

Wallace, S. (1998). *Stress* [On-line]. Available: http://www.virtualpsycho.com/stress/challange-beliefs.htm.

4 Mental and Emotional Problems

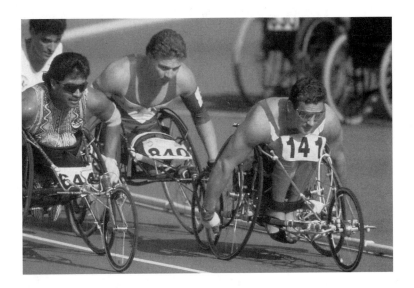

Behavior Pathology Defined, Described

The primary purpose of this book is mental health and the methods of promoting a positive mental health status. However, it is important to discuss various departures from health in order to comprehend more completely the presence of comprehensive mental health. As discussed in earlier chapters, there is often no clear or distinct line between illness and wellness. Rather, the human condition is more of a spectrum with the obviously healthy having a greater number of the characteristics of well-being and the obviously ill having many fewer of these characteristics. Human beings generally move freely along this spectrum or continuum. When someone is considered to have a departure from mental health, they have a significant absence of the characteristics of well-being or remain at a position on the spectrum not indicative of health for prolonged periods of time. There are many and, at times, conflicting views regarding what constitutes the limits and dimensions of mental health. For the purpose of this chapter, standards of mental health or psychiatric illness are based upon the American Psychiatric Association's publication *Diagnostic and Statistical Manual of Mental Disorders, 4th Edition* (*DSM-IV*). This publication is used as the basis for defining departures from mental health and is generally referred to in the United States and in many other countries as the "psychiatrist's bible."

Criteria of Mental Illness

According to the *DSM-IV*, certain criteria must be present to indicate the occurrence of mental illness. The first is that it must be a behavioral or psychological *syndrome*—a group of symptoms that tend to occur together—that causes present distress, disability, or increased risk of death, pain, disability, or loss of freedom. Thus, the disorder must cause noticeable symptoms, and, quite possibly, it may prevent the person from engaging in normal, day-to-day activities. It may also encourage behavior with serious consequences. The *DSM-IV* further states that this syndrome must not be a cultural response to an event. For instance, a person with all the symptoms of depression might not be considered (according to the *DSM-IV*) to be displaying clinical depression if that person recently experienced the death of a close family member. The second condition is that the current behavior must be a symptom of a "behavioral, psychological, or biological dysfunction in the individual" (American Psychiatric Association, 1994, pp. xxi–xii). This is perhaps the key, albeit an enigmatic one, to the entire definition. The *DSM-IV* clearly states that mental disorders are always the product of *dysfunctions*, and that these dysfunctions arise in individuals. Therefore, there are no *mentally disordered* groups by definition, although there may be groups with a large proportion of individuals displaying a mental disorder (Carson, Butcher, & Mineka, 1996).

To determine if there is a departure from mental health, it is important to ascertain the extent of interruption in lifestyle, how long the interruption has existed, and if it is getting worse or better. In addition, it is important to recall if this interruption has occurred in the past and just how extensive and/or prolonged it was. If a physical illness or medication use associated with an illness is present, either or both of these could be responsible for a problem that might be considered to be mental or emotional in nature. Many psychiatric illnesses seem to run in families. This is not to imply that the genetics of an individual clearly defines whether or not the person will develop mental illness. Genetic predisposition is an area that biologists are still attempting to understand; however, in most cases, genetic predisposition simply means that an individual has an increased risk. A simple analogy for this is that fair-skinned individuals are more likely to sunburn. This does not mean, however, that a fair individual will sunburn each time he or she goes outside, or that the individual cannot take steps, such as applying sunscreen, to protect his or her skin. Nor does it mean that a dark-skinned individual will never sunburn. Genetic predisposition must be looked at in the same way. Finally, an awareness of past family life, education, success in dealing with others, patterns of success or failure, interest and goals in life, and so on can all shed light into the nature of a condition that may seriously disrupt a person's life or be termed a departure from mental health. Clinicians trained in diagnosing mental health problems would likely consider how a person looks, acts, and thinks. Appearance regarding personal care and hygiene is only one aspect. The nature of a person's response to others or events, facial expressions, outlook on life, and so on are all important clues. Finally, thinking patterns can serve to reveal if an individual is in touch with reality or is reacting in an inappropriate or potentially harmful manner.

A Multiaxial Method of Assessment

The *DSM-IV* employs a *multiaxial method*—each axis represents a broad area of human function that might be affected by mental disorder—to incorporate the diverse factors involved in departures from mental health. Each of the five axes describes a potential dimension of the combination of factors and circumstances that are involved in human mental health. *Axis I* considers clinical disorders such as those associated with impulse control, sleep, eating, anxiety, mood, drug abuse, problems with cognition, or psychotic conditions.

Axis II considers the impact of mental retardation or one of the varied forms of personality disorders (formerly referred to as neurosis). *Axis III* considers such general medical conditions of the various organ systems of the human body as blood and circulation, the nervous system, respiration, digestion, and reproduction, to name a few. *Axis IV* considers the psychosocial and environmental influences of or in the human condition. Some of these include the primary support group, educational deficiencies, housing, economic impacts, the legal system, access to health care, and other environmental and social problems. *Axis V* considers how well a person is able to function. This multiaxial approach to assessing departures from mental and emotional well-being is very representative of the complex nature of comprehensive mental health. Representative constituents and components of Axes I and II are described in this chapter. Unless otherwise noted, the material presented reflects the acumen and orientation of the *DSM-IV.*

Impulse-Control Disorders

While there are many instances where human beings must act very rapidly in order to avoid harm, impulses that allowed for survival in the past have become less necessary to ensure survival today. In modern society, behavior that involves acts that might prevent harm or serve to propagate the species need not be as impulsive in nature as it was in earlier times. Contemporary society neither requires nor values such behavior. Individuals who are unable to manage or control impulses to act face many difficulties in today's world.

Gambling

With the rise of legitimate avenues for gambling ranging from casinos to state lotteries to bingo parlors, people in the United States have greater opportunity to gamble than any time in recent history. Social gambling seems to be on the rise as a form of recreation. A smaller segment of society earns their living gambling. Professional gamblers generally have a system based on probability or hunches that is often calculating and logical. Another type of gambling takes control of the lives of individuals. This is known as *pathological gambling.* The pathological gambler may have a strong family history of gambling, and often there is a history of other types of addictive behavior. Pathological gamblers generally need to increase the size of their wagers to maintain the exhilaration resulting from betting. Often, they will attempt to stop or reduce their gambling practices, especially if there are heavy losses or debts.

Pathological gamblers may have to lie to family members and others regarding their gambling practice. Even in light of heavy losses and the need for deception, pathological gamblers may find gambling to be the preferred means of escaping from problems or pressures in life. An important sign of pathological gambling is when an individual commits crimes such as theft or fraud and puts family relationships and career at risk to continue gambling.

Explosive Disorder

While it could be argued that violence is an innate human trait, it is becoming less accepted and tolerated in today's world. Whether acceptable by modern standards or not, most acts of violence have a purpose such as protection, domination over another, revenge, or efforts to have financial gain, as in a robbery. Violent attacks that arise without one of these sources of motivation are even more difficult to comprehend. Such "unreasonable" or "unmotivated" forms of violence are termed *intermittent explosive disorder.* Such episodes are characterized by rage and aggression disproportionate to any insult or wrong committed against the attacker. These outbursts are not brought on by alcohol or other drugs. Such outbursts do not fit the personality of the individual but may be so severe and ungoverned that they destroy relationships or cause extreme fear and discomfort in relatives and co-workers. Even the individual suffering from this disorder feels sorry, foolish, and disbelieving after the anger has subsided.

Trichotillomania

Trichotillomania is an incessant pattern of pulling out one's own hair. It is common for individuals to fuss with, pull, twist, tangle, or even pull the hair in various regions of their bodies on occasion. If this hair pulling results in significant hair loss and the person cannot stop because the activity relieves stress or provides a stimulating reaction, then there may be a problem. Often, the person experiencing this disorder attempts to pull out the entire hair follicle. Most common sites of concentration include the scalp and eyelashes and eyebrows, although any hairy region of the body can become the point of focus. Often, the region becomes completely devoid of hair.

Pyromania

Some individuals experience a release of tension or some form of gratification when observing fires or the aftermath of fires that they themselves have started. Much of the pleasure involved is in the act of actually setting the fire. There is usually an indifference to the risk or harm to property or even individuals affected by the fire. These are not acts of vandalism, arson, or expressions of social or political convictions. The person suffering from *pyromania* does not commit these acts while under the influence of drugs, alcohol, or delusions. Some varieties of conduct disorders may include fire setting as a means to gain attention, but this is something different and is not an impulse-control issue. Fire-setting activities for the individual suffering from pyromania usually begin in the adult or young adult years and are more often episodic than frequent or regular in occurrence.

Kleptomania

Most acts of theft are committed to gain something of value to the thief. In some cases, individuals steal because of anger toward a person, organization, or society in general. None of the aforementioned is *kleptomania*. This disorder involves stealing to provide either a relief of tension or a thrilling sensation. Individuals suffering from kleptomania generally have no use for or place any real value in the objects they steal. More often, they experience a sense of tension before and relief or gratification following the theft. Very frequently, the act of theft is precipitated by a particular environment or setting such as a bookstore or a supermarket. Specific objects may also trigger the sense of tension that precedes the theft.

Eating Disorders

Food is vital to the survival of human beings. The drive to search for food is as old as the human race. For some, involvement with food becomes more than an issue of providing sufficient nutrients to maintain life, and food tastes and preferences become the principal motivation in feeding. Further, human beings' primitive ancestors did not have adequate means to process and store food so their bodies have become very efficient at food storage, especially in the form of fat. In the industrialized nations of the world, malnutrition generally takes the form of overnutrition. Eating disorders arise as a result of a combination of overnutrition or excess calorie consumption and contemporary images of an ideally shaped body.

Bulimia

Bulimia literally means "eating like an ox." During a given period of time, those suffering from bulimia will consume a quantity of food much larger than most people would. This is referred to as *bingeing*. Food binges may involve certain favorite foods like pie, ice cream, or cakes but may also include super meals containing an array of nutrients. Many experience an inability to control the amount of food they eat or are unable to stop eating after a given period of time. This is not a matter of "grazing" or snacking continuously during the day but, rather, entails the consumption of a very large amount of food in a particular interval of time. In most cases of bulimia, the bingeing is followed with an effort to negate any weight-gaining effect of the food eaten. This behavior is generally inappropriate and is often potentially harmful. These compensatory measures are termed *purging*. Purging most often involves self-induced vomiting brought on by placing the fingers or an object to the back of the throat to stimulate the gag reflex. Some individuals with bulimia develop the skill of vomiting at will. Other, less frequently employed purging techniques include the use of laxatives or enemas. There is a nonpurging variety of bulimia where fasting, exercise, or a combination of both is employed to compensate for the binge eating. Most sources (including the *DSM-IV*) indicate that about 90 percent of those who suffer from bulimia are females.

Anorexia

Anorexia nervosa, a condition in which a person endeavors to avoid gaining weight or even maintaining normal body weight, is primarily a disorder affecting women. Generally, those with anorexia nervosa do not have an accurate or realistic perception regarding the dimension of their bodies. Weight loss is usually accomplished through a significant reduction of food intake (restricting type) but may also involve eating followed by the use of vomiting or laxatives to avoid weight gain (binge-eating/purging type). This eating disorder can seriously damage the physical health of individuals and can even be life threatening. Those with anorexia nervosa weigh only 85 percent (or less) of the expected body weight and possess a distorted image of their body shape. In spite of weighing much less than their optimum weight, there is constant belief or concern that they are fat or look fat. This often accompanies failure to recognize the consequences of the weight loss such as cessation of menstruation, skin problems, and reduced tolerance to cold. Untreated, the person suffering from anorexia nervosa runs the risk of premature death.

Problems with Alcohol and Other Drugs

Alcohol and other drug use are widespread in contemporary society. Drug use seems to predate written history and will likely continue to be a part of the human experience for the foreseeable future. The majority of recreational drug use is to promote relaxation, enhance sociability, aid performance, or to simply add to the enjoyment of life. When such relaxation or enjoyment exceeds other sources of satisfaction, the drug user often moves toward a drug-centered life. While many people are able to use drugs with no severe negative effect, a certain segment of society is damaged severely by drug use. While there are obvious possibilities of damage to physical health associated with drug use, there are likewise potential threats to mental health. According to the *DSM-IV*, mental health is most negatively impacted by two drug-related phenomena. These are *substance-use disorders*—dependence and abuse—and *substance-induced disorders*—intoxication, withdrawal, delirium, psychosis, mood disorder, anxiety disorder, sexual dysfunction, or sleep disorder.

Substance-Use Disorders

Abuse. Drug *abuse* implies use that is harmful to the user. Signs that an individual is abusing drugs include

1. Missing work or school, failure to meet obligations, or receiving poor evaluations at work/school because of drug use
2. Being arrested or getting into legal trouble as a result of drug use
3. Operating a motor vehicle while under the influence of drugs
4. Getting into fights while under the influence of drugs
5. Experiencing disruption of family or social relationships due to drug use

Dependence.   The *DSM-IV* suggests that a cluster of three or more of the following symptoms occurring during a twelve-month period defines drug dependence:

1. *Tolerance*—the need for a greater amount of the chemical to achieve the desired effect
2. *Withdrawal*—a configuration of symptoms that arise when the drug is not ingested and that are sufficiently severe or uncomfortable to cause the individual to repeat drug-taking behavior to prevent or relieve them
3. *Increased dosage*—when the user takes a larger amount or continues taking the drug for a longer time than was intended
4. *Unsuccessful cessation*—when attempts to "cut back" or stop the use of the drug are not successful
5. *Modified lifestyle*—when much or all of the individual's life is involved in obtaining or using the drug
6. *Damaged lifestyle*—when, in spite of the obvious negative impact of the drug, the individual is unwilling or unable to discontinue use

Even though the science involving brain chemistry and addiction makes it rather clear that chemical dependency is an illness, many in society still equate drug use with character weakness and a lack of self-control. However, combining consideration of the multiaxial view of mental illness to the newer findings regarding the neurochemistry of addiction may enhance understanding of this extensive and intense problem in today's society.

Substance-Induced Disorders

The use of recreational chemicals can either magnify preexisting psychiatric disorders or bring about a drug-induced disorder that mimics any of a wide range of psychiatric problems (Cohen, 1995; Washton, 1995). Individuals with these types of problems are often referred to as *dual-diagnosis* or mentally ill/chemically dependent (MI/CD) clients because they have coexisting substance-abuse and mental illness problems. These individuals are at higher risk for suicide than chemical abusers or other psychiatric patients (Osher et al., 1994), have more difficulty abstaining from drug use (Osher & Drake, 1996), and tend to be *binge* users of recreational chemicals (Riley, 1994). A common theory is that these individuals develop a substance-abuse disorder in an effort to self-medicate their existing psychiatric illness. However, current literature has revealed mixed results in the examination of this theory; and, while the hypothesis is exceedingly difficult to test, it is apparent that other factors, including the availability of certain drugs (Mueser, Bellack, & Blanchard, 1992), strongly influence the development and course of these disorders.

Sleep Disorders

The quality of sleep in human beings is studied via *polysomnography*. Polysomnographic testing involves a series of measures including electrooculography, electroencephalography, electromyography, airflow, chest wall movement, and other procedures to determine human activity during sleep. There are five stages of sleep, including the rapid-eye movement (REM) sleep associated with dreaming and four types of non-rapid eye movement (NREM) sleep. REM sleep occupies 20 percent to 25 percent of normal sleep, and the various NREM activities—such as transition from wakefulness to sleep, light sleep, deep sleep (where sleepwalking and nightmares may occur)—occupy the remainder of the sleep period. While sleep is a very easy, rewarding, and natural thing for many, some experience problematic and disturbing sleep patterns.

Hypersomnia

Hypersomnia is a condition in which the individual cannot seem to get enough sleep. This does not include those whose schedules limit them to insufficient amounts of sleep each night; rather, it involves a situation in which, after sleeping as much or more than would be adequate for most people, someone is still tired and difficult to awaken. In addition to the excessive night sleeping, an individual with primary hypersomnia may feel drowsy or fatigued during the day and even conduct routine uncomplicated behavior and not be able to remember being engaged in the activity. According to the *DSM-IV,* those with primary hypersomnia often exhibit symptoms of depression and are also at risk for drug abuse related to stimulant use.

Insomnia

People who have trouble getting to sleep or who fail to sleep for a sufficient portion of the night are described as suffering from primary *insomnia.* This condition is not caused by the alterations in circadian rhythms caused by shift work or travel across multiple time zones. Further, it is not as a result of drugs interfering with sleep. Individuals may wake up part way through the night and not be able to fall back to sleep or may repeatedly wake up during the night. In some cases, it is a matter of not gaining rest or restoration as a result of sleep. Negative conditioning may be involved when, due to a medical condition or a psychological problem, an individual has difficulty falling asleep or maintaining sleep throughout the night. Following resolution of the problem, the individual may anticipate not being able to sleep and this negative association with poor sleep may cause anxiety and arousal that act to prevent sleep. Lack of sleep can in turn make people irritable and uncommunicative and can promote poor performance, adding to the problem that may have precipitated the primary insomnia in the first place.

Nightmares

A prolonged dream that frightens or produces such anxiety in a person that the person awakens to full alertness still filled with fear may be described as a *nightmare.* Sometimes a nightmare involves an actual experience that put the individual at risk or caused embarrassment. On other occasions, it is an elaborate dream involving being persued or attacked. REM sleep occurs every ninety to one hundred minutes during typical sleep periods, so the nightmare can take place at any time during the night. However, humans tend to sleep more heavily during the later part of the sleep period, so the nightmares generally appear later at night. In some cases, withdrawal from drugs that suppress REM sleep can result in a "REM sleep rebound" with accompanying nightmares. Nightmares often commence in childhood and may continue throughout life, although most children tend to outgrow them.

Sleep Terror Disorder

The individual with *sleep terror disorder* suddenly awakens in a highly aroused state feeling frightened. The person usually sits up in bed and cries or screams. If the individual awakens, he or she does not remember the contents of the dream and remains confused and disoriented. Often, the individual returns to sleep before awakening fully and does not remember the incident in the morning. Sleep terror disorder differs from nightmares in several ways. If it begins in childhood, it often resolves itself by the adolescent years. It has also been observed to begin in the early adult years. There is some indication that it is more frequent among biological relatives.

Personality Disorders

The *DSM-IV* does not include the term *neurosis* anywhere in its 886 pages. That term has been replaced with the description of a series of behaviors and "inner experiences" that place the individual at odds with the expectations of the surrounding world. These behaviors and inner experiences, if they have an enduring pattern, are collectively termed *personality disorders*. Personality disorders are manifested in individuals by the way they perceive themselves and others, how they respond emotionally, how they interact with others, and how they control impulses. Those exhibiting one of the various types of personality disorders would be likely to be rigid, steadfast, and unable to adapt or modify their behavior in light of the needs of others. These behaviors often impede the development of effective relationships or hinder achievement and are generally long-standing and not the result of some other disorder. The ten different personality disorders described in the *DSM-IV* are summarized in the following sections.

Paranoid Personality Disorder

Paranoid personality disorder involves suspicion and distrust of other people and their motives. Those suffering with this disorder may exhibit hostility toward those for whom they hold suspicion. This may be manifested through aloofness, a pugnacious nature, and a propensity to complain. Due to the high level of suspicion regarding the motives of others, individuals with this disorder may seem to be devious, guarded, or secretive in their dealings. These behaviors may cause a hostile reaction from others, which only serves to convince the individuals that their suspicions were justified. Those experiencing this disorder continue their suspicions even if no evidence exists to support such feelings. There is often a preoccupation with thoughts of being wronged by others, and the loyalty and integrity of even close associates come under suspicion. In such circumstances, even harmless or positive things such as questions regarding well-being or compliments are misinterpreted or considered to have a hidden meaning. Forgiveness for such perceived wrongdoing is not easily given, and those with this disorder often bear grudges. A reluctance to confide in others due to a belief that such information may be used against them makes it difficult for others to communicate or attempt to offer support. There may be counterattacks on perceived insults, and there is often suspicion regarding the fidelity of partners.

Schizoid Personality Disorder

Individuals with *schizoid personality disorder* seem almost the opposite to those with paranoid personality disorder in that neither praise nor criticism from others has any impact upon them. These individuals rarely demonstrate strong emotions such as joy or anger and give the impression that they lack emotion. They are socially detached and do not seem to desire close or interpersonal relationships. If they do form any sort of emotional bond or loving connection, it may be with a pet. Few activities seem to produce pleasure in those suffering from schizoid personality disorder, and sensuous activities including sexual experiences seem unimportant or unrewarding. There seems to be little or no interest in interaction with others, and they may freeze or react inappropriately in social situations. Because of the desire to be alone, they may find successful and rewarding employment that involves social isolation such as night-shift work or long-distance driving.

Schizotypal Personality Disorder

Schizotypal personality disorder differs from schizoid personality disorder in that the individual's appearance and/or behavior may be noticeable due to its peculiar, odd, or even eccentric nature. While those with schizotypal personality disorder usually lack close friends, that may be the only major thing in common with schizoid behavior. This disorder includes suspicious and paranoid thinking along with intense social anxiety that does not seem to diminish as familiarity develops. Beliefs, thinking patterns, and even mannerisms of speech may be difficult for others to comprehend. There may be belief in the supernatural, magic, or telepathy accompanied by preoccupation or odd fantasies.

Antisocial Personality Disorder

Psychopathy, sociopathy, or *dyssocial disorder* are terms that have also been utilized to describe *antisocial personality disorder,* which features a pattern of infringement on the rights of others without any regard for the consequences. Indications of this disorder begin prior to fifteen years of age with a pattern of behavior that includes violation of societal norms, convention, or laws. Unlawful behavior may lead to repeated arrests, patterns of avoiding arrest, or illegal occupations. Individuals with this disorder may be deceitful and manipulative. Impulsivity may lead to poor decision making in such areas as employment, risk taking, or relationships. Aggressive and irritable mannerisms can lead to assault, fights, reckless driving, or high-risk sexual behavior or drug abuse.

Lack of responsibility includes defaulting on debts or failing to provide adequate financial support for dependents. There is generally little remorse for any hurtful behavior, and the attitude expressed is that those harmed or victimized are weak, foolish, or in some way deserving of their fates. An individual with antisocial personality disorder may impulsively quit a job without any prospect of another one or make a whimsical move to a new location without any prior planning. As those with this disorder age, there is often a history of such things as personal injury, poverty, homelessness, and incarceration.

Borderline Personality Disorder

Individuals with *borderline personality disorder* fear rejection, separation, or abandonment. There are great fluctuations in mood with regard to relationships. Periods of intense happiness or of a sense of closeness and commitment in relationships are generally of short duration and followed by real or imagined rejection. Often, individuals with this disorder make a commitment to "get serious" very quickly and may frighten a partner or prospective partner off. There is generally an overreaction to someone "cooling" or ending a relationship. Fear of abandonment is realized, and reaction to it may go as far as self-mutilation or feigned or attempted suicide. The overpowering fear of abandonment may cause unreasonable response to such simple things as a change in plans or someone being late for an appointment. These behaviors yield a pattern of unstable relationships that include rapid idealization followed by devaluation of a partner. There may be intense and frequent mood shifts. Anger is directed toward someone who is suspected of abandoning or contemplating to abandon a relationship and is severe and accompanied by displays of temper. Impassivity is often manifested in the form of binge eating, unsafe driving, overspending, drug abuse, or high-risk sexual behavior. Passing through these "roller coaster" relationships and reactions to them is a chronic feeling of emptiness in the individual with borderline personality disorder.

Histrionic Personality Disorder

The *DSM-IV* characterizes *histrionic personality disorder* as featuring excessive emotionality and attention-seeking behavior. Individuals with this disorder strive to be the center of attention and tend to be extremely dramatic or even theatrical when expressing their emotions. Individuals with this disorder may consider relationships to be more intimate than they actually are. There are consistent attempts to employ physical appearance to attract attention. Provocative and sexually seductive behavior—often inappropriate to the circumstances—is common, and same-sex friendships are difficult because of perceived competition for attention. Emotional responses tend to be shallow and inconsistent, and it is common for individuals with this disorder to alienate or lose the support of friends.

Narcissistic Personality Disorder

The self-esteem of individuals with *narcissistic personality disorder* may be quite fragile. They are very sensitive to criticism or evaluation by others. It is likely that they overestimate their achievements or potential and may seem to be arrogant and boastful as a result of constant discussion of their accomplishments or importance. Such individuals often actually believe that they are exceptional and that only others with similarly high standards and capabilities can appreciate or understand them. Time is often devoted to anticipating or seeking the admiration of others. It can become a problem when someone with narcissistic personality disorder is seeking service. The inflated opinion of their importance may cause them to assume that they do not have to wait in line or follow rules or procedures designed for "ordinary" people. They may be patronizing or disdainful in their treatment of food servers or salespeople. Further, they may not feel inclined to recognize the value of the needs or feelings of others. Interpersonal relationships may suffer due to a need on the behalf of someone with this disorder to have their accomplishments recognized as best or to have their needs addressed first. Failure or criticism is not taken well and may cause an inappropriate reaction, ranging from aloof indifference to defiant counterattack.

Obsessive-Compulsive Personality Disorder

Obsessive-compulsive personality disorder *should not be confused with* obsessive-compulsive disorder, *which is discussed later in the chapter.* Individuals with this disorder are engrossed with flawlessness, control, and orderliness at the expense of flexibility, openness, or productiveness. There may be stubbornness to their rigidity and adherence to rules and regulations. Adherence to rules has more to do with the fact that they are rules than with whether they make sense or apply in a particular instance where an exception might be appropriate. Things must be done their way, and so it is difficult for them to delegate responsibility. There is often checking and re-checking of details to the extent that a task may not ever be completed. Individuals with this disorder regard moral and ethical issues as "letter-of-the-law" issues. Rule bending or the application of situational ethics is out of the question. There is excessive devotion to the completion of tasks, and even recreation and hobbies are approached with a high degree of organization and precision that would negate the joy in the activities for most people.

Dependent Personality Disorder

Those with *dependent personality disorder* often have others make decisions for them or direct other aspects of their lives. This develops due to an extreme need on behalf of the person to be directed and cared for. Often they will only make decisions with extreme difficulty and many times require advice and assurance from others that the decision was correct. Individuals with this disorder avoid disagreeing with others out of concern that they may lose the approval and support they desire. Relationships are sought and fostered for the potential care and support they offer. This is important to those with dependent personality disorder due to the need to have others assume direction of life's decisions. They often lack the self-confidence to initiate things on their own, and they assume others have more skill or ability. This causes them to wait for someone else to begin to do something or to be around to offer the support or help they are certain will be needed. In some cases, there is an unrealistic fear of finding themselves in a situation in which there is no one to make decisions for or take care of them.

Avoidant Personality Disorder

Individuals with *avoidant personality disorder* feel inadequate and socially inept. Due to a fear of disapproval, rejection, or criticism, work that puts performance on display is avoided. The assumption is always present that others will be severely critical of their performance. They avoid making friends unless there is some assurance that they will meet the approval of others and be accepted. Close personal and intimate relationships are restrained out of fear of inadequate or unacceptable behavior. The *DSM-IV* suggests that there is a "low threshold" for detecting what might be criticism of their behavior or performance. Meeting strangers is particularly difficult, and there is a tendency to exaggerate the risk in ordinary endeavors such as applying for a job, meeting new people, or even just dressing up and going out in public.

Anxiety Disorders

All human beings experience anxiety to some extent. In a mild form, anxiety may serve to promote caution and prudence in human behavior. Anxiety becomes a problem for individuals when it begins without a reasonable stimulus. Some of the anxiety disorders can seriously disrupt a person's life. The discomfort may be so intense that it promotes harmful patterns of drug or alcohol use or other self-destructive behavior. Some anxiety disorders are characterized by the presence of a panic attack.

Panic Attack

The *DSM-IV* describes the *panic attack* as a discrete period of intense fear or discomfort accompanied by specific cognitive or physical symptoms. Panic attacks fall into three distinct subtypes. One subtype is the unexpected or uncued panic attack. In this instance, there is no specific or easily identified cause of the attack. Rather, it is described as occurring spontaneously and unexpectedly. The second subtype is the cued or situationally bound panic attack. In such instances, the attack is preceded by a specific situational cue or by anticipation of such a cue or trigger. Situationally predisposed panic attack is the third form. In such cases, exposure to a situational cue may or may not immediately trigger a panic attack. The cue is generally involved, but the reaction may not occur until some time has passed since exposure.

Panic attack develops very rapidly once the symptoms begin, may reach a height of intensity in ten minutes or less, and may last for as long as two hours. Symptoms may include

- Sweating
- Pounding or rapid heart rate
- Shaking or trembling
- A shortness of breath
- A choking sensation
- Chest pain
- Upset stomach or nausea

- Lightheaded, dizzy, or faint sensations
- A feeling of unreality or separation from oneself (depersonalization)
- Fear of going "crazy"
- Fear of dying
- Tingling sensations or numbness
- Hot flashes or chill

The *DSM-IV* suggests that the occurrence of four or more of the preceding symptoms would suggest a panic attack.

Panic attacks generally accompany such anxiety disorders as panic disorder, social phobia, specific phobia, and post-traumatic stress disorder. These and other forms of anxiety disorder—including agoraphobia and obsessive-compulsive disorder—are discussed in the following pages.

Panic Disorder

Panic disorder is described as occurring with or without agoraphobia. *Agoraphobia* means fear of the market or open spaces and has been recognized for centuries. The term *phobia* implies an unreasonable and unwarranted fear of an object or a situation that is far in excess of any risk or danger actually involved. When *panic disorder without agoraphobia* occurs, there are recurrent panic attacks that may be unexpected. This is followed by unremitting concern that another one will occur. The individual involved may also engage in significant changes in behavior as a result of the attacks. Some of the attacks are unexpected, but others may be associated with a cue or environmental trigger. Patterns of attack may be frequent and regular or intermittent. These repeated attacks might cause fear of an undiagnosed physical illness or of declining mental health. Frequently, major depressive disorder occurs in individuals with panic disorder. In about 30 percent of the cases where both conditions exist, depression precedes the panic disorder.

Panic disorder with agoraphobia might be best described as the result of an effort to control the onset of panic attacks. In an attempt to avoid the cues that are suspected of triggering the panic attacks, the individual begins to avoid certain environments. Places avoided become more numerous until the only "safe" haven is home. Riding public transportation, driving an automobile, visiting a supermarket or shopping center, or attending public functions all become feared and avoided. On occasion, an individual with panic disorder with agoraphobia may develop "safe zones" around home. Familiar streets or a specific pattern of travel to another safe area may be possible. Others, however, become trapped within the walls of their homes or apartments.

Phobias

At one time, over two hundred different phobias were classified. The *DSM-IV* has condensed this list to three: agoraphobia (already mentioned), social phobia, and specific phobia. Characteristics of *agoraphobia* include concern about being in places that might bring on a panic attack. Specific places may be feared such as bridges, crowds, travel of some distance from home, and so on. A major concern seems to be the ability to withdraw from a situation if panic begins. If travel away from home is necessary, it may involve significant worry amounting to torment that a panic attack will occur.

Social phobia involves fear of being evaluated by others, meeting strangers, or being called on to perform in public. There is an underlying fear on the part of the individual that something humiliating or embarrassing will happen to them. A situationally bound panic attack can occur if the individual with this type of phobia is exposed to a social situation that he or she fears. Generally, social situations or opportunities to perform are avoided, or they are endured under extreme fear. Patterns of distress, avoidance, or anxious participation in events can exert a negative influence on such things as social life, schooling, work, or even family life when normal routines become unbearable.

In cases of *specific phobia,* anxiety generally follows exposure to a specific object or situation (phobic stimulus). The reaction follows the pattern of either situationally bound or situationally predisposed panic attack. Unreasonable, unwarranted, and excessive fear results when the individual with specific phobia encounters or anticipates an encounter with the phobic stimulus. Those with specific phobia practice avoidance of phobic cues. They suffer extreme anxiety in anticipation of phobic cues or distress upon encountering one. There are four subtypes of specific phobia: (1) animal type, which is unreasonable fear of certain insects or animals (this generally begins in childhood); (2) natural environment type, which includes fears cued by such things as storms, water, heights, or other things associated with the natural world; (3) blood injection injury type, which includes fear of blood, receiving an injection, surgery, or injury; and (4) situational type, which involves cues received from specific things such as flying, highway traffic, enclosed spaces, and elevators.

Obsessive-Compulsive Disorder

Obsessive-compulsive disorder *should not be confused with* obsessive-compulsive personality disorder, *which is discussed earlier in the chapter.* This disorder involves recurring obsessions or compulsions that occupy a significant portion of a person's day or cause impairment or distress in the individual. Obsessions are disturbing thoughts, images, ideas, or impulses that intrude in inappropriate ways into some individuals' thought patterns. Despite efforts to block them, they seem to reoccur—and often at highly inappropriate times. These thoughts may range from thoughts of saying something embarrassing, such as swearing in public, to stealing something or telling an "off-color" joke at work. Obsessions may also manifest themselves as fear of germs, impressions of being dealt with dishonestly, or fear that a family member is in danger or already harmed. There may be attempts to block or neutralize these obsessive thoughts with other thoughts or specific actions. An obsession regarding contamination with germs may be managed by repeated hand washing, sterilization of personal objects, or avoiding crowds. Thoughts of a pornographic nature may be avoided by reciting a poem or humming a song. Someone obsessed with the thought of sleeping in and being late for work may repeatedly check the alarm clock throughout the night. This is referred to as *obsessive doubting with compulsive checking.* When an action designed to overcome the anxiety of an obsession becomes excessive, it is termed a *compulsion.* Compulsions may be behavioral as in the example of checking the alarm clock or hand washing, or they may be mental such as attempting to distract the mind with alternative thoughts or actions. Individuals with obsessive-compulsive disorder eventually realize that either or both of these are unreasonable.

Attempts to resist a compulsion often produce anxiety that may continue until the individual resumes the behavior or mental act. These behaviors can be highly disruptive to normal life and may require a significant amount of time each day. Some individuals are able to incorporate compulsive behavior into everyday living, but generally there are disturbances in the performance of tasks that require focus or attention. Attempts to avoid the triggers that stimulate the obsessions or compulsions can likewise be distracting and interfere with normal daily routines.

Post-Traumatic Stress Disorder

Memories of distasteful, dangerous, or undesirable events can offer motivation to avoid such things in the future. If such thoughts or memories are extreme, they can be very troubling. These recurring memories, thoughts, or dreams can be distressing to both children and adults. *Post-traumatic stress disorder* develops following exposure to a traumatic event that involved real or imagined threats of death or serious injury and where the individual was horrified, felt at extreme danger, or was helpless to assist. These traumatic events are experienced in a variety of ways. Vivid memories or dreams may recur and intrude into the individual's life. Persons with post-traumatic stress disorder may feel as if they are reliving the event. Repeated vicarious experiences can produce intense distress. Individuals with this disorder attempt to avoid anything that reminds them of the event, and they may attempt to avoid whatever seems to arouse the vivid recollections. The need for repeated diligence in coping with these memories can create the impression that things will never get better. Reactions such as sleep disturbances, poor concentration, jumpiness, and a low threshold for irritability may ensue. If it continues, this disorder can have significant negative impact on home, school, work, friends, and family.

Mood Disorders

There are two general categories of mood disorders, the depressive disorders and the bipolar disorders. The first of these is characterized by a depressed mood that does not feature any episodes of elevated mood (unipolar). A bipolar disorder, on the other hand, features up and down periods in which depressed mood periods are punctuated with elevated or manic episodes.

Depression

Depression is an illness with the potential to cause great suffering and serious harm. As many as one person in ten experiences severe depression during their lifetime. Depression, like other aspects of health and illness, has a wide range in both severity and type and should not be considered a single illness. Two varieties of depression-related disorders discussed in the *DSM-IV* are presented here.

Major Depressive Episode. Characteristics of *major depressive episode* vary among individuals. There are several symptoms that are indicative of this disorder, and, thus, two individuals suffering from depression may exhibit differing characteristics. There may be thoughts of death, ideas about death, or notions about suicide. Attempts at suicide or elaborate plans to commit suicide may be present. Some individuals with major depression begin to believe that they would be better off dead. This could be because their emotional state just feels too painful or that the demands and complications in life seem impossible to overcome. The individual with depression may report, or others may observe, a diminished capacity to concentrate, make decisions, or even think effectively. This can interfere with success in school or performance at work or result in poor decision making. It could be reasoned that such examples of unsuccessful performance might further complicate life and add to the burden of the already depressed status. Most days may find the individual suffering from a lack of energy or experiencing fatigue. This fatigue may be more psychological than physiological in nature since it is often reported even if there has been little or no physical exertion. Some individuals with major depression may begin to experience guilt feelings. These feelings of guilt may have no basis in fact. Further, a sense that they are of little worth to themselves or others may develop. An actual—not imaginary—disturbance of psychomotor function may occur. Psychomotor retardation implies a slowing of activities to a rate far below that of noninvolved persons. Agitated psychomotor activity can bring on restless feelings or purposeless movements. These changes could involve speech or various forms of body movement such as fidgeting, pacing, or hand wringing. There may be a marked fluctuation in body weight. In some cases, there will be a loss of appetite producing a loss of weight; but, in other instances, there will be an increased desire for food with an accompanying weight gain. Things that normally motivate attention or enjoyment are ignored or hold little interest to the individual with major depressive disorder. Interest in recreational pursuits, hobbies, and family activities may dwindle.

There may be a depressed mood for most of the day nearly every day. Individuals with this disorder feel like they are under the proverbial "dark cloud"; they are sad and often see situations in their life as hopeless. Some may not verbally express their sadness, but it is often noticeable to observers. There may be reports of aches and pains, outbursts of anger, exaggerated frustration, or irritable crabby moods. If some of these symptoms continue, there is almost always a negative interruption of performance in school or work and a negative impact on family and social life.

Dysthymic Disorder. *Dysthymic disorder* is a depression that is of a lower intensity but lasts for a longer period of time. It may begin in childhood or adolescence (early onset) or in the adult years (late onset). In either case, the depression is present in chronic form more often than it is not for many years. It may interfere with a child developing any notion regarding the positive prospects offered by opportunities in life. Many of the symptoms indicative of major depressive disorder—hopeless feelings, over or under sleeping and/or eating, fatigue or low energy, poor self-esteem, ineffective decision making, and inability to concentrate on tasks—apply to dysthymic disorder. One prime difference that serves to distinguish between the two is that the "low-grade" long-lasting mood disturbances associated with dysthymic disorder are not too dissimilar to the usual functioning of the individual. Individuals with dysthymic disorder develop thinking patterns that reflect low levels of self-confidence and self-esteem. Due to the chronic nature of this condition, an individual may not have experienced or remember ever feeling upbeat or positive about things. Because of the continual "downer" outlook, individuals with this disorder may have trouble making friends or being included in social activities. The individual who always sees and points out the down side to every scenario is not much fun to be around.

Bipolar Disorder

In earlier times, *bipolar disorder* was called *manic-depressive illness.* The individual with this disorder alternates between periods of depression and manic highs. The rhythm or meter of the pattern of highs and lows plus the variations in the height of the highs (mania) and the depth of the lows (depression) serve to differentiate between three general forms of bipolar disorder: bipolar I disorder, bipolar II disorder, and cyclothymic disorder. To understand the forms of bipolar disorder, there must first be an understanding of manic episodes.

The *DSM-IV* describes a *manic episode* as a period of abnormally and persistently elevated, expansive, or irritable mood that lasts for one week or longer. The manic episode will interrupt normal activities associated with work, school, family, or friends. This elevated mood state may be intense enough to require hospitalization to prevent individuals who are experiencing the manic episode from harming themselves or others. Often, there is grandiose behavior and unwarranted high self-esteem, often causing the individual to imagine that he or she have superior knowledge or ability. A highly talkative state may occur with manic speech patterns that are difficult to comprehend or interrupt. Flights of fanciful thought may race through the person's mind causing rapid and tangential changes of subject. The individual is easily distracted and not able to focus thoughts or hold attention very long. The need for sleep is often markedly diminished. Goal-directed behavior increases, and the individual experiencing the manic episode may engage in multiple activities without regard for the risk involved or the probability that they will not have the time to ever complete them. When a person experiences some of the symptoms described, it is understandable that he or she may exercise poor judgment and become involved in uncontrolled self-indulgent or high-risk activities. Shopping sprees, unwise business investments, dangerous driving, and atypical social activity all may occur. Be aware that something very similar to the manic episode—the *hypomanic episode*—may also be involved in bipolar disorder. The hypomanic episode differs primarily in duration and intensity. While most of the behaviors manifested are very similar to those described for a manic episode, they last for a shorter period of time and are not so dramatic as to interfere with the normal business of the individual. Those experiencing a hypomanic episode do not pose the danger to themselves or others that is possible during a manic episode.

Bipolar I Disorder.   In *bipolar I disorder,* the mood swings between mania and depression are relatively equal in that the depression and the mania are both quite severe. The depression reaches the level of major depression, and the up phase is of true mania proportions.

Bipolar II Disorder.   In *bipolar II disorder,* the up phase only reaches hypomania proportions but the down phase reaches the extreme levels of a major depressive episode. So, while the individual with this disorder is not at as great a risk during the hypomanic phase, that person is at risk of suicide while depressed.

Cyclothymic Disorder.   The individual with *cyclothymic disorder* experiences cyclical ups and downs in mood, but the swings are less severe. The up phase may only reach hypomanic levels, and the down phase does not reach the depths of major depression. In spite of the relatively mild swings in mood, they are still swings and can be upsetting to both the individual with this disorder and those with whom that individual interacts. Further, there are indications that those with cyclothymic disorder have an increased risk of developing bipolar I disorder.

Summary

Mental and emotional problems exist at one end of the continuum of mental health. While some of these problems may have a genetic component, the majority are of unknown cause. The *Diagnostic and Statistical Manual of Mental Disorders,* 4th edition, *(DSM-IV)* is the book mental health professionals use to diagnose these problems. The *DSM-IV* defines mental disorders as follows: "conceptualized as a clinically significant behavioral or psychological syndrome or pattern that occurs in an individual and that is associated with present distress or disability or with a significantly increased risk of suffering death, pain, disability, or an important loss of freedom" (American Psychiatric Association, 1994, p. xxi). Certain problems are related to difficulty in the control of various impulses. These include gambling, explosive disorder, trichotillomania, pyromania, and kleptomania. There are also eating disorders, including bulimia nervosa and anorexia nervosa, as well as overeating disorders and other disorders of eating patterns. Other disorders related to alcohol and drug use include substance-use disorders (substance abuse and substance dependence) and substance-induced disorders. Sleep disorders include hypersomnia, insomnia, nightmares, and sleep terror disorder. The *DSM-IV* includes the broad category of personality disorders, which include paranoid personality disorder, schizoid personality disorder, schizotypal personality disorder, antisocial personality disorder, borderline personality disorder, histrionic personality disorder, narcissistic personality disorder, obsessive-compulsive personality disorder, dependent personality disorder, and avoidant personality disorder. Another broad category the *DSM-IV* recognizes is anxiety disorders. This includes panic attack, panic disorder, phobias, obsessive-compulsive disorder, and posttraumatic stress disorder. The last category discussed is mood disorders, which encompasses unipolar disorders—including major depressive episodes and dysthymic disorder—and bipolar disorders—including bipolar I and II as well as cyclothymic disorder.

DISCUSSION QUESTIONS

1. Considering the difficulty in defining *mental disorder,* what do you believe is a workable definition? What problems do you see with the *DSM-IV*'s definition?

2. The *DSM-IV* definition of mental disorder creates the idea that mental disorders are limited to individuals and that there are no disordered groups. There may, however, be groups composed of a high percentage of disordered individuals. It also brings into play the idea of a "cultural response," stating that the disorder is not such if it is a normal cultural response to an event. How does the idea of "cultural response" and the basis of the disorder resting solely on the individual create problems?

3. Impulse-control disorders, like many other mental disorders, are controversial issues. For example, if a person with a diagnosed impulse disorder such as kleptomania steals small items of little financial worth, should that person be held criminally responsible? What if a person with pyromania commits arson? Should that person be held responsible? What if a person with explosive disorder commits a violent crime?

4. Eating disorders are serious illnesses that can severely damage the physical and mental health of diagnosed individuals. Some people argue that the media and popular culture fuel eating disorders by creating a culture that favors "thin only." Do you agree? What can be done to mitigate these effects?

5. People in the United States treat persons with alcohol and drug dependence largely as criminals. There is an argument that these individuals should be treated as people with a disease—patients rather than convicts. Do you agree? What are the consequences of this change in perspective in terms of public policy?

6. Personality disorders are often unrecognized, and most people at times show slight characteristics of all of these. If all of these disorders have a biochemical basis and can be treated medicinally, are these drugs ethical? What dilemmas do they pose?

7. Much discussion has been given to the overprescription of anti-anxiety drugs. What issues are raised by the prescription of medication to regulate emotions? Is this ever a good idea? When?

8. What special issues in the area of mental disorders are important during adolescence and young adulthood? What would be effective ways of intervening for adolescents with depression, anxiety disorders, and other mental disorders? How would these methods differ from those used with adults?

9. MI/CD treatment has become a "turf battle" between chemical dependence professionals and mental health professionals. Individuals with MI/CD disorders present a unique treatment challenge. What is the best way of handling this? How would their treatment differ from individuals with chemical dependency alone, or those displaying mental disorders without associated chemical problems?

10. Post-traumatic stress disorder gained popular notice after the Vietnam War, when many veterans were diagnosed with the disorder. How has public perception of the disorder changed since then?

RELATED WEBSITES

Impulse Control Problems
Gamblers Anonymous: http://www.gamblersanonymous.org
Gam-Anon Services: http://wwwgamblersanonymous.org/gamanon.html
Trichotillomania Learning Center: http://www.trich.org/

Eating Disorders
Overeaters Anonymous: http://www.overeatersanonymous.org/
National Eating Disorders Society: http://www.laureate.com/
American Anorexia/Bulimia Association: http://members.aol.com/AmAnBu

Alcohol and Drugs
Alcoholics Anonymous: http://www.alcoholics-anonymous.org/
Al-anon/Alateen: http://www.al-anon.alateen.org/
Narcotics Anonymous: http://na.org
Cocaine Anonymous: http://www.ca.org/
Marijuana Anonymous: http://www.marijuana-anonymous.org/
Co-Dependents Anonymous: http://www.ourcoda.org/

Sleep Disorders
American Sleep Disorders Association: http://www.asda.org/
National Sleep Foundation: http://www.sleepfoundation.org/

Anxiety Disorders
Anxiety Disorders Association of America: http://www.adaa.org/
National Victim Center: http://www.nvc.org/
Obsessive-Compulsive Center: http://www.deancare.com

Mood Disorders
Emotions Anonymous: http://www.mtn.org/EA
National Depressive and Manic-Depressive Association: http://www.ndmda.org/
National Mental Health Association: http://www.nmha.org/
National Alliance for the Mentally Ill: http://www.nami.org/
Anxiety Disorders Association of America: http://www.adaa.org/

Phobias
The Phobia List: http://www.sonic.net/~fredd/phobia1.html

REFERENCES

American Psychiatric Association. (1994). *Diagnostic and Statistical Manual of Mental Disorders* 4th Ed.). Washington, DC.: Author.

Carson, R., Butcher, J., & Mineka, S. (1996). *Abnormal Psychology and Modern Life* (10th Ed.). New York: HarperColllins.

Cohen, S. (1995). Overdiagnosis of Schizophrenia: The Role of Alcohol and Drug Misuse. *Lancet, 346,* 1541–1542.

Mueser, K., Bellack, A., & Blanchard, J. (1992). Comorbidity of Schizophrenia and Substance Abuse: Implications for Treatment. *Journal of Counseling and Clinical Psychology, 60,* 845–856.

Osher, F., & Drake, R. (1996). Reversing a History of Unmet Needs: Approaches to Care for Persons with Co-occurring Addictive and Mental Disorders. *Journal of Orthopsychiatry, 66,* 4–11.

Osher, F., Drake, R., Noordsy, D., Teague, G., Hurlbut, S., Biedsanz, J., & Beaudett, M. (1994). Correlates and Outcomes of Alcohol Use Disorder Among Rural Outpatients with Schizophrenia. *Journal of Clinical Psychiatry, 55,* 109–113.

Riley, J. (1994). Dual Diagnosis. *Nursing Clinics of North America, 29,* 29–34.

Washton, A. (1995). Clinical Assessment of Psychoactive Substance Use. In A. Washton (Ed.), *Psychotherapy and Substance Abuse.* New York: Guilford Press.

CHAPTER

5   Self-Esteem

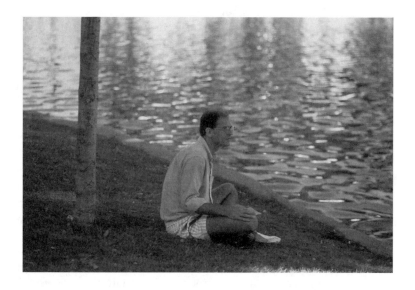

Self-Esteem: A Solid Foundation

Just what is self-esteem? Coopersmith (1981) defined it as "an expression of approval or disapproval, indicating the extent to which a person believes himself or herself competent, successful, significant, and worthy" (p. 415). Crandall (1973) defined self-esteem as "liking and respect for oneself which has some realistic basis" (p. 98). Rosenberg (1979) described self-esteem as "the product of some complex combination of judgments about the self occurring outside the individual's awareness" (p. 132). There are many definitions of self-esteem used interchangeably in the literature, such as self-acceptance, self-like, self-love, self-respect, self-regard, and self-worth. To put it more simply, if self-esteem were to be defined in two words, they would be "feeling good" (Coopersmith, 1981).

Self-esteem is important throughout one's life, but it is particularly important during developmental or impressionable years of childhood and adolescence.

It is important for youngsters to feel good about themselves to have a strong foundation of self-esteem. The ability for youngsters to learn life skills in school—cope with stress, communicate with others, solve problems, and cope with emotions— enables them to promote their own well-being (Weisen & Orley, 1996). Because self-esteem is so important to young people, and because it is a learned concept, it is finding its way into curricula and schools across the country (Gurney, 1987).

Although there are many terms for self-esteem that researchers use interchangeably, as already noted, there are distinct differences that the reader should be aware of. Within these theories, other concepts such as self-concept, self-esteem, self-efficacy, and self-image are involved. Before discussing each term in detail, it is important to discuss at this point the differences between these four concepts. Each of these terms represents a different idea. *Self-concept* can be defined as the perceptions people have about themselves in terms of personal attributes and roles they fulfill (King, 1997). This does not include value judgments or attitudes toward self. Instead, it is more of a description of what actually exists. *Self-esteem*, on the other hand, is the evaluation people make of their self-concept descriptions and the extent to which they experience satisfaction or dissatisfaction with them (King, 1997). This refers more to people's feelings about themselves and their attributes. Self-esteem is usually thought of as being either positive or negative, whereas self-concept is a relatively neutral concept. For example, individuals may describe themselves as overweight, which is their perception or self-concept. This is different, however, from having negative feelings about being overweight, which is related to self-esteem.

The third concept, *self-efficacy*, differs from self-esteem in that it refers more specifically to the degree to which an individual possesses confidence in his or her ability to achieve a goal (Greene & Miller, 1996). It is similar to self-esteem in that there is a value judgment being made; however, this judgment is specifically related to ability to achieve a goal. Therefore, it follows that self-esteem is a more general and global concept and self-efficacy is more domain specific. For example, a person may have a generally high self-esteem in which the person has positive attitudes toward himself or herself as a person. However, this person can have both high and low self-efficacies. The person might very competent in the area of math, thus creating a high self-efficacy in this area. On the other hand, this person may have trouble with writing, thus creating a low self-efficacy in this area. Finally, *self-image* can be described as how people see themselves. Often times, this perception is based on the perception that others have of the person. Therefore, self-image can be considered extrinsic in nature, whereas self-concept and self-esteem are considered intrinsic. The term *self-efficacy* can be considered both intrinsic and extrinsic depending on who is determining the quality of the outcome.

The distinction between these four terms is an important one. Given this information, it is easy to understand how self-efficacy is more directly related to the process of goal setting and goal attainment.

Although there is evidence that self-esteem has an effect on the types of goals people choose (Adler & Weiss, 1988), examination of self-efficacy may make more sense. Greene and Miller (1996) support this concept. They found that perceived ability, or self-efficacy, relates to goal orientation. Both of these affect cognitive engagement during a task and are linked together. People who adopt learning goals engage in more self-regulation and use more cognitive learning strategies. It has also been supported that students with a high self-efficacy use more cognitive strategies and have a higher level of cognitive engagement in a task. General self-esteem may also be an important predictor of goal-setting behavior (Adler & Weiss, 1988). Together, these concepts are essential in creating happiness and fulfillment. A person needs to have both a positive self-esteem and a feeling of self-efficacy in certain areas to feel competent and gain self-acceptance.

As already noted, there are many definitions of self-esteem. Self-esteem can be thought of as existing beneath a continuum or range of emotional states. It provides a stable foundation for this range, so that someone who has a solid self-esteem is more likely to experience balance within his/her emotional states. Certainly, a person with high self-esteem is not always "up," but, even on the bad days, he/she is able to eventually reach emotional homeostasis.

One way to better understand self-esteem is to explore the concept of the *reflexive self*. Sociologists often look at the self as a continuous process that takes place in interactions with others and in self-reflection. This self-reflection—communication with the self about the self—is an important part of self-esteem. In fact, one can argue that it is this *self-talk* that determines how people feel about themselves and influences their self-esteem. The *reflexive self*, therefore, can be defined as the ability to engage in an internal conversation with self as both the subject and the object (Falk & Miller, 1997). It includes the concepts of self-image, self-efficacy, self-recognition, self-perception, self-concept, and self-esteem. As a person grows, these dimensions of the self become more complex and intertwined. This definition of the reflexive self, however, also implies that the responses of others are crucial in the development of the self. The *object* refers to how people think or believe other people perceive them. It is this combination of views about self and beliefs of how other people view individuals that drives the development of self-esteem.

Concepts Related to Self-Esteem

Studies have shown that self-esteem has an effect on the type of mate a person chooses, how people interact with others, careers chosen, and success within those careers. A person who has high self-esteem generally exhibits happiness and is able to look at the world in a positive but realistic light. That person is able to relate well with others and not be threatened by the success of friends and colleagues.

Poor self-esteem, on the other hand, affects so many other aspects of people's lives, the choices they make, and the way they behave. The ripple effect is phenomenal. Low self-esteem has been associated with poor school performance and a high dropout rate. Additionally, those with a low self-esteem are more likely to indulge in the use of alcohol and controlled substances and to become prematurely sexually active. These behaviors, in turn, often lead to a higher number of sexual partners and increased chances of getting sexually transmitted diseases (STDs) which can affect fertility, inflict recurrent pain, and, in the case of AIDS, be life threatening. In addition, negative self-esteem is tied in with many aspects of mental dysfunction, such as loneliness. Lonely people often feel worthless, incompetent, and unlovable (Brage & Meredith, 1994).

Coopersmith (1981) found low self-esteem to be related to depression, sadness, and lethargy. In the extreme, it can even lead to suicide or suicide attempts (Carlson & Cantwell, 1982). Other less extreme, but equally negative, characteristics include conceit, the tendency to over-inflate strengths, and a controlling or pushy nature. Although these characteristics may at first seem counterintuitive, people with low self-esteem, as already discussed, feel that negative things in their lives are a result of a quality they possess and cannot change, while positive things are simply a result of luck. Because they do not feel personally responsible for the positive experiences they have, it is necessary for a person with low self-esteem to "put others down" to create an experience that allows them to feel good about themselves.

Sellers and Waligroski (1993) found that depression was associated with weight gain, but self-esteem was not. Self-esteem was, however, associated with perceived attractiveness. This association highlights the personal nature of self-esteem. Because self-esteem is the way people feel about themselves, factors that affect self-esteem can vary greatly highly from person to person. For instance, one person might value intelligence highly and may therefore have low self-esteem when confronted with poor academic performance. Another person might value athletic ability and find it very difficult to deal with losing an important game.

What makes a person have a good or bad self-esteem? The answer to this question can lead to an awareness that can help people experience the benefits of a positive self-esteem through the creation of interventions. This is an elusive question to answer, however, because self-esteem is intertwined with many other central ideas. Often, it is difficult to distinguish a cause-and-effect model. Instead, it is useful to have an understanding of some of the more important concepts to fully understand the makings of self-esteem.

Cognitive Distortions

One concept that is crucial is that of *cognitive distortions*. Remember the reflexive self and how perceptions affect self-esteem? Well, often a problem occurs when a person's beliefs are irrational. If people have beliefs about themselves that are irrational and faulty, then self-esteem can suffer. These irrational beliefs can be called *cognitive distortions*. In a way, they are bad habits. When people engage in cognitive distortions, they interpret reality in an unreal way. These are negative because they are often judgmental and inaccurate. In addition, people tend to apply labels to other people and events before they are able to really evaluate them. Following is a list of the nine most common cognitive distortions that can affect self-esteem (McKay & Fanning, 1987):

1. *Overgeneralization* involves taking one event or fact and making a general rule of it. This rule is never tested. However, it is applied to future situations. This creates a sort of absolute reality that makes life confining. Often, people fall prey to this distortion. They might make one mistake in a certain area, and suddenly this mistake determines their success in that area.

2. *Global labeling* is applying stereotyped labels to whole classes of people, things, behaviors, and experiences. This is similar to overgeneralization, except here the distortion takes the context of a label instead of a rule. This not only creates stereotypes, but it also cuts a person off from experiencing the variety of life.

3. *Filtering* can be defined as the process of selectively abstracting certain facts from reality and paying attention to them. By doing this, a person ignores the rest. This creates blind spots and interpretations that are biased. (If you can only remember the times in school when you received a bad grade, then you are guilty of filtering information.)

4. *Polarized thinking* occurs when a person lives in a black and white universe where there are no shades of gray. This is a true all-or-nothing situation; a person is either smart or stupid. This creates problems because usually people associate themselves with the negative side of the spectrum because no one is perfect all the time.

5. *Self-blame* involves literally blaming self for everything whether or not it is an accurate assessment. (Any shortcomings are your fault regardless of the amount of control you have over the situation. If you find yourself constantly apologizing, you probably fall into this category.) This type of distortion is dangerous because it blinds people to their strengths and accomplishments.

6. *Personalization* refers to the belief that everything that happens is somehow related to self. It is a narcissistic quality in which people constantly compare themselves to other people. This has two major drawbacks. First, it creates a constant feeling of pressure and being observed. Second, it often makes people overreact and act inappropriately.

7. *Mind reading* happens when a person thinks everyone in the world thinks like he or she does. This is a type of projection in which people assume that others feel the way they do and that there is a commonality of human nature that may or may not be true. This can hurt self-esteem in that people are likely to think that everyone agrees with their negative opinions of themselves.

8. *Control fallacies* deal with control over the world. People can see themselves as in charge or just the opposite—everyone but themselves is in charge. Overcontrol can result in false feelings of capabilities, whereas undercontrol can result in feeling as if events are out of a person's control. Undercontrol feelings are harmful to self-esteem in that they create feelings of helplessness and hopelessness.

9. *Emotional reasoning* results when a person relies on emotions to interpret reality and direct action instead of thoughts and rational laws. This can be disastrous to self-esteem because it holds the notion that if a person *feels* useless, then the person must *be* useless.

All of these cognitive distortions are important in that they can negatively affect self-esteem. It is essential that people be aware of and understand the different ways they can create irrational thoughts. Knowing this information can help people to recognize when they are engaging in such distortions and to make the first steps in changing thoughts to be more accurate and rational.

Attribution Theory

Another concept related to self-esteem is *attribution theory.* Attribution theory deals with examining how people attribute their successes and failures. This is related to the idea and perception of control. Generally, people can be classified as having either an internal or external locus of control. People who have an internal locus of control view their successes and failures as a direct result of their thoughts and actions. On the other hand, people with an external locus of control view their successes and failures as a result of their environment. The extent to which a person aligns himself or herself within this spectrum affects self-esteem.

People with good self-esteem believe in themselves. They view the world in a fundamentally different way than those with low self-esteem. If they have a negative experience, they attribute it to a simple cause that they can remedy. If they experience a positive event, they attribute it to a fundamental personal characteristic. For instance, if a person with high self-esteem fails a test, that person simply attributes it to the fact that he or she did not study and decides to study harder in the future. If a person gets an *A,* that person attributes it to a belief that he or she is intelligent. If people with high self-esteem stumble over some problems in life, they fix the problems or seek help in fixing them. Bolstered with this belief in themselves, they aim high in life, making choices they find mentally stimulating and fulfilling (both in terms of career and personal issues); and, typically, they are quite successful. This success, in turn, feeds into their self-esteem, contributing to what studies have shown—that people who generally are happier in life are more mentally and physically healthy.

People with low self-esteem, on the other hand, attribute positive experiences to a universal cause beyond their control, such as luck. They attribute negative experiences to intrinsic personal characteristics. People with low self-esteem who fails tests tell themselves that they are stupid, and if they get good grades, they guessed well or some other chance intervened.

Chandler, Lee and Pengilly (1997) offer support for attribution theory and its relationship with self-esteem. Their findings suggest that causal cognition on performance may either enhance and maintain or threaten self-esteem. Students with higher self-esteem attributed their success to a more controllable dimension than those with lower self-esteem. These students were also more accepting of favorable feedback and less accepting of unfavorable feedback as opposed to their counterparts. Generally, internal, stable, and controllable dimensions were associated with self-enhancement. In addition, self-esteem affects expectancy of success, which contributes to causal attributions. These findings suggest that expectancies are related to the direction of performance outcome and level of self-esteem. It would hold, therefore, that increasing expectancies of success might result in modifying student cognitions that, in turn, will increase self-esteem.

Learned Helplessness

Related to attribution theory is the theory of *learned helplessness.* Learned helplessness is a phenomenon that refers to a thought process in which people "learn" through their experiences that nothing they can do will affect their situation. According to this theory, the reason for this effect is motivational. Failure causes an expectation of uncontrollability that if persistent, leads to a withdrawal of effort. This is often seen in students with learning disabilities. It is also one of the reasons given for people remaining in poverty for so long. Recently, researchers have begun to look at these phenomena in terms of attribution theory. They hold that expectations of uncontrollability depend on the attributions people make for their failure (Witkowski & Stiensmeier-Pelster, 1998).

One of the outgrowths of this line of thinking is the possibility that the performance deficits seen in learned helplessness studies may be due to a desire to protect or enhance self-esteem. This suggests that one strategy to deal with failure consists of the attempt to diminish its effect on self-esteem by attributing failure to specific instead of global causes. Witkowski and Stiensmeier-Pelster (1998) found support for this self-esteem protection theory as opposed to learned helplessness. They found that subjects withdrew effort on a test of intelligence and performed poorly after experiencing failure only when they thought the results would be publicly available. Further, the subjects used several self-protection strategies including attributing the failure to specific, unstable causes and viewing the test given as an inadequate measure of intelligence. These findings add to the learned helplessness theory by adding a new variable that influences performance—public or private knowledge.

Attribution theory, along with the learned helplessness phenomenon, has contributed greatly to the study of self-esteem. The information in these two concepts helps explain how a person can have a positive or negative self-esteem. Together, all the information in this section gives way to a more complete understanding of self-esteem. It is this information that will help people develop programs and strategies for increasing self-esteem.

Changes in Self-Esteem

Self-esteem is not static. Just like emotions, self-esteem is so fluid that it changes on a daily basis. For example, you may start out feeling good about yourself on a given day, and then you get a C on a paper you thought had deserved much better. Later in the day, a fight with your significant other further dampens your spirit. Now, you can not help but focus on some of the less-than-perfect aspects of your body, and, before you know it, your self-esteem is much lower than it was at the start of the day.

Self-esteem can be perceived as a continuum, and factors both intrinsic and extrinsic constantly feed into it. These factors move self-esteem along the continuum, either raising it or lowering it. However, it is up to the person to decide exactly *how much* these factors affect self-esteem. A person who feels worthy intrinsically will always have that belief as a support and will be able to withstand the fluctuations self-esteem succumbs to throughout the day and throughout life.

Developmental Changes

Just as self-esteem can change from day to day as a result of events, self-esteem changes over the life span. In general, self-esteem is expected to be somewhat stable over time within developmental periods; however, it is less stable between developmental periods such as middle childhood to adolescence. Self-esteem begins to develop in early childhood. As a child grows, there is an increasing ability to take the role of specific others. This allows a child to view himself or herself through the eyes of others, which leads to reflection and the evaluation of behavior. Self-esteem begins to develop based on the feelings the child experiences based on these perceptions. The gaining of peers and social environments increases these opportunities to judge their capabilities. When a child enters school, a new stage begins in which feelings become generalized and self-esteem becomes more stable and transsituational. In adolescence, dramatic shifts in self-esteem occur. Self-esteem becomes increasingly important as peers become significant others. These changes during adolescence may be disruptive to the self-concept as teenagers attempt to bring together discrepancies in the way they view themselves (Falk & Miller, 1997).

Research supports the notion that even young children expect that self-liking will affect one's thoughts, feelings, and behavior. In addition, research suggests that as children grow older they attribute and explain self-esteem more in terms of psychological concepts (Daniels, 1998). The results of Daniels' (1998) study indicate that there is a shift in the cognitive process of self-esteem between the ages of five and nine. During this time, the child begins to understand that personality is not simply a mood that is shaped and changed by trying hard. Rather, it is a way of shaping and interpreting events and is difficult to change.

Gender and Self-Esteem

Only one major pattern of self-esteem acquisition throughout life has been noted. In grammar school, females tend to have higher self-esteem than males; but, by adolescence, the trends reverse. These findings are suspect, however, because it has been found that males are more likely to embellish or exaggerate their answers on self-esteem measuring instruments. They also are open to interpretation (Schwalbe & Staples, 1991). It may be that adolescent girls experience a shift in the factors that affect their self-esteem; the most important factors become extrinsic, as opposed to intrinsic. Adolescent girls may not necessarily suffer from a developmentally necessary decrease in self-esteem, but they experience this decrease as a result of developmentally necessary changing of priorities (Josephs, Markus, Tafarod, 1992).

Sidebar: Self-Esteem and Gender

Much research has investigated the question of the differences in self-esteem among men and women. The overwhelming consensus is that there is no significant difference between levels of self-esteem in men and women; however, there are a number of differences in the factors that relate to self-esteem as they affect men and women (Josephs et al., 1992). Women are more likely to develop what has been called a *collectivist self-esteem*, which means that they view relations with other people—especially those they value and consider important—as vital to their self-esteem. Men are more likely to develop *individualist self-esteem*, meaning that their self-esteem is based almost entirely on personal, internal attributes and has little to do with others. Women are more likely to view academic work and self-perceived competence as important to their self-esteem than are men (Schwalbe & Staples, 1991). Additionally, men ascribe more importance to being independent, autonomous, and separate than most women do.

What are the reasons for these differences? Most researchers believe that social cues and cultural expectations are more responsible than inherent biological differences. For a biological difference to be part of the explanation, many people look to the gene as the answer. However, this is only partially correct when it comes to complex concepts such as self-esteem. There is not a known mechanism for a genetic difference between men and women accounting for their differences in self-esteem (Sapolski, 1997). Thus, environmental and cultural factors are considered. Schwalbe and Staples (1991) suggest that these differences may exist because society prescribes different levels of competence for social behaviors to the sexes. As an example, women communicate better than men do and men are better competitors. These differences in perceived competence could translate eventually into actual differences because the person begins to emphasize what he or she perceives as his or her strength. This leads to practice—in communication or competition in the preceding example—that in turn increases actual competencies. These competencies then become a source for self-esteem.

It is possible that there are evolutionary reasons for these differences in self-esteem. If the assumption is accepted that humans are more likely to survive and prosper if they cooperate with each other, it seems logical for people to have developed the traits that cause them to favor and prosper in these types of situations. This ensures cooperation with each other. It is possible that self-esteem is related to the ability or perceived ability to complete the tasks associated with participation in society. These tasks might differ for men and women, and this may explain the reasons for the differences in male and female self-esteem. While it is difficult to ascribe these differences to a given gene, it seems likely that there is some mechanism for maintaining them in the population, a mechanism that most likely involves a combination of genetic factors and environmental cues. Whatever the possible reasons for differences are, it is important to remember that self-esteem is not an intrinsic trait and *can* be changed.

Once a person becomes a young adult, self-esteem becomes more of an intrinsically generated characteristic. It is at this point in life that adults begin to make choices and enjoy or suffer the consequences associated with them. The foundation of self-esteem plays a big part in decision making. It should not, however, be misconstrued that one can be "stuck" with a certain level of self-esteem. This is a characteristic that is pliable. The ability to choose esteem-building exercises and behaviors or be controlled by the externals of society is in the hands of those who want to take control of their mental well-being.

Give Yourself a Little Credit

Look around you at the room in which you are sitting and take special note of anything that is red. Look around again so that you can memorize a list of all red things around you. Now, close your eyes and list all things that are blue.

This exercise is often given to students in one of the authors' classes. It is designed to demonstrate that when a person focuses on one thing (in this case, the category of red items), it becomes difficult, if not impossible, to notice other items (such as anything in the room that is blue).

And so it is with self-esteem. If individuals focus on the negative aspects of themselves, it becomes increasingly difficult, if not impossible, see the positive. And, as has already been discussed, a low self-esteem can lead to a world of other problems.

Developing High Self-Esteem

Self-esteem is an attribute whose foundation is laid by parents or other caregivers. The single most important aspect of parental effects on self-esteem is the amount of physical affection the child receives. The amount of punishment a child receives is insignificant, as is feeling "favored" above other siblings (Felson & Zielinski, 1989). Parental effects are stronger in earlier years and are cumulative. However, it is unclear whether a distinction can be made between actual parental behaviors and perceived behaviors. Hence, if a child feels that he or she receives a substantial amount of physical affection, even when objectively the level of affection is average, there is a positive increase in self-esteem (Felson & Zielinski, 1989). There are several suggested tips on how parents can help increase their child's self-esteem (Daves, 1999; Appell, Hoffman, & Speller, 1999):

1. Support and encourage.
2. Lead by example.
3. Encourage peer relationships.
4. Provide a home environment where stress is held to a manageable level.
5. Keep expectations high by consistently offering new challenges to your child.

6. Allow your child to assume personal responsibility by gradually giving up a small portion of your control.
7. Provide feedback.
8. Provide a structured, coherent, and consistent plan of discipline within the family.

However, the foundation possessed as one emerges from childhood is only the beginning. As an adult, new responsibilities of nurturing self-esteem come into play. Often, people who are suffering from a low self-esteem want very much to change their outlook. A lament often heard is, "I just want to feel good about myself." Unfortunately, many people who actively seek to change their self-esteem try to do so overnight. However, just as a person's current level of self-esteem was not created overnight, it cannot be changed instantly.

"One-shot" self-esteem enhancing seminars simply do not work (Donnelly & Procaccino, 1993). Self-esteem is simply too complex of a concept to change in one day. It is a learned behavior that must be changed slowly, as changes in other learned behaviors must be made. The negative habit (low self-esteem) must be eliminated and replaced by a positive habit (high self-esteem). This is not a process that is easy, quick, and painless. It is a complicated journey that occurs in small steps, little by little.

Consider another example that most people can relate to. It is estimated that 60 percent of the adult population are considered overweight. When someone decides to lose weight, he or she is often tempted by weight-loss systems that advertise a quick loss. However, this is not the most effective way of losing weight. If a person is fifty pounds overweight, certainly he or she did not gain that weight in one week. Therefore, no one can expect to lose that amount of weight in such a short period of time.

Whether the reference is to a physical shift (as in losing weight) or a psychological shift (such as increasing self-esteem), changes are programmed within the body and mind over time. Although it is not what people want to hear, worthwhile things often take time.

Daily Recognition

Building self-esteem is based on giving daily doses of praise and recognition. If you are pursuing better self-esteem yourself, you can start by asking yourself a few pertinent questions. What did you accomplish today? What have you done well? How will you improve those things that did not turn out to your satisfaction? What will you do to remind yourself that your goals are attainable? These are all important questions that should be addressed every day.

Your daily dose of praise and recognition is like money in the bank. In fact, it helps build your "self-esteem account." And, like a bank account, if you contribute to it on a regular basis, it will be there for you when you need it on those bad days when you need an extra boost of self-esteem.

Difficulty of Change

When faced with this advice, many people feel it is unrealistic. To request that people with poor self-esteem praise themselves and provide self-recognition may seem a little strange. But, like many things in life, people become that which they pretend to be. There is a process of resistance that occurs whenever people try to change something about themselves. However, this process is normal and an important part of change. To illustrate this, fold your hands. Which thumb do you have on top? The right or the left? In a large group of people, a certain percentage of people will have the right thumb on top, and another, the left. Which of these is right? If you are laughing because there is no right or wrong answer, you are correct. There is no right thumb to have on top, just the one that feels best for you—just as there is no right or wrong way to view the world. Outgoing is no better than shy, and liking sports is no better than liking music.

Now, refold your hands so that the other thumb is on top. It probably feels awkward, strange, and even unnatural. But, realize that about half the people you know find this comfortable. Remember that there is no right or wrong way—just whatever works best for you. If you unfold your hands and refold them, you will probably find that they go back to the first position. Most people find change and growth uncomfortable, like folding your hands backward.

Accurate Self-Assessment

Self-esteem is dependent on the perception and interpretation of daily events. This leads to an assessment of self worth and abilities. A common problem for most people is an inability to accurately conduct a self-assessment. Often, people view or evaluate themselves inappropriately. This leads to problems with self-esteem. It is important for people to learn how to think about themselves and how to assess their strengths and weaknesses in a way that will facilitate a good self-esteem.

Describing Strengths and Weaknesses

The first step is being able to accurately state your weaknesses. To begin, take out a piece of paper and make a list of the *weaknesses* or things you would like to change about yourself. Take a look at your list. How did you describe your areas of weakness? Everybody has faults, and that is okay. What is not okay is when people think and talk about their faults in a nonbeneficial way. McKay and Fanning (1987) discuss several ways to change negative self-evaluations. The following list is taken from their book:

- *Use nondisparaging language.* Eliminate words and descriptors that have a negative connotation. For example, "lousy on the phone" can be changed to "I feel somewhat nervous on the phone."

■ *Use accurate language.* Deal with facts only and do not exaggerate the negative. For example, it is more accurate to state "I would like to lose ten pounds" than "I'm a cow."

■ *Use language that is specific rather than general.* This translates to eliminating words such as *everything, always, never, completely.* Limit your descriptions to particular situations, settings, or relationships. For example, "I occasionally lose my car keys" can be substituted for "I lose everything."

■ *Find exceptions or corresponding strengths.* This is most important with items that make you feel the worst about yourself. For example, an appropriate way to describe being "lousy at arguing" is "I do not have a killer instinct, but I like that I do not have to be right all the time."

These tips are essential for being able to conduct an accurate self-assessment. Learning to explain your weaknesses in an appropriate way will set the stage for a positive self-esteem. This requires a major commitment to stop negative ways of talking about yourself. Take some time to look at each weakness you listed. Try to rephrase it with the preceding guidelines. How does your new list compare to the old?

Analyzing weaknesses is only one part of a self-assessment. Another important step involves strengths. It is important to acknowledge your strengths. On a piece of paper, make a list of your strengths or things you find pleasing; use complete sentences and elaborate using adjectives and synonyms. This is helpful, because people often downplay their strengths. It is important to take credit for things done well. In addition, strengths should be celebrated through repeating positive statements and thinking about specific examples when they have been demonstrated (McKay & Fanning, 1987).

Regular Tune-Ups

The relationship of self-esteem to the self can be likened to the relationship of oil to a car. Oil is essential to the smooth running of any car, so part of a car's maintenance includes regular oil changes every three thousand to five thousand miles. When the oil is not changed occasionally, the car will start to sputter and it simply will not run well. Similarly, people start to sputter if they are not encouraged throughout the day. Regular doses of self-esteem help to ensure smooth running throughout the day and throughout life.

Pearls of Self-Esteem

As the following story illustrates, a person can only offer esteem-building actions to others if a person's own self-esteem is functioning well. The story discusses mental well-being and strong self-esteem through five *PEARLs:* purpose, enthusiasm, attraction, responsibility, and love. These PEARLs impact not only the individual but also each person with whom the message and its meaning are shared (Donnelly, 1998).

The PEARLs of Self-Esteem

The Pearl of Purpose

We are born to this earth with all of the world's promises in the palm of our hand. Each day of our lives is an expression of our unique purpose and an extension of our potential. You and only you possess the ability to establish purpose in your life. A vision that lies in your heart and soul is yours to seek and lies inside of yourself. Remember, the ancestor of every action is a thought, and, as you think, so shall you be.

You possess these amazing attributes and myriads more, even if you have not yet chosen to apply each one's potential in your life. The secret is to fix your purpose and to set your course to its completion, knowing that you, in your infinite intellect and perception, are at the helm. Everyone has met individuals who for inexplicable reasons have chosen to release themselves from the responsibility of seeking solutions. Instead, their energy is wasted on blaming others or society for the ills plaguing their progress, not realizing that they are the sole possessors of the key to their success. The difference between you and them might be as thin as the wing of a dragonfly or the wing of an eagle. The choice is yours. Remember, the Creator's greatest gift to you is You.

Fulfill your promise to greatness by firing your strength to surpass the limits of mediocrity. Step forward from the stagnation of routines that have entangled you in your relationships and yourself. The fear that binds you can be released with the resources you have been given if you condition your mind to attain prosperity. The greatest influence on your path to success is the power of the simple word.

The Pearl of Enthusiasm

Enthusiasm is the effervescence of life. As single droplets of water wear away the rock, practice faith in yourself by wearing away obstacles once recognized as fear. Fire up your energy and strive forward to perform each of your daily tasks with total commitment to pursuing your goals. A child does not consider defeat. He tries to fly by flapping his arms like imaginary wings. He knows after awhile that his form was not made for flight and goes off in pursuit of other amusements, knowing that at least he tried. Act now in pursuit of your dreams with child-like enthusiasm. You will never fly unless you try.

Enthusiasm for living is the celebration of people's divine nature, for the word itself means *God-within*. For children, the contents of their world consist of new discoveries and fantastic tales filled with wonder and excitement. Each day beckons with laughter and hope. Boundless hopes in the future rise up to sustain the dreams of youth as yet unhindered by the tether of adult sensibility.

Once mature, people often distill the essence of wonder into the bitterness of cynicism or indifference. These negative feelings undermine their vitality and tranquillity and prevent them from living each day to the fullest. Preserving an enthusiastic outlook can diffuse the anger and disillusionment that everyone experiences in the occasional drudgery of life. Engage fully in the pageantry of living your dreams. You are a child of the universe created in a miraculous mold from which no other living being can claim identity. Yours is the only life that you will lead, so live it justly, wisely, and earnestly. Reach out boldly to make your contribution, for, as once was noted, "Every man is worth just so much as the things are worth about which he busies himself." Greet the day with enthusiasm, for another precious day of life has been given to you.

The Pearl of Attraction

Minds are like magnets attracting the metals of thoughts. Experiences of today are expressions of countless thoughts throughout people's lives. Thoughts of today are considered previews of tomorrow's coming attractions. Attract yourself to what it is you desire and deflect thoughts of dissatisfaction and doubt. Remember, dreams are thoughts of tomorrow's reality.

You are limited by the degree to which your faith in your ability dictates. Allow no constraints on your aspirations. As was written centuries ago, "Whatever you desire, believe that you will receive, and you shall have." You deserve the fulfillment of all of your dreams. Direct your thoughts to trusting your abilities and your knowledge to attain your aspirations.

Discern your strengths and make them stronger. Seek out your weaknesses and make them strengths. In this way, you verify the value of your self-worth and are not bound by anyone else's plan. Your power lies in the possibilities aroused by tapping these inner resources of your potential. Conceive the idea of what you expect to achieve and imagine that you have already attained it. You may learn by observing success in other people's lives and then by applying the techniques to your experience, but understand that the path to your destination can only be walked by you.

The Pearl of Responsibility

"The true measure of a man is not how he behaves during times of comfort or convenience but how he behaves during times of challenge and controversy" (Martin Luther King Jr.). The circumstances in life that create challenge are those that possess the greatest opportunities for growth. They who excuse themselves from progress are shunning self-responsibility. This resolve to accept self-discipline and responsibility strengthens the integrity of a person's character. Remember, you will succeed even if the step in the direction of your dream is as slow as that of a snail.

Learn from your shortcomings and do not dwell on misfortunes. Failure is guaranteed if you project your past errors into the future without having solved the problems of the present. Forgiving yourself for failures is less difficult when you know that your next success will be due in part to learning from these struggles.

Only you have the power to attain the prosperity that you deserve through your own merits. Never allow the inner conflict that is a part of all decision making to dampen your resolve. Realize that achieving your goal will have to take as long as it is necessary, but act on your goal now. Do it now! Action is the only means by which you attain prosperity. There once was a man who had the blues, because he had no shoes, until, upon the street, he met a man who had no feet. You deserve better. When you shift the responsibility for improving your circumstances squarely on your shoulders, you break the cycle of disillusionment. Instead of blaming others or outer circumstances for your stagnation, admit that it is in fact you who are the only real force with influence in your life.

Face the reality that is the truth. Only you can initiate the change necessary for self-improvement. Ask yourself the question, "What is it that I can change about myself, my habits, and my interactions with others that will produce positive results?" Study how others have made remarkable strides in their lives. Read stories about those who have succeeded, and make the effort yourself to experience similar success. Become an expert on your dream. Expend the time and effort necessary to gain knowledge and experience. Confidence is bred of learning and sustains your hopes and beliefs.

Exact the discipline required for progress whether it is in the physical, psychological, or spiritual realm. By developing these three areas, you alter your present set of conditions forever and have already invested in your success. Responsibility is a necessity for those who aspire to fulfill their ambitions. And remember that you were given all of the gifts with which to seek and gain happiness. Act now.

(continued)

The Pearl of Love

You are a wonderful person, worthy and deserving of love. Delight in your distinction and appreciate the unique qualities of others. Encourage another's growth toward self-fulfillment by acknowledging their progress and effort. A bloom blossoms with the sun's masterful touch but withers without water's gentle brush. Deflect the barbs of your enemies with a shield cast from your abundance of love. Greet each one you meet with love in your heart, and you will have the power to withstand the harshest critics. Love protects you from discouragement and uplifts you in your triumphs. With love in your heart, nothing can disturb you.

It is said that Abraham Lincoln was criticized for being too close to his enemies. His councilmen encouraged Lincoln to destroy his enemies. Lincoln responded by simply saying, "Do I not destroy my enemies by making them my friends?"

In the course of daily living, challenge yourself to be noncritical of those with whom you come into contact. If criticism weighs your tongue, imagine delivering the message to yourself. Judge others against a yardstick of lengthy measure so that they will apply a comparable standard of mercy to your words and deeds. Pardon to the extent that you love. The act of forgiveness lifts the burden of another's anger from your shoulders, freeing you to move ahead on your spiritual journey.

Before reading the remainder of this chapter, spend a few moments reflecting on each of these PEARLs. Think about how purpose, enthusiasm, attraction, responsibility, and love play a role within your life. Then, spend a few moments thinking of how each of these areas is related to self-esteem. What is suggested within this section, as within all areas of this book, is to insightfully apply this material. Keep in mind that there are three steps to changing behavior: Step 1: awareness; Step 2: reflection; and Step 3: application.

Self-Esteem and Mental Functioning

Because self-esteem is at the core of so many other aspects of self, it has a profound effect on mental functioning. Someone who has a strong and positive sense of self is able to concentrate or focus better and able to think more clearly in general than someone with low self-esteem.

Low self-esteem emotionally affects individuals because it brings about higher stress levels, depression, and a myriad of negative thoughts and emotions that must be contended with on a daily basis. The person with low self-esteem is so busy constantly dealing with these thoughts and emotions—in essence, battling with self—that it leaves less time to deal with other issues in life. A person plagued with low self-esteem, therefore, is less able to concentrate on the problem at hand because the problems with self keep creeping into the picture.

Self-Assessment: Improving Self-Esteem

On a sheet of paper, write down something positive about yourself. It can be something that reflects a physical aspect of yourself, the way you behave, or an attribute that you possess. Anything goes, as long as it is positive and it reflects part of you. Now read that item aloud, and do so again before you go to bed tonight. Tomorrow morning, add another item to the list, and read the entire list aloud. Do it again before going to bed, then repeat the process every day for a total of twenty-one days.

At the end of this exercise, you will have a lengthy list of some of your positive aspects. Reading these items aloud helps your mind to more fully assimilate what is on your list, because you are using two senses: sight and hearing. Also, timing is important. By reading this list aloud just after waking in the morning and just before going to bed at night, you will conduct the exercise when your brain is producing the greatest amount of alpha waves. Psychologists indicate that a person's mind is most receptive when these waves are most abundant. So, completing this exercise is one way in which you can reinforce positive, strengthening messages and help build your self-esteem.

Techniques, Exercises, and Esteem Enhancers

Ten Steps to High Self-Esteem

Improving your self-esteem is a slow process, but it is composed of small steps, just like any other process. What follows is a list of simple changes people can make that will help in improving self-esteem (Burns, 1990):

1. *Accept who you are.* Develop an appreciation of yourself as a person, including both your physical attributes and your emotional and mental characteristics. For instance, if you want to lose weight, you must learn to accept yourself at a higher weight first, so that you can like yourself enough to want to change because it will benefit you. Accepting yourself allows you to develop intrinsic motivation for change.

2. *Give yourself credit.* As in the self-assessment activity, you should gain an understanding of the positive things that you do. Make lists of accomplishments; if necessary, make a shift in perspective—parent, student, teacher, worker, and so on. These are all worthy things that take a level of skill and should give you a sense of accomplishment.

3. *Develop your own values.* Do not let other people's expectations or beliefs control your priorities. Allow yourself to make decisions based on your own beliefs and values, and have the courage to stand behind those convictions.

4. *Accept your strengths and weaknesses.* Weaknesses are part of the human condition, and, although you should consider constructive ways to improve, you definitely should not allow yourself to concentrate on all the things that you feel you "cannot" do. It is counterproductive and harmful.

5. *Do not be afraid to take risks.* Like weaknesses, failures are a mark of being human. If you never fail, you have never done anything. Whatever you want to do, go for it. You will spend your entire life wondering what could have happened if you do not sometimes risk things.

6. *Turn failures into successes.* A situation or circumstance that does not turn out the way you expect often leads to a dead end. However, all failures are opportunities to learn, to change perspective, to gain something that was not available before the endeavor began. The old adage, "that which does not kill us makes us stronger," is true. If you always succeed, you are not moving forward in life.

7. *Join groups that will promote your self-esteem.* If you enjoy music, join a club that focuses on jazz. If tennis is your strength, go out and play. If you do not practice those things you enjoy, you cannot experience the good feelings that come along with them.

8. *Demand respect by respecting yourself.* If you feel that someone is treating you unfairly, let them know. People who value themselves treat themselves and others with kindness. Anyone who consistently treats you with disrespect does not deserve to be in your life.

9. *Seek fulfilling relationships.* Do not allow yourself to be abused or taken for granted. Too often people settle in relationships, whether friendships or romantic relationships, out of habit or fear. Relationships are work, but they can be improved. The best relationships help to teach people that they are worthy of all the positive things love can offer.

10. *Avoid being judgmental.* If you make negative criticisms, you are likely to be criticized. Remember the Golden Rule, and realize that if you are constantly feeling negative about those around you, it will not seem odd to constantly feel negative about yourself. Everyone deserves a chance!

Seven Steps to Building Self-Esteem

According to the National Council of Self-Esteem, seven steps to building self-esteem are:

1. *Love yourself properly.* Then and only then will you be able to love others.

2. *Guide people away from believing they must compare themselves to others.* Everyone is the very best "them."

3. *Recognize that you are not actions or decisions.* Self-worth is innate. Because a person fails in a relationship does not make that person a failure. Sometimes things simply do not work. Events are outside of yourself and sometimes outside of your control.

4. *Help people to become more responsible by encouraging them in their own growth.* Individuals become more responsible by accepting choices and consequences and by making decisions and accepting accountability.

5. *Help people to understand that mistakes are only stepping stones for growth and opportunity.*

6. *Help people to recognize that life is a journey to be embraced and enjoyed one day at a time.*

7. *Help people to recognize that praise pays.*

Summary

This chapter explores self-esteem as the foundation of who you are, how you behave, and most importantly, how you feel about yourself. There are countless characteristics that make up who you are, which is what contributes to the beautiful uniqueness of individuals. However, you all possess characteristics that are perceived as positive and others that are perceived as less favorable, and these contribute to your self-esteem.

Although there are those who doubt whether it is possible to alter self-esteem, this chapter takes the opposite stance. This philosophy can be exemplified within one statement: Who controls your thoughts? Most would agree that you control your own thoughts. Then, quite obviously, you have the opportunity to build up or break down your sense of self. As Ralph Waldo Emerson once said, "The ancestor of every action is a thought." In other words, your behaviors are a mere extension of your thoughts.

There are several exercises within this chapter designed to help the reader become more aware of existing levels of self-esteem and to demonstrate how to modify existing behaviors and thoughts through esteem-building exercises. Through positive thoughts and enhanced self-esteem, individuals can feel better about themselves and extinguish undesirable behaviors. This process is not simple, but, like love, it is an essential element of life.

DISCUSSION QUESTIONS

1. Self-esteem has been coined the buzz word of the 1990s. How has this heightened awareness of self-esteem created a negative image surrounding self-esteem?

2. Define and describe three actions you can personally take within the next twenty-four hours to enhance your self-esteem and that of someone you know.

3. Some people contend that happiness revolves around them and has nothing to do with how they feel about themselves. Defend the notion that happiness and self-esteem

come from within. Then, discuss how perceptions of situations far outweigh situations themselves.

4. Imagine that a close friend of yours tells you he has a very low opinion of himself and he does not know what to do about it. According to him, his self-esteem has "spun out of control."
   a. How would you respond to this friend?
   b. How can you help him to begin feeling better about himself without simply placating him with false assurances that "things will get better"?

5. Some people have contended that public schools should strive to foster self-esteem in students and that currently many schools encourage competition and unhealthy behaviors because of the evaluation process that is inherent to assigning grades. Discuss how schools could work to improve student self-esteem without sacrificing honest indicators of achievement and progress.

6. Self-esteem is a personal quality, and factors that are important to one person's self-esteem, such as academic achievement, might be unimportant to another person's self-esteem. With this in mind, can an accurate measure of self-esteem ever be created for standardized testing? If so, how?

7. How does perception of "normalcy" affect self-esteem throughout life? Are there any points during a person's life when feeling "different" from others is more or less likely to affect self-esteem? When, and why?

8. What special self-esteem issues confront minorities of all types? Consider individuals who are gay and lesbian; racial and ethnic minorities; people with physical and mental disabilities; and persons performing jobs unusual for their gender, such as a female truck driver or a male kindergarten teacher.

9. What factors are most important to *your* self-esteem (job, school, relationships)? Why? Are these factors within or outside of your control? How has this changed over your lifetime?

10. See the movie *The Breakfast Club*. In what ways do the students in this movie relate to each other differently at the end of the day as compared to the beginning? What caused these changes? Do you label yourself or feel labeled by others? How could changing your own perception of yourself raise your self-esteem?

RELATED WEBSITES

http://www.bsos.umd.edu/socy/rosenberg.html   The University of Maryland's site discussing and including the Rosenberg Self-Esteem Scale

http://www.geocities.com/CollegePark/Union/4617/67.html   Minnesota Education Association self-esteem enhancement suggestions for students

http://barksdale.org/   The Barkdale Self-Esteem Organization's page, including various assessment scales and suggestions for self-esteem enhancement:

http://www.coachbarnett.com/articles.html   Articles about self-esteem chosen by Dr. Cynthia Barnett

http://www.utexas.edu/student/lsc/handouts/1914.html   A list of strategies for improving self-esteem from the University of Texas

http://www.ksu.edu/wwparent/courses/ip/esteem.html   I'm Positive—a course on self-esteem from Kansas State University

http://www.kidstrek.com/star.html   Designed for young children, this website focuses on familiarizing them with the concept of self-esteem and includes some books and articles

http://www.geocities.com/Athens/6042/selest.html   A very thorough self-esteem bibliography for those interested in doing some research

http://www.ptc.tec.mn.us/programs/osp/iosp1228/ slideshow/selfest/sld001.htm   Slide show about self-esteem and its importance, including some interesting discussions about self-image and self-concept

http://barksdale.org/Evaluation/eval69.html   Another self-esteem evaluation, with on-line forms to fill out

http://self-esteem-NASE.org   This website provides a thorough bibliography for research, as well as articles and books focusing on self-esteem

REFERENCES

Adler, S., & Weiss, H. M. (1988). Criterion Aggregation in Personality Research: A Demonstration Looking at Self-Esteem and Goal Setting. *Human Performance, 1*(2), 99–109.

Appell, D., Hoffman, M., and Speller, N. (1999). Get Your Daily Dose of Self-Esteem. *Exceptional Parent, 29*(9), 55.

Brage, D., & Meredith, W. (1994). A Causal Model of Adolescent Depression. *The Journal of Psychology, 128*(4), 455–468.

Burns, M. (1990, August). Steps to Self-Esteem. *Essence;* 37–38.

Carlson, G., & Cantwell, D. (1982). Suicidal Behavior and Depression in Children and Adolescents. *American Academy of Child Psychology, 21,* 361–368.

Chandler, T. A., Lee, M. S., & Pengilly, J. W. (1997). Self-Esteem and Causal Attributions. *Genetic, Social, and General Psychology Monographs, 123*(4), 479–491.

Coopersmith, S. (1981). *Self-Esteem Inventories.* Palo Alto: Consulting Psychological Press.

Crandall, R. (1973). The Measurement of Self-Esteem and Related Constructs. In J. Robinson & P. Shaver (Eds.), *Measures of Social and Psychological Attitudes* (pp. 45–168). Ann Arbor: Institute for Social Research.

Daniels, D. H. (1998). Age Differences in Concepts of Self-Esteem. *Merrill-Palmer Quarterly, 44*(2), 234–258.

Daves, J. L. (1999). Improving Your Child's Self-Esteem. *Exceptional Parent, 29*(9), 52–54.

Donnelly, J. (1998). PEARLS of Self-Esteem: Five Stages to Self-Empowerment. *Self-Esteem Today 10*(1), 8–11.

Donnelly, J., & Procaccino, A. T. (1993). Effects of a One-Time Self-Esteem Enhancing Seminar on Students: Are We Wasting Our Time? *Health Educator, 24*(2), 17–20.

Falk, R. F., & Miller, N. B. (1997). The Reflexive Self: A Sociological Perspective. *Roeper Review, 20*(3), 150–153.

Felson, R., & Zielinski, M. (1989). Children's Self-Esteem and Parental Support. *Journal of Marriage and the Family, 51,* 727–735.

Greene, B., & Miller, R. (1996). Influences on Achievement: Goals, Perceived Ability, and Cognitive Engagement. *Contemporary Educational Psychology, 21,* 181–192.

Gurney, P. (1987). Self-Esteem Enhancement in Children: A Review of Research Findings. *Educational Research, 29* (2), 130–136.

Josephs, R., Markus, H., & Tafarodi, R. (1992). Gender and Self-Esteem. *Journal of Personality and Social Psychology, 63*(3), 391–402.

King, K. A. (1997). Self-Concept and Self-Esteem: A Clarification of Terms. *Journal of School Health, 67*(2), 68–70.

McKay, M., & Fanning, P. (1987). *Self-Esteem, the Ultimate Program for Self-Help,* New York: MJF Books.

Rosenberg, M. (1979). *Conceiving the Self.* New York: Basic Books.

Sapolski, R. (1997). A Gene For Nothing. *Discover, 18*(10), 40–46.

Schwalbe, M., & Staples, C. (1991). Gender Differences in Sources of Self-Esteem. *Social Psychology Quarterly, 54*(2), 158–168.

Sellers, M. I., & Waligroski, K. (1993). Factors Related to Depression and Eating Disorders: Self-Esteem, Body Image, and Attractiveness. *Psychological Reports,* 1003–1010.

Weisen, R. B., & Orley, J. (1996). Mental Health Promotion in Schools. *World Health, 49*(4), 29.

Witkowski, T., & Stiensmeier-Pelster, J. (1998). Performance Deficits Following Failure: Learned Helplessness or Self-Esteem Protection? *British Journal of Social Psychology, 37,* 59–71.

OTHER RESOURCES

Aron, E., & Aron, A. (1996). Love and Expansion of the Self: The State of the Model. *Personal Relationships, 3,* 45–58.

Aron, A., Paris, M., & Aron, E. (1995). Falling in Love: Prospective Studies of Self-Concept Change. *Journal of Personality and Social Psychology, 69(9),* 1102–1012.

Bandura, A. (1997). Self-Efficacy: Toward a Unifying Theory of Behavioral Change. *Psychological Review, 84*(2), 191–215.

I Hate Myself . . . I Love Myself. (1993, February). *Good Housekeeping,* 88–92.

Johnson, C. (1993, February/March). Self-Esteem: From the Inside Out. *Momentum,* 59–62.

King, K. (1997). Self-Concept and Self-Esteem: A Clarification of Terms. *Journal of School Health, 67*(2), 68–70.

McMillan, J., Singh, J., & Simonetta, L. (1995, March). Self-Oriented Self-Esteem Self-Destructs. *The Education Digest,* 9–11.

Mills, R. (1993). A New Understanding of the Self: The Role of Affect, State of Mind, Self-Understanding, and Intrinsic Motivation. *Journal of Experimental Education, 60*(1), 67–81.

6 Communication and Social Well-Being

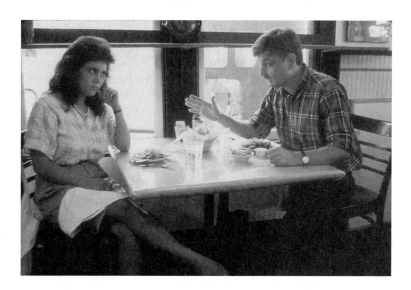

Importance of Communication

All species communicate; it is nature's way of identifying needs, desires, or interests to other species. Yet, among humans, communication is often viewed as the killer of relationships: too little communication, inappropriate communication, misinterpreted communication. The major focus of this chapter is on the latter of these—misinterpreted communication. There is a popular saying that "the road to hell is paved with good intentions." Perhaps it is more appropriate to say, "The road to hell is paved with communication misinterpretation."

It is clear that humans cannot function fully by themselves. Both Umberson (1987) and Verbrugge (1985) have shown that people who have multiple roles in life and who are involved with others tend to be healthiest. Men especially benefit from relationships, for married men have a substantially longer life span than single men. Chapter 7 highlights the importance of social support in dealing with stress. It is obvious that positive mental health requires strong ties with friends, family, and loved ones. Yet, for many, the inability to communicate effectively drains such relationships (Tannen, 1986). Individuals must be able to communicate effectively to maintain mental health. However, it is easier said than done.

According to Blonna (1996), communication takes place on two different levels—what is actually said (the content) and what is going on between the individuals. Both are very important issues in effective communication. The relationship between the people can either be referred to as *symmetrical* or *complementary* (Watlawick, Beavin, & Jackson, 1967). *Symmetrical relationships* are based on equality, whereas *complementary relationships* are unequal, possibly resulting from the perceived power of one of the parties. It is the latter type of relationship that tends to cause stress and problems in communication.

Effective communication involves both the sending and receiving of the messages. It is possible that an innocent message being sent to somebody could be greatly misinterpreted. For example, in a complementary relationship where one person has power over another, even the simplest comments can be taken out of context. Individuals often take great precautions in making sure what they say is exactly what is intended, yet these same individuals often fail to recognize that, if there is an unequal component in the relationship, misunderstanding may still take place.

Another major factor that allows miscommunication is the process that males and females use to interpret comments or actions. John Gray's book *Men Are from Mars, Women Are from Venus* (Gray, 1992) was one of the most popular books on the market during the late 1990s. The assertion from Gray is that men view things differently than women, and, to avoid problems, both sexes need to realize this distinction. For example, it has been understood by people for decades that men (generally) view sex differently than women do (generally). Sex is more of a physical outlet for men, whereas women view it as more of an emotional experience.

The movie *Grease* has a classic song where Danny (John Travolta) and Sandy (Olivia Newton-John) sing about their summer. In a nutshell, Danny and Sandy met during the summer in the late 1950s. At the end of the summer, Sandy was supposed to have gone back home to Australia. However, unbeknownst to both Sandy and Danny, she has mysteriously been able to stay in the states and go to the same school as Danny. On the first day of school, both Danny and Sandy are separately talking to their friends about how their summer went. The movie shows Danny and Sandy talking to their friends via a song. Danny had a slightly different version than Sandy. Now, part of that may have been to boost his image among his pals, but some of it was also how people interpret events. The point here is that a person's perceptions can influence communication. Many relationship problems stem from miscommunication. For relationships to flourish and continue to grow and for people to maintain mental health, the lines of communication must remain open. As Blonna (1996) stated, "Rarely do unresolved issues clear up without any attempts to clarify and fix them" (p. 251).

Keep in mind that the term *relationship* is not just referring to two people who are involved romantically and physically. It also refers to other intimate relationships, such as work-related relationships (employer-employee), relationships between parent and child, and relationships between friends.

Components of Effective Communication

There is more to effective communication than just merely giving a statement. Truly effective communication must deal with a number of related issues. Two of the most important include nonverbal communication and listening (Egan, 1988; McKay, Davis, & Fanning, 1983).

Nonverbal Communications

In addition to the verbal aspect of communication, there are also nonverbal aspects of communicating needs, desires, and wants. These could be through facial expressions or body position. Some people wear their emotions outwardly, that is, it is obvious when something has happened even though they have said nothing. For instance, reading excitement, joy, sadness, or anger on a person's face is not uncommon. Sometimes people are not even aware that they are sending such clear messages. For example, rolling of the eyes is one way to indicate one's displeasure. A furrowed forehead is a good indicator of confusion.

Body language can be another barrier to effective communication. As with most aspects of communication, body language is interpretative, but it can still have an impact on a person's ability to communicate. It is up to a person to ask for clarification. For example, when somebody does not make eye contact during a serious conversation, it is easy to feel that the person is not listening. In this case, it is easy to clarify by asking whether the person is listening or just diverting his or her eyes for some other reason.

Finally, the space between individuals can have an impact on communication. Hall (1973) has demonstrated that four space zones exist. (a) *Intimate space* allows close proximity and is limited to those who are intimate partners. (b) *Personal space* is primarily reserved for close relationships in which touching may or may not take place. (c) *Social/constructive space* is for less intimate involvement. (d) *Public space* is for formal gatherings and involvement with large groups.

Listening

Seaward (1997) uses the analogy of communication being a two-sided coin. He states that listening is one of those sides. Three major issues are associated with listening: (a) not correctly hearing what the person is saying, (b) not paying attention, and (c) being interrupted. These latter two can be very frustrating for people.

Facial Expressions

As an activity, stand in front of a mirror and observe your face. First, smile and look at your appearance. Note the look of your mouth, eyes, and what wrinkles or creases are created. After smiling, act angry. Again, observe your facial expressions. One often can tell what one is feeling just by looking at their face. Now try the following: confused, ecstatic, exhausted, sad, confident, happy, depressed, bored, lonely, surprised, and anxious. Again, how do these appearances look on your face? Some of these feelings are very obvious, but let's try some that are often difficult to impersonate.

Try the following feelings in the mirror: hopeful, jealous, smug, frustrated, guilty, lovestruck, embarassed, ashamed, and shy. Note the slight differences in the way that the eyes appear. . . the use of the mouth. . . eyebrows, and even the way that the nose may be flared. These are often more difficult to demonstrate and often one cannot distinguish between them.

As obvious as it may seem regarding these facial expressions, sometimes it's not as easy as it may seem. How many times have you misinterpreted somebody's feelings by just looking at their face and how did that effect your ability to communicate with that person? Some facial expressions may mask the true feelings, or it may be misinterpreted as a different feeling. It is critical that one uses facial expresses as only a guide and not as a certainty on how one is feeling.

Reflect on what it is like to have a conversation with someone who constantly interrupts the conversation. Also reflect on what it is like to speak to somebody who does not listen. It does not allow for effective communication. In fact, for many, it may make them feel like "second class" citizens whose concerns are not viewed as important enough to warrant the attention of the other person. Many things in life are allowed to interrupt communications; television, phone calls, cell phones, beepers, E-mails, and call waiting are some of the more prevalent offenders. Most people can accept some level of interruptions, but if the topic is really important, such interruptions can cause a serious problem. At times people need to ensure that the conversation is not interrupted. Let the voice mail/answering machine pick up the message. The E-mail can wait. Turn off the cell phone and/or beeper. Do not answer the call waiting.

In addition, it is important for the listener to provide some indication that, indeed, he or she is listening. Essential behaviors such as eye contact help ensure the talker that the listener is listening. Periodic nods or comments ("aha, I see") also let a person know that the other person is listening. Even occasional completing of sentences can tell a person that someone is listening—although too much of it can be even more irritating than not listening at all.

The first issue, not correctly hearing what the person is saying, takes a little more work. Think back to the childhood game called *telephone,* in which one person whispers a statement into another person's ear, that person passes the comment to the next person, and it continues until all people have received the comment. Typically, when the last person repeats the message to the entire group, the story is very different than the original statement. It illustrates that communication is more than just talking and/or listening; it is a blend of both. It is easy to misinterpret what somebody says. To avoid that, experts in communication encourage people to use what is referred to as *active* or *reflective listening* (Greenberg, 1999). This means that the *listener* periodically *restates* what he or she has just heard. It is hoped that if there is any confusion or misunderstanding then it can be addressed at that time.

Imagine that Joan is talking to Beth about the problems she is having at work. Throughout the conversation, Joan is explaining how her boss does not appreciate her work. Periodically, Beth needs to restate for clarification purposes what Joan has said. For example, Beth could restate, "So, you think the boss doesn't like you?" If this is true, Joan could reinforce it. However, if it is not true, Joan could then correct it. If it is not true, Joan can say, "No, it's not that he doesn't like me, it's just that he wants too much from me."

The importance of active listening is two-fold. First, it lets people know they are being heard. Second, it allows both people to clarify what is being said. The importance of this can not be stressed enough. Too many interpersonal relationship problems take place because of misinterpreted statements. Oftentimes, even the phrase used may be affected greatly by the tone or inflection of the voice. Depending upon which word is emphasized, the meaning can be completely different. Active listening can assist in clarification.

The Risk-Taking Aspect of Effective Communication

Whereas many of the ideas stated elsewhere in this chapter are common in various stress management and/or communications books, this section presents a rather unique and different approach, which is basic to the function of communication. For effective communication to take place, a person needs to take a risk.

First, what is a risk? A *risk,* according to *Merriam-Webster's Collegiate Dictionary* (1993), is the "possibility of loss or injury." Thus, if people take risks in relationships, they are possibly exposing themselves to some problems (i.e., arguments, breakups, or even the truth). Before looking at risk taking in the area of effective communication, consider risk taking in general.

The word *risk* can bring a number of ideas to mind. Insurance companies ascertain the risks they are willing to take to insure a person. Risk can also be viewed in the business sense; starting a new business can be a risk. However, insurance companies, businesses, and banks take risks all the time. In these examples, risk taking is a *calculated*—rather than a *blind*—*approach* to doing something.

Risk Taking in Mental Health

Risk taking has certain characteristics that are applicable to mental health. First, risk takers hardly become bored. Risk taking prevents stagnation. Second, risk takers have the attitude, "Let's see what happens." They realize that they may fail, but they are willing to try. This "not-afraid-to-fail" strategy is an important element to remember. Finally, after a decision has been made, a risk taker often exhibits confidence—(albeit a conservative confidence)—in participating in the event that may be risky.

A person who is mentally healthy is able to understand the risks, the advantages and disadvantages of the risks, and some safeguards to prevent these risks from turning into daredevil or suicidal activities. Risk taking is not often discussed in the context of mental health. Yet, certain elements of excitement and enthusiasm exist in risk takers, which can be positive attributes for mental health.

For some reason, risk taking is becoming somewhat of a lost art in our society. It is relegated to only a few people, and the mainstream society looks upon these people with perhaps some admiration but usually with trepidation. When people think about risk takers, they are usually thinking of those individuals who participate in certain sports, such as rock climbing. Though it is true that these physical risks can be an important element of mental health, risk taking is not restricted to just physical activities. People can also take risks intellectually and emotionally.

Physical Risks.   Physical risks are probably the best known of all risks. There is something unique about those individuals who participate in such risks. Have you ever talked to somebody who has parachuted? Have you ever talked to somebody who has climbed a mountain? Have you ever witnessed individuals who have completed a major event such as a marathon or a "century" (100-mile) bicycling event? If you have not, try it sometime. Ask why they did it.

Answers such as "Well, it was there," or "I just had to do it," or "I had to prove to myself that I could do it" are just some of the answers that may be received. But try to look beyond such answers to see what truly lies beneath that person's response. It is very difficult to describe, which is why many individuals respond by saying, "I don't know."

Another approach might be to ask the risk taker how he or she felt during the event. A rock climber, when reaching the summit, has a tremendous feeling of exhilaration. Many feel that they have overcome certain obstacles to complete the task. Anytime a person completes a goal or task, a certain amount of pride and sense of accomplishment sets in—certainly something that improves self-esteem.

When pressed for more details, people often respond that during the risk-taking activity they use a tremendous amount of concentration effort. When Frank Shorter won the 1972 Gold Medal in the Olympic Marathon in Munich, Germany (which started the running fad in the United States), he was asked how he was able to stay focused for so long. He responded that the race only seemed about twenty minutes in length. His concentration was so intense that everything else passed by without notice.

When life seems to hang in the balance, other things seem trivial. In other words, it puts things in perspective for the risk taker. When a group of risk takers get together, they know what these experiences are—for they have all experienced them at some time. People who have never partipated in such activities have a very difficult time understanding what is so alluring about them.

Risk takers also have their own language. It is not unusual for them to say, "Let's get scared." What does this mean? It means that they want to challenge themselves to reach out to a new dimension that they have not yet experienced—for they believe that they cannot grow unless they are willing to move into that uncharted zone.

Note that physical risk taking is very subjective. Being in a canoe is not much of a risk for a person who has "shot the white-water rapids." However, for some, just getting near the water is a personal victory. Climbing a steep hill may be nothing to an accomplished rock climber, but, for the average person, it may be sufficiently risky. The point is that risk taking is measured not in what a person does but in the perception of the doer.

So, what should an individual know about physical risk taking and its role in his or her mental health? Several suggestions probably need to be heeded. The first is that physical activity should not be attempted unless the person is physically fit. This does not mean that it is necessary to be a world-class athlete, but beware of falling into the "couch-potato-who-suddenly-has-a-desire-to-be-ambitious" mode. Becoming minimally physically fit may be a risky adventure.

Second, whatever the risk, be sure of the safety aspects of the activity. Taking physical risks is not equivalent to taking suicidal risks. Jumping from an airplane at 10,000 feet with only a parachute on your back is risky enough. To not have been trained in the proper landing procedure, what to do in emergencies, or other precautions is just plain foolish.

White-water rafting appears to be one of the most popular risk-taking activities among "average" physically fit people. But, going white-water rafting without proper gear and training is going beyond risk taking—it probably involves an underlying death wish. Risk-taking activities are really calculated risk taking. Risk takers do everything in their power to protect themselves. Yet, no matter how well they prepare, they are still "on the edge." It is much the same with auto insurance companies. They take a calculated risk with people. They want people who are well prepared to drive. Yet, when they insure a person, they know that, no matter how well prepared that person is, there is always the chance of something happening.

Another factor to consider is the way the person actually participates in such activities. Most physical risk-taking activities occur in groups. Very few are single events, and those that are single events typically are for the advanced person. Participating in a risky activity with a group allows for a sharing of experiences. People who have participated in a group activity together can share similar thoughts and experiences. An equally important part of the risk-taking adventure goes beyond the actual activity to the group processing of feelings afterward. This sharing allows people to share their feelings with others in a sort of social support system that is so important to their lives.

Intellectual Risks.   Do all risks have to be physical? Of course not. There are some people who should not be involved with physical risks. That does not mean that risk taking cannot take place. Intellectual risks are a possibility.

An *intellectual risk* is a "thinking" risk. Perhaps it is something that challenges common beliefs; perhaps it exposes something that had not been considered previously; perhaps it attempts to stretch intellectual ability. These risks are similar to the physical risks that were already discussed. A certain sense of satisfaction can take place from such experiences.

What are some examples of intellectual risks? As with physical risks, some preparation for intellectual risks should be taken. It could be something as straightforward as enrolling in a course to ensure proper safety knowledge. It could be a willingness to listen to a speaker presenting a different point of view. It can be considered risk taking because this person *could* change an existing belief system. Keep in mind that one of the goals of risk taking is to keep the person from becoming "stagnant"; being exposed to a new idea could "shock" the system.

In the mid-1970s, the first miniseries appeared on television. *Roots* was a multiday series of movies depicting the life of a young African in the 1700s who was kidnapped and brought to the United States as a slave. The movie was graphic; it portrayed how slaves were *really* treated. It made people uncomfortable to watch—even more uncomfortable because they were from a nation that had tried to put that type of treatment of slaves behind them. It was a risk because it challenged people to rethink a certain belief.

A popular intellectual risk on college campuses is that of people coming back to college after having careers already established. Today *nontraditional students* are heard of frequently. The percentage of nontraditional students (for the sake of argument, those who are over twenty-five) has risen dramatically over the past twenty years. Think about the risk that these individuals are taking. Many are leaving a comfortable life (both intellectually and financially) to do something else. Starting college around age thirty is risky. Fortunately, most of these students are outstanding students, possibly because they feel that they have more to lose if they do not succeed.

Other intellectual risks may include reading books, viewing television shows, and participating in activities in which there are many differing views. Again, the idea is not "suicidal" risks but calculated risks. Quitting a job and starting college without assessing the financial picture is not necessarily risky but could, in fact, be foolhardy.

How does this tie into mental health? As with physical risks, the idea that intellectual risks promote positive mental health is paramount to this theory. Risk taking keeps people off guard. It prevents them from becoming stagnant. People who are mentally unhealthy are often boring (or bored), depressed, and not interested in a lot of things. One way to prevent that from happening is to occasionally take risks. An intellectual risk can keep a person mentally sharp.

Emotional Risks. So far, the risks that have been discussed have consisted of physical and intellectual dimensions. This chapter's topic is effective communication, so how does risk taking affect communications? It has a great deal of impact. Emotional risks are needed to maintain relationships with others and with self. Remember that most people's relationships with others are guided by two basic fears:

1. The fear of being hurt
2. The fear of hurting others

These two fears direct how people deal with each other. Everyone has experienced being hurt by someone else. In addition, everyone has hurt someone at some time, and it is not a good feeling. Once someone has been hurt or has hurt someone else, it may take years to trust or believe that person again.

Another factor that affects relationships is a person's practice of "pretending not to know what one really knows." What this means is that too often people know what is happening in a particular situation, yet, to avoid any pain, they pretend to not know it. For example, parents may know that their adolescent child is engaging in sex. They can confront the child to address their concerns, or they can ignore the fact and pretend that it does not exist. In many instances, it may be entirely appropriate to "pretend" that something is not really happening, but there are times when it is absolutely critical to address the issue. Again, people often hesitate because they allow the two fears to get in the way.

For a relationship to grow, these fears need to be overcome. These fears can actually prevent growth. Unless individuals are willing to risk overcoming these fears, growth will not take place. Reread this statement, for this is the foundation upon which the rest of this chapter lies.

Many people allow these two fears to obstruct their relationships with their spouses, children, loved ones, friends, and colleagues. The fears can become so much of an obstacle that a buildup of resentment or anger can take place. When that anger is finally released, it often appears irrational because the underlying cause is not identified. So, how do people overcome these fears? It is risky to say something to somebody that may hurt him or her, because knowledge of having hurt someone does not feel very good. It is also risky to say something because the other person may say something in return that hurts. That does not feel very good either. So what do people do? They tend to overlook things. They pretend to not know what is going on. Instead of getting to the root of the issue, they decide to just overlook it, thinking that eventually it will pass away. The particular event probably *will* pass away, yet the concern, anger, or fear that has occurred can be buried deep in the person's psyche and may not emerge for years to come.

So, how do people overcome these two fears? There are three basic approaches. The first is to *ask brave questions;* the second is to *give brave answers;* and the third is to *give brave statements.* Though these approaches seem easy enough, in reality they are risky because they may violate one of those two fears that control relationships.

Ask Brave Questions.   Select a person for whom you care a great deal. It can be a spouse, lover, close friend, parent, or child. Keep that person in mind as you read this section.

What could be the bravest (or riskiest) question that you could ask that particular person? Since you are not being asked to repeat this to anybody, think long and hard about this question. What *could* be the riskiest question that a person could ask somebody that *might* elicit one of the two basic fears? Here are some examples of such questions:

- Do you love me?
- What can I do to be a better husband (or spouse/lover/parent/child)?
- Where do you see this relationship going?
- Is there somebody else in your life?
- Will you marry me?
- Do you want a divorce?

These are brave questions.

Assuming you do get brave, be prepared for risky answers. The answers might, if honestly answered, hurt both people involved. Imagine two individuals, Chris and Pat, who are in a relationship. Chris says, "Pat, do you love me?" That could be a brave (and risky) question. What if Pat did not love Chris? Would Pat lie and say "yes" just to avoid hurting Chris's feelings (because Pat has hurt others before—and it does not feel good)? And if Pat does not love Chris and yet tells Chris, "Yes, I do love you," how is that going to affect their relationship?

This is not to say that hurting somebody is good, but people cannot be so obsessed with fear that they will not allow relationships to move forward. Relationships must be continuously worked on to improve. Once they become stagnant, they tend to slip backward. People often talk about the lack of any personal involvement in a relationship. The reason is, partially, that they are afraid to ask brave questions.

Give Brave Answers.   Giving brave answers is easier said than done. Bear in mind that all relationships are limited by two fears and that someone's brave answer may hurt someone else. But, as indicated earlier, sometimes the risk is necessary for that relationship to flourish and grow. Using Chris and Pat as an example, if

Pat says, "No, I don't love you, Chris," it is definitely going to impact the relationship. On the other hand, perhaps it will help clarify in both of their minds where each person is coming from. In turn, the relationship may grow stronger.

Obviously, asking brave questions is not of any value if the question does not receive brave answers. Look at this from two aspects: What if a brave answer is not given in response to a brave question? What if the question is ignored or ridiculed or causes outrage? Then, one of the first reactions should be reconsideration of the relationship. Perhaps this individual is not serious about the relationship. A brave question deserves a brave answer. After all, a brave answer may serve as an example for the other person.

Give Brave Statements.   On the other hand, what if people do not give others the chance to give brave answers because they fail to ask brave questions? It should be obvious that brave questions and brave answers go hand in hand. However, a related approach, yet very much independent of the other two, is giving brave statements. Brave statements are specific and clear descriptions that another person can understand. Again, think back to the two fears—a person who allows those fears to exist may be too afraid to give brave statements.

One of the greatest barriers to communication occurs when people feel that they are being *blamed* for something. It is only natural for a person's defenses to step in to try to dispel such blaming. Thus, when giving a brave statement, and to prevent the person who is receiving the message from feeling blamed, the use of *I statements* is recommended by most communications experts. I statements take the blame out of statements and focus on the *feelings* of the person giving the message. Feelings are often perceived thoughts, and people are more tolerant of discussing their perceptions and less likely to have a major argument (Schafer, 1999).

For example, Joe and Kate have been seeing each other for nearly a year. They are living together, and everybody thinks it is just a matter of time before they get married. When Joe has his buddies over, Kate feels ignored. Whether or not she *is* being ignored is not the issue. What is the issue is that Kate *feels* she is being ignored, does not like it, and wants to express her dissatisfaction to her partner. If she said something like "You ignore me when your friends are over," that would be an accusation that Joe would need to address. When a person is accused of something (especially if that person thinks he or she is wrongly accused), statements fly without much thought.

On the other hand, if Kate uses an *I statement*, she gives Joe a statement that is less threatening to him. For example, consider the phrase, "I feel ignored when you are around your buddies, and I do not like that feeling." The statement does not *blame* anybody, but it tells him what she feels. She also indicates when this feeling takes place (". . . around your buddies . . ."). The second phrase ". . . and I do not like that feeling" is hard to argue about. What is open for dialogue is the first phrase: "I feel ignored when you are around your buddies." By stating it as an *I statement*, Kate is telling Joe how she is feeling about a certain action (". . . being around your buddies . . ."). The discussion can now focus on her interpretation of that event.

Perhaps Joe just thought that Kate would not be interested in the guys' conversations. Perhaps Joe thought he was doing her a favor by not including her in the conversation. Because the *I* statement is less threatening, it is hoped that the couple can discuss their feelings about this issue. If Joe comes back with a statement such as "I do not ignore you . . . ," he can indicate that he is giving his interpretations and/or perceptions. It may not be true but it is how he felt.

Other issues with brave statements include making sure that the word *but* is minimized. Greenberg (1999) indicates in his book that when the person uses the word *but* it negates all the words prior to it. He uses the example, "Yes, your needs are important, but . . ."; What the person is actually saying is "Although your needs are important, something else [apparently] is more important." Greenberg encourages people to use the word *and* instead of *but*. The statement would now read, "Yes, your needs are important, and . . . ," allowing the person to confirm the importance of the first aspect but also recognizing the importance of another issue.

Assertiveness

Greenberg (1999) uses the terms *passive, assertive,* and *aggressive* to categorize people's actions. Keep in mind that rarely does a person consistently represent only one type. The other person in the interaction, the task that is being discussed, or the mood of either person can all play important roles. Greenberg encourages people to try to remain *assertive,* because assertiveness allows people to express themselves and get what they want but not at the expense of others. Being *passive* allows people to feel like they are being "used," whereas being *aggressive* results in people tending to "use" others. People sometimes become aggressive if being assertive is not effective, but, generally speaking, being assertive prevents people from moving to the aggressive stage. *Assertiveness training* teaches people how to become assertive.

So how can you express yourself, satisfy your own needs, and not hurt others in the process? It is tough, but there are some basic policies to follow. First, you can complete various assessments to determine your type of approach.

How do you become more assertive? It takes a great deal of practice, but there are some general tips that can be of value. Blonna (1996) identifies several ways to be assertive when refusing an offer:

1. Face the other person from a normal distance. Being too close can be misinterpreted as being aggressive; being too far away may be viewed as timidity.
2. Look the person directly in the eyes.
3. Keep your head up.
4. Speak clearly, firmly, and at a volume that can be heard.
5. Just say no.
6. Be prepared to repeat the no—some people are persistent.
7. Stick to your guns. If this is something that you do not want to do, maintain your decision.

Finally, Bonna (1996) offers the following suggestions for when you feel compelled to explain the decision:

1. Thank the person for the offer.
2. Express appreciation for their confidence in you.
3. Affirm your friendship with the person.
4. Reject the offer, not the person.

When dealing with an employer request, a person may feel even more awkward. The old adage is, "To truly get something done, give it to a person who is busy." Typically, the boss will give important items to those people who they know will get it done. It is frustrating to know that if you are good at your job, you will be *rewarded* by being given more work. One suggestion is to prioritize the important items that you are working on.

Suppose that you have five major projects/responsibilities that you are working on. If the boss approaches you for additional work, it is time to sit down with the boss, indicate appreciation of the trust he or she has in you, and ask the boss specifically which of the other projects you need to de-emphasize. It not only provides the boss with an idea of how busy you are, but it also allows the boss to reassess the many different projects that are of value to the workplace. This approach lets your boss know that you want to be a team player but have limited resources, time, and energy. The boss can then offer you suggestions for handling this new responsibility. This helps by not making you feel that you are being taken advantage of, allowing the boss to know what you are doing, and providing new ways to illustrate to your boss that you may need assistance.

Conflict Resolution

Related to both assertiveness and the issues of stress is being able to resolve problems in a relatively peaceful matter without loss of dignity for either party. Seaward (1997) notes that conflicts tend to focus on content, values, or ego. *Content conflicts* result from misinterpretation of information. *Value conflicts* tend to result from differing values or beliefs that people may possess. Finally, *ego conflicts* (often the hardest to deal with) result in a win-lose approach in which each tries to prove that he or she is correct and the other is wrong. This can get very personal.

How do people resolve conflict? Basically, people want what is fair (in their minds). Thus, it is important to clearly describe what it is you want and why you feel you deserve it. Remember, there are two sides to all stories. You need to allow the other side to give his or her viewpoint as well. Refusing to listen to both sides of the story discourages people from being interested in your perspective.

Some tips for conflict resolution follow:

1. Make sure that you get the name of the person to whom you are talking. People like to be called by their names. In addition, in the event that you call back, you can indicate that you spoke to Mrs. Smith about this issue.
2. Make sure that you speak to somebody who has the authority to address your needs. If you call a number, immediately ask for the person in charge.

Typically, the first person you talk to does not have the authority to make any major decisions. Nothing is more frustrating than to speak at length about an issue only to be passed on to repeat the story. For example, if you have some problems with financial aid at your university, chances are that you will initially speak to a student worker when you call. Instead of wasting your time (and theirs), ask to speak to the office manager or director of financial aid about a problem that you have.

3. Beforehand, make a written list of your concerns and what you feel should be done to resolve the issue. Think of all the possible reasons why the other side will not give in, and then think of your comeback so that you are not at a loss for words when the other person comes up with an item that you are not prepared to deal with.

4. Understand that there are two sides to the story, and let the other side know that you want a peaceful resolution to the problem. Ask what that person would do in your position.

5. If you are still not satisfied, ask the person who his or her supervisor is. This should not be used as a threat but rather to let the person know that you are not satisfied with the resolution and that you intend to pursue this until an acceptable resolution takes place. Do not threaten to call an attorney or boycott the store, and do not call anyone names. People are more likely to deal with people who are keeping their temper and are willing to negotiate.

6. Keep a notepad nearby to keep track of important names, ideas, phone numbers, and so on.

7. Remember that most companies want to maintain their good reputation and want their customers satisfied. Thus, beforehand make a list of what you would settle for. For example, imagine that you have purchased a television that has a warranty of one year for parts and labor. At 370 days, the television's picture tube burns out. Obviously, you would like a new television, but, technically, this one is out of warranty. If you cannot obtain a brand new television, what would be an acceptable settlement? Perhaps the company will pay for a new tube, and you will be responsible for the labor. You would probably be wise to "shoot for the moon" first and then, when you are left with the impression that nothing is going to be done, resort to your alternatives.

Many of these same principles apply not only to business problems but also to interpersonal problems (i.e., the financial aid situation). Most universities are under increasing pressure to retain students at their college. Most administrators also are aware that if students feel they are getting the runaround they are likely to drop out. Thus, such administrators have let it be known to directors of various departments (i.e., financial aid, registration, records) that it is important to resolve problems as quickly as possible.

Self-Assessments

To determine your general pattern of behavior, indicate how characteristic or descriptive each of the following statements is of you by using the codes that follow. Rathus (1973) developed this scale.

+3 = very characteristic of me, extremely descriptive
+2 = rather characteristic of me, quite descriptive
+1 = somewhat characteristic of me, slightly descriptive
−1 = somewhat uncharacteristic of me, slightly nondescriptive
−2 = rather uncharacteristic of me, quite nondescriptive
−3 = very uncharacteristic of me, extremely nondescriptive

_____ 1. Most people seem to be more aggressive and assertive than I am.

_____ 2. I have hesitated to make or accept dates because of shyness.

_____ 3. When the food served at a restaurant is not done to my satisfaction, I complain about it to the waiter or waitress.

_____ 4. I am careful to avoid hurting other people's feelings, even when I feel that I have been injured.

_____ 5. If a salesperson has gone to considerable trouble to show me merchandise that is not quite suitable, I have a difficult time saying no.

_____ 6. When I am asked to do something, I insist upon knowing why.

_____ 7. There are times when I look for a good, vigorous argument.

_____ 8. I strive to get ahead as well as most people in my position.

_____ 9. To be honest, people often take advantage of me.

_____10. I enjoy starting conversations with new acquaintances and strangers.

_____11. I often do not know what to say to attractive persons of the opposite sex.

_____12. I hesitate to make phone calls to business establishments and institutions.

_____13. I would rather apply for a job or for admission to a college by writing letters than by going through with personal interviews.

_____14. I find it embarrassing to return merchandise.

_____15. If a close and respected relative were annoying me, I would smother my feelings rather than express my annoyance.

_____16. I have avoided asking questions for fear of sounding stupid.

_____17. During an argument, I am sometimes afraid that I will get so upset that I will shake all over.

_____18. If a famed and respected lecturer makes a statement that I think is incorrect, I will have the audience hear my point of view as well.

_____19. I avoid arguing over prices with clerks and salespeople.

_____20. When I have done something important or worthwhile, I manage to let others know about it.

_____21. I am open and frank about my feelings.

_____22. If someone has been spreading false and bad stories about me, I see him (her) as soon as possible to have a talk about it.

_____23. I often have a hard time saying no.

_____24. I tend to bottle up my emotions rather than make a scene.

_____25. I complain about poor service in a restaurant and elsewhere.

_____26. When I am given a compliment, I sometimes just do not know what to say.

_____27. If a couple near me in a theater or at a lecture were conversing rather loudly, I would ask them to be quiet or to take their conversation elsewhere.

_____28. Anyone attempting to push ahead of me in a line is in for a good battle.

_____29. I am quick to express an opinion.

_____30. There are times when I just cannot say anything.

For items 1, 2, 4, 5, 9, 11, 12, 13, 14, 15, 16, 17, 19, 23, 24, 26, and 30, reverse the score (thus, –3 is actually +3). Final score can range from –90 to +90. The higher the score to +90, the more assertive you usually act. The lower the score to –90, the more passive you are.

Source: "A 30-Item Schedule for Assessing Assertive Behavior," by S. A. Rathus, 1973, _Behavior Therapy, 4,_ pp. 398–406. As found in _Comprehensive Stress Management,_ by J. S. Greenberg, 1993. Madison, WI: W. C. Brown Publishers.

If you are effective in resolving conflict, your interpersonal relationships will be improved. The result of this improvement will be a decrease in the number of stressors you experience. Less conflict of shorter duration resolved to your satisfaction will mean a less stressed and healthier you.

You might be interested in an identification of your typical modus operandi, that is, how you usually deal with conflict situations. To make this determination, circle the answer that best describes how you would react to each of the following situations:

1. If a salesgirl refused to give me a refund on a purchase because I had lost the sales slip, I would tell her,
    a. "I'm sorry—I should have been more careful," and I would leave without the refund.
    b. "You're the only store in town that handles this brand of merchandise. I demand a refund, or I'll never shop here again."
    c. "Look, if I can't have a refund, can I exchange it for something else?"

2. If I had irritated a teacher by questioning his/her theoretical position, and he/she retaliated by giving me a D on an excellent paper, I would
   a. Not say anything; I would realize why it happened and be quieter in my next class.
   b. Tell him he was dead wrong and that he could not get away with being so unfair.
   c. Try to talk to him to see what could be done about it.
3. If I worked as a television repairman and my boss ordered me to double-charge customers, I would
   a. Go along with him; it is his business.
   b. Tell him he is a crook and that I would not go along with his dishonesty.
   c. Tell him he can overcharge on his calls, but I am charging honestly on mine.
4. If I gave up my seat on the bus to an older woman with packages, but some teenager beat her to it, I would
   a. Try to find the woman another seat.
   b. Argue with the teenager until he moved.
   c. Ignore it.
5. If I had been waiting in line at the supermarket for twenty minutes and then some woman rushed in front of me saying, "Thank-you—I'm in such a hurry!" I would
   a. Smile and let her in.
   b. Say, "Look, what do you think you're doing? Wait your turn!"
   c. Let her in if she had a good reason for being in such a hurry.
6. If a friend was to meet me on a street corner at 7:00 P.M. and at 8:00 P.M. he still was not there, I would
   a. Wait another thirty minutes.
   b. Be furious at his thoughtlessness and leave.
   c. Try to telephone him, thinking, "Boy, he'd better have a good excuse!"
7. If my wife (or husband) volunteered me for committee work with someone she (or he) knew I disliked, I would
   a. Work on the committee.
   b. Tell her (or him) she (or he) had no business volunteering my time, and I would call and tell the committee chairperson the same.
   c. Tell her (or him) I want her (or him) to be more thoughtful in the future and then make a plausible excuse she (or he) can give the committee chairperson.
8. If my four-year-old son refused to obey an order I gave him, I would
   a. Let him do what he wanted.
   b. Say, "You do it—and you do it now!"
   c. Say, "Maybe you'll want to do it later on."

To score your responses for each item except Number 4, give yourself 1 point for an *a* answer, 5 points for a *b* answer, and 3 points for a *c* answer. For Number 4, give yourself 3 points for an *a*, 5 points for a *b*, and 1 point for a *c*. Add up your points. The total should fall between 8 and 40.

Your score should give you a hint regarding your usual manner of dealing with conflict. The closer you are to a score of 8, the more submissive (nonassertive) you are when involved in a conflict; the closer you are to a score of 40, the more aggressively you respond. A score near the midpoint (24) indicates you generally compromise as a means of dealing with conflict.

Techniques/Exercises

1. Have the class break into groups of three. Have one person be the *listener*. Have the second person *take notes and observe*. The third person is to *describe* how to get from his or her home to a hospital (or any other type of location). At the conclusion, have the listener tell these same directions. This is to practice active listening.

2. Practice asking brave questions and giving brave answers/statements to the following scenarios:
   a. Person asking somebody he or she loves to assess their relationship
   b. Person seeking his or her value as an employee
   c. Child seeking opinion of parent on his or her homework

3. In gender-specific groups, ask a series of questions and have the groups answer them independently. Then ask the groups to share their answers. See if there are any patterns of differences in the answers between males and females. Such questions could include:
   a. What is the role of sex in a relationship?
   b. What is the role of money in a relationship?
   c. What is the one thing that bothers males/females about the opposite sex?
   d. What are the advantages of being the opposite sex?
   e. What are the advantages of being the sex you are?

4. Using the theory of the two fears in all relationships (the fear of being hurt and the fear of hurting others) in small groups, have each person identify times when he or she has hurt someone and has been hurt by someone and identify the thoughts and feelings that each had surrounding those events.

5. In small groups, have each person identify a problem that he or she has encountered with a product he or she has purchased. Without indicating how they attempted to resolve the issues, have the groups role-play or brainstorm their strategies.

Summary

Effective communication is paramount to maintaining mental health. The entire gamut of a person's life is focused around dealing with others (home life, work life, friendships), and, if communication is not maintained, problems can exist. Such problems can result in unhappiness, depression, lowered self-image, and a loss of control.

For communication to be effective, the dynamics of effective communication must be understood. Active listening is critical, along with the willingness of individuals to not allow interruptions to interfere with efforts. This chapter discusses the role of risk taking in relationships. Since all relationships are based on two fears (the fear of being hurt and the fear of hurting others), it is imperative that individuals attempt to overcome such fears by asking brave questions and giving brave answers and statements.

Finally, the chapter discusses the importance of dealing with conflicts and offers suggestions for resolving problems with people in personal conflicts, professional conflicts, or consumer conflicts.

DISCUSSION QUESTIONS

1. Describe the role that risk taking plays in effective communication.

2. List five strategies for attempting to deal with conflict.

3. For active listening to be effective, what specific strategies should be incorporated?

4. Discuss the various types of communication, the importance of each, and how to ensure that the true message is being delivered.

5. What risk-taking strategies can be incorporated to ensure that relationships will continue to grow and flourish?

RELATED WEBSITES

http://www.phy.mtu.edu/apod/mind   Dialectical Behavior Therapy: includes mindfulness, interpersonal effectiveness, emotion regulation, and distress tolerance. A great focus of this site is borderline personality disorder.

http://www.counseling.com/Ccom/reference.html   This site addresses reference and resource information regarding alcohol problems, chemical dependency, emotional/mental health, and family problems and provides crisis hotlines from the American Counseling Association.

http://www.hcn.net.aul—Health communication network- offers media releases, sources, career opportunities, and knowledge resources.

http://www.region.peel.on.ca/health/commun/cmintro.htm   This site emphasizes building communication skills for healthy relationships, and discusses how to communicate effectively.

http://www.integrocanada.com/index.html   This site is dedicated to development and improvement of interpersonal skills, communication skills, and leadership skills.

http://www.interpersonalo-skills.com/briefings/fiftyreasons.html   Offers the latest briefings, programs and services, and professional staff to help improve interpersonal communication skills.

REFERENCES

Blonna, R. (1996). *Coping with Stress in a Changing World*. St. Louis: Mosby.

Egan, G. (1988). *You and Me: The Skills of Communicating and Relating to Others*. Monterey, CA: Brooks/Cole.

Gray, J. (1992). *Men Are from Mars, Women Are from Venus: A Practical Guide for Improving Communication and Getting What You Want in Your Relationships*. New York: Harper Collins.

Greenberg, J.S. (1993). *Comprehensive Stress Management*. Madison, WI: Wm. C. Brown.

Greenberg, J. S. (1999). *Comprehensive Stress Management (6th Ed.)*. Columbus, OH: McGraw-Hill.

Hall, D. (1973). *The Silent Language*. Garden City, NY: Doubleday/Anchor Press.

McKay, M., Davis, M., & Fanning, P. (1983). *Messages: The Communication Skills Book*. Oakland, CA: New Harbinger Press.

Merriam-Webster's Collegiate Dictionary (10th Ed.). (1993). Springfield, MA: Merriam-Webster.

Rathus, S. A. (1973). A 30-Item Schedule for Assessing Assertive Behavior. *Behavior Therapy, 4,* 398–406. In J. S. Greenberg (1993), *Comprehensive Stress Management*, Madison, WI: Wm. C. Brown Publishers.

Schafer, W. (1999). *Stress management for wellness*, (4th Ed.). Orlando: Harcourt Brace College.

Seaward, B. L. (1997). *Managing Stress: Principles and Strategies for Health and Well-Being*. Boston: Jones and Bartlett.

Tannen, D. (1986). *That's Not What I Meant: How Conversational Style Makes or Breaks Relationships*. New York: Ballantine Books.

Umberson, D. (1987). Family Status and Health Behaviors: Social Control as a Dimension of Social Integration. *Journal of Health and Social Behavior, 28,* 306–319.

Verbrugge, L. M. (1985). Gender and Health: An Update on Hypotheses and Evidence. *Journal of Health and Social Behavior, 26,* 156–182.

Watlawick, P., Beavin, J. H., & Jackson, D. D. (1967). *Pragmatics of Human Communication*. New York: W.W: Norton.

CHAPTER

7 Stress

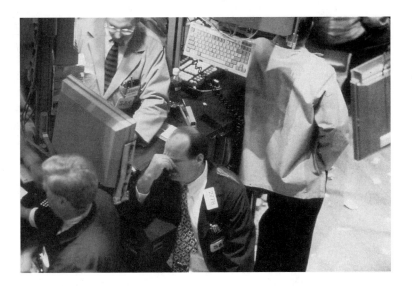

Stress and Its Effect on Mental Health

It is not the intent of this chapter to replace the many fine stress management books on the market. However, it is important to address the issue of stress and its effect on mental health. Perhaps no topic better lends itself to discussing the multidimensional view of health than stress. Stress affects the physiological, emotional, sociological, and spiritual aspects of health.

When going through a stressful period, family and friends may offer a phrase such as "Get it off your chest. You'll feel better." Typically, they are right. Other times, a sense of nausea may develop from worrying too much about some issue (most of the time the issue is not really worth getting that worked up about). The mind-body connection is a very sensitive relationship, and it can easily be thrown out of equilibrium. Fortunately, however, the body is extremely flexible and adaptable and can often take a lot of abuse. However, if a person's body is *abused* long enough, problems occur.

Although Selye has been credited as being a pioneer of stress, it wasn't until the late 1970s and 1980s that a great amount of work was done on how stress caused problems. (Rice, 1999) During the last twenty years, investigators have developed a better understanding of the role that stress plays in affecting the various physical components of the body. These physical components include the immune system, the endocrine system, and the many neurotransmitters that are found in the brain. While it is not the intent of this chapter to provide a detailed account of the physiology of the body under stress, it is important to understand the basics.

Terminology

First, some key terms. A *stressor* is anything that causes stress. *Stress*, from a physiological standpoint, is described as the "rate of wear and tear on the body" (Seaward, 1997, p. 5). Seaward states that, psychologically, stress is the "inability to cope with perceived or real (or imagined) threat to one's mental, physical, emotional, and spiritual well-being, which results in a series of physiological responses and adaptations."

A stressor is anything that threatens, prods, scares, worries, or even thrills a person. Thus, it is important to understand that stress does not have to be the result of a negative event. For instance, getting married and having a child are among the more stressful events in a person's life. Individuals are under stress everyday. However, stress has an important function. It helps people function properly during change; when under stress, the body is easily able to deal with change. However, too often people are exposed to too many stressors and their bodies are under constant "alert."

Many body systems experience significant reactions when they are under stress. However, generally speaking, the body does not distinguish a real threat from a perceived threat. For example, suppose someone was out walking and a very mean dog appeared and started snarling; that person would probably become quite nervous. The heart would start to pound; muscles would tense up; vision would become clearer; the person's blood pressure would increase; and respiration would become more concentrated. Many parts of the body would partially slow down because the body needs to reserve its energy and distribute blood to those parts that are in greater need. For example, during stress, the intestinal tract slows down.

However, imagine yourself walking along a path at night and hearing some movement of the bushes. You cannot see or hear anything except for the bushes that are being pushed aside. You recall hearing in the news that there was a wolf that had been spotted throughout the area and you start to believe that this movement is being caused by a wolf. You quicken your pace and give nervous glances over your shoulder, wondering when the wolf is going to attack you. The noise becomes more obvious, and you realize that you have no place to go to escape. Physiologically, your heart quickens, your blood pressure rises, your muscles tense, and your vision becomes more focused. Even though you do not know exactly what the problem is, you sense that you are in danger. As you stand waiting for the impending attack, you look up and notice a mother deer and her fawn coming through the bushes. You breathe a large sigh of relief, realizing that the noises you heard were these gentle animals and not a vicious wolf. The wolf was perceived and was not in reality there; yet, your body reacted the same as if a snarling wolf were at your heels.

Take it one step further. You come into work, and your secretary tells you that the boss wants to see you right after lunch. The secretary has no additional information except that the boss cannot be reached before that time. Throughout the morning, you may wonder what the boss wanted. As you continue thinking, you might conjure up ideas that perhaps the boss is mad at you and that you have done something wrong. You start thinking that maybe you said something to a client that was inappropriate. Throughout the morning, you allow yourself to be consumed by this concern. Your heart is racing, your blood pressure has risen, your stomach is churning, you are nervous, and you find it hard to concentrate. After an excruciating morning and an almost nauseous lunch, you meet with the boss. It is only then that you discover that the boss wants to commend you for doing a fine job with a particular client.

You are so relieved that you cannot even bask in the glory of the moment, for your mind is racing with a million thoughts about how relieved you are. That is *perceived stress*. It would be inaccurate to suggest that this stress does not exist. It exists in the mind, and it causes the body to react (maybe even more intensely) as if there were a real stressor. In fact, perceived stress often exists for a much longer time period than that caused by a real threat. Sure, you may be really stressed that a dog is nipping at you, but, once you make it to safety, your body returns to normalcy relatively quickly. However, with perceived stress, a person's body is at a heightened state—on alert—for hours. According to Girdano, Everly, and Dusek (1997), stress caused by *symbolic threats* tends to last longer because of the incredible amount of internal dialogue that goes on inside a person's head. It is often difficult for people to *let go* of a statement that somebody makes—even a stranger. For example, if you are driving and a complete stranger gestures angrily, you may think about it for hours afterwards—perhaps thinking "I didn't do anything wrong" or "What did I do wrong?" In reality, you may not have done anything wrong, but hours later you are still letting it bother you.

People are under a lot of stress these days, and much of that stress is *perceived*. This is not to diminish the importance of such stress but to illustrate that people do not have those "snarling dog" issues on a daily basis. They are often dealing with stresses that they allow to creep in and bother them. Usually, these perceived stressors take the form of threats to security, self-esteem, way of life, or safety. Uncertainty is another critical issue that leads to stress, and, finally, change also is a major contributor to stress. Many times, change, uncertainty, and threats go hand in hand. Chapter 8 discusses how to reduce or dissipate these stressors, but Chapter 7 primarily focuses on how stress affects physical and mental health.

The level of perceived stress can be determined by completing Assessment 1 (Table 7.1). This instrument is highly regarded among mental health specialists. Its primary focus is people's perceptions and how they relate to day-to-day living.

TABLE 7.1   Assessment 1: Perceived Stress Scale

	Never	Almost Never	Sometimes	Fairly Often	Very Often
1. In the last month, how often have you been upset because of something that happened unexpectedly?					
2. In the last month, how often have you felt that you were unable to control the important things in your life?					
3. In the last month, how often have you felt nervous and "stressed"?					
4. In the last month, how often have you dealt successfully with day-to-day problems and annoyances?					
5. In the last month, how often have you felt that you were effectively coping with important changes that were occurring in your life?					
6. In the last month, how often have you felt confident about your ability to handle your personal problems?					
7. In the last month, how often have you felt that things were going your way?					
8. In the last month, how often have you found that you could not cope with all the things that you had to do?					
9. In the last month, how often have you been able to control irritations in your life?					
10. In the last month, how often have you felt that you were on top of things?					
11. In the last month, how often have you been angered because of things that happened that were outside of your control?					
12. In the last month, how often have you found yourself thinking about things that you have to accomplish?					
13. In the last month, how often have you been able to control the way you spend your time?					
14. In the last month, how often have you felt difficulties were piling up so high that you could not overcome them?					

For questions 1, 2, 3, 8, 11, 12, 13, and 14, assign the following scores:

Never = 0   Fairly Often = 3

Almost Never = 1   Very Often = 4

Sometimes = 2

For questions 4, 5, 6, 7, 9, and 10, assign the following scores:

Never = 4   Fairly often = 1

Almost Never = 3   Very Often = 0

Sometimes = 2

Total your score. Your range will be from 1 to 56. If you scored under 20, you can be classified as having low stress; between 20 and 36, you have moderate stress; above 36, you have high stress.

Source: From S. Cohen, T. Kamarck, & R. Mermelstein, "A Global Measure of Perceived Stress," *Journal of Health and Social Behavior, 24,* (1983):385–396.

Recognizing Stress Symptoms

When examining a person's ability to deal with problems, it is evident that people handle obvious dangers and visible threats better than invisible, elusive, or embarrassing day-to-day irritations. Yet, these latter items cause the most people the most stress. Unfortunately, there is no simple way to determine if a person is overstressed. The symptoms are often varied, but what is important is for people to know what is normal for them. The problem with symptoms related to stress is that sometimes they are disguised by other symptoms. Individuals may not know if their symptoms are stress induced or if they are actually injured. For example, back problems are often related to stress. However, back problems should not be ignored. A physician should be consulted to rule out factors such as herniated disks.

Tense Muscles; Sore Neck, Shoulders, and Back

Symptoms involving sore muscles could be the result of some injury obtained through lifting, movement, or some other involvement. Yet, in most instances, muscle problems in the neck, shoulders, and back can be traced to excessive stress. The backbone has hundreds of thousands of nerves running to and from it. When under stress, muscles contract, so it is no wonder that stress may result in neck or back pain.

Insomnia

Trouble falling asleep, trouble staying asleep, and early waking are examples of how excessive stress can affect a person's sleep. It is important to note that sleep in itself is not sufficient to combat stress, although, without sufficient sleep and rest, the body is much more vulnerable to the effects of stress. Everyone has had an occasional bout of sleeplessness, and, in many instances, individuals can trace it back to some issues that are causing them problems. When people are dealing with excessive stress, such sleep difficulties are exaggerated.

Fatigue

With the possible exception of the exhaustion experienced by someone who has just completed a running marathon or some other physically exhausting activity, fatigue is one of the classic symptoms of stress. If a person wakes up from a regular night's sleep and is exhausted, there is a good chance that that person is dealing with some major stressors in life. Of course, it is advisable to discuss this with a physician to rule out any anemia or other disease (i.e., mononucleosis). Fatigue is one of the most common complaints in medicine (McGuigan, 1999). Ruling out any physiological problems, most fatigue complaints can be traced to stress.

Boredom, Depression, Listlessness, Dullness, and Lack of Interest

People who exhibit these characteristics may be overstressed. When the body has to be constantly activated to deal with stress, it can become drained of energy (thus the fatigue). When people are fatigued, they are more vulnerable to problems associated with boredom, depression, and so on. Again, people have all been occasionally bored. They have all been depressed. The critical issue is a person's ability to snap out of it after a short time period. People who are under a great deal of stress have a difficult time snapping out of it.

Drinking Too Much

Obviously, drinking too much can be a sign of other problems (i.e., alcoholism); however, assuming that individuals are not alcoholics, stress can lead people to drinking more than they intend, drinking at inappropriate times, or drinking when they really do not want to. Again, many of these "symptoms" are classic alcoholism symptoms, but it should also be pointed out that a person does not need to be an alcoholic to have problems with alcohol. A person who is under a great amount of stress may, indeed, experience some temporary relief with alcohol. The problem is dealing with the aftereffects of the alcohol once the buzz has worn off. Unfortunately, the stressor that caused the drinking probably has not gone away. And, unless a person is careful, a whole new series of stressors can result from inappropriate drinking.

This is not to say that people cannot enjoy alcohol. Millions of people in the United States relax at dinner or with friends while having a drink. However, people need to know their drinking patterns; it is important for them to literally write down when they consume alcohol. People could discover that they are likely to consume more alcohol when they have specific problems in their lives. They may want to make a special effort to avoid using alcohol during those times.

Eating Too Much or Too Little

A great deal of research on obesity indicates that many people eat to relieve their stress. Others lose their desire to eat when stressed. Be aware that high amounts of stress could have an impact on a person's eating habits.

Diarrhea, Cramps, Gas, and Constipation

A person's digestive system is one of the best indicators of the amount of stress he or she is currently dealing with (Greenberg, 1999). As indicated earlier, people know their own bodies best; they know what is normal. So, a deviation from that could be an indication of the person's inability to adequately deal with the stress in that individual's life. When a person is stressed, the intestines seem to be "low priority." This means that blood is drawn from that part of the body (which normally uses a great amount of blood) and is sent to those areas where it is needed more (i.e., brain, muscles, heart, lungs), which, in turn, affects the delicate balance of the intestines.

The small intestines are lined with small, finger-like structures called *villi* that help move the digested foods along. This motion is called *peristalsis*. In the large intestines, these villi do not exist, but the colon does have contractions that move the fecal matter through the intestines. The large colon absorbs much of the water from this fecal matter before allowing it to be emptied out.

Peristalsis (movement) of the small and large intestines is a finely tuned activity. If stress affects this movement and slows it, an excessive amount of liquid will be removed from the fecal material, resulting in constipation. However, if stress affects the peristalsis so that it becomes very active, the fecal material will be moved along the intestines at a very fast pace, resulting in diarrhea (Whitehead, 1998). According to McQuade and Aikman (1974), diarrhea is more likely to occur when a person is in a panic mode, whereas constipation is more evident among those individuals suffering from depression.

Gas is another indicator of stress. Everybody produces gas in the intestines, and most of this gas is reabsorbed back into the system. However, some people expel large quantities of gas because of the excessive movement of the large intestines. This movement prevents the intestines from reabsorbing this gas.

Keep in mind that other factors may result in constipation, diarrhea, or gas. Certainly a flu bug or food poisoning could result in diarrhea. Not eating enough fiber could result in constipation, and dining at the "all-you-can-eat taco restaurant" may result in gas.

Tics, Restlessness, and Itching

When a person is under stress, blood flow to the skin is reduced and sensitivity to this large organ is affected. Thus, some people under stress experience a host of irritating, but fortunately not too serious, episodes of itching or small muscle movements (tics). Restlessness is also a common trait of stress. Individuals experiencing restlessness cannot get comfortable, no matter what they are doing or where they are. They may be tossing and turning while in bed; they may not be comfortable sitting or standing. Everything seems to be a struggle for them.

Finally, rashes are often associated with stress. A young woman in a freshman health class indicated that the audiotape that was played for class for relaxation purposes was almost identical to the one she had received from Dr. "X." Dr. X was a dermatologist, and this student had gone to him for a problem rash that she had developed right after she started her freshman year. After exhausting all other possible explanations (laundry detergent, food, clothing, etc.), the dermatologist came to the conclusion that the rash was stress induced.

Indeed, after thinking about it, the young woman realized that she was in a very stressful situation. She was the first in her family ever to go to college; her parents had always pressed her to be a "great" student; they wanted her to go to medical school. They wanted her to live at home so they could monitor her lifestyle. All of these issues lead to a stressful situation, which resulted in the young woman developing a rash. The dermatologist gave her an audiotape and told her to listen to it twice a day. Within two weeks of starting this physician-directed stress-management program, her rash started to disappear, and it was completely gone within a month.

A rating scale using more possible symptoms of being overstressed is provided in Assessment 2 (Table 7.2). The problem is to identify those particular symptoms that you have experienced over the past two weeks. It is difficult to isolate a particular symptom and then state that it is stress induced, because people are different in how they perceive stress and how they react. It is important for people to become conscious of themselves and how their bodies react during certain times.

TABLE 7.2   Assesment 2: Symptoms of Stress

Within the past two weeks, how often did each of the following events occur?

Event	Did Not Occur	Occurred 1 or 2 Times	Occurred Several Times	Occurred More Than 10 Times
Difficulty falling asleep				
Emotional tension				
Emotional ups and downs				
Impulsive, spur-of-the moment actions				
Talking faster than usual				
General fatigue or heaviness				
Feelings of being emotionally unstable				
Decreased interest in sex				
Feelings of anxiety				
Difficulty organizing thoughts				
Inability to concentrate				

Event	Did Not Occur	Occurred 1 or 2 Times	Occurred Several Times	Occurred More Than 10 Times
Difficulty sleeping through the night				
Grinding teeth				
Verbal attack on someone				
Nightmares				
Headache				
Diarrhea				
Easily startled				
Feelings of hopelessness				
Chest pain				
Significant interpersonal conflict				
Feeling that things are "out of control"				
Slow recovery from a stressful event				
Loss of appetite				
Difficulty staying with an activity for long				
Pounding of heart from tension				
Strong urge to cry				
Increased appetite				
Forgetful				
Upset stomach				
Neck pain				
Pain in back				
Trembling or nervous twitch				
Stuttering or stumbling in speech				
Difficulty sitting still				
More impatience than usual				
Hostility				
Dryness of mouth or throat from tension				
Irritability				
Fuzzy, foggy thinking				
Strong urge to "run away from it all"				
Strong urge to hurt someone				
Feelings of joylessness				
Feelings of being "overwhelmed by it all"				
Depressed feelings				
Short-tempered				

Analysis:

High-Distress Symptoms: 50 or higher   Did not occur: 0 points
Medium-Distress Symptoms: 20–49   Ocurred 1–2 times: 1 point
Low-Distress Symptoms: 0–19   Ocurred several times: 5 points
After completing, identify what you can do   Occurred more than 10 times: 10 points
to reduce such stress, thus reducing the symptoms.

Source: From Schafer, W. , (1992) *Stress Management for Wellness,* (2nd Edition) Fort Worth: Harcourt Brace Jovanovich College Publishers.

Stress and Disease

Stress has historically been thought to cause a particular problem, for example, ulcers. For many years, the term *psychosomatic* (mind-body) has been used; more recently, the term *psychoneuroimmunology* has been used, indicating the study of the interactions of the conscious mind (psycho); the brain and central nervous system (neuro); and the body's immune system. Basically, the implication is that the mind-body connection is so strong that the mind can cause certain physical ailments (Jermott, 1985). Although recently there has been some research to show that ulcers have some viral connections, generally speaking, people still think of ulcers as being caused by stress. When an individual is under chronic stress, it changes the lining of the stomach wall, allowing for more production of gas and less protection of the stomach wall; thus, the wall of the stomach gets irritated and becomes ulcerated.

It also seems apparent that if people are under a great deal of stress and their blood pressure remains high that certain long-term problems could result (i.e., stroke or heart attack). Greenberg (1999) refers to this type of stress-induced illness as *psychogenic psychosomatic illness.*

However, Greenberg (1999) goes on to state that, theoretically, it is possible that exposure to chronic stress can lead to future problems caused by the effects of stress on the immune system. The theory behind this is that people are constantly bombarded with various viral and bacterial infections. Yet, they are mostly healthy. When a person's body is exhausted through stress-inducing actions, the immune system is weakened and less likely to resist such viral or bacterial invaders. Greenberg refers to this as *somatogenic psychosomatic illness.*

For example, consider finals week. Students manage to make it through the entire time period, probably skipping meals, skimping on sleep, and running themselves ragged. They each complete three or four major final exams, a major report, and several other items before they can leave for the semester break. They go to bed on Thursday evening with all of their work completed, and, although they are exhausted, they lie down feeling good that they have accomplished all that they set out to do. They wake up Friday morning, and they are sick with bad colds. Now, why did this happen? Was it coincidence? Possibly, but chances are that they allowed their bodies to deplete their ability to fight outside invaders and, when they finally "let their guard down," they succumbed—in this case to colds. The somatogenic psychosomatic theory suggests that chronic stress starts "chipping away" at a person's resistance and that eventually something will "break." The example given was a cold, but it is theorized that, exposed to enough stress *and* not taking steps to try to relieve that stress, the "problem" could be a heart attack, a cancer formation, or an accident. This is still completely theoretically, but increased understanding of the immune system can only lead to better understanding of the body's ability to maintain resistance.

The Nervous System

The central nervous system (CNS) is comprised of the brain and the spinal cord. Basically, the central nervous system consists of a voluntary component (people can think before something happens—like reaching out and picking up a pencil) and an automatic system called the *autonomic nervous system* (ANS). The ANS consists of two sections, the *sympathetic nervous system* and the *parasympathetic nervous system.* The ANS allows the body to maintain homeostasis or balance.

The Sympathetic Nervous System

The *sympathetic nervous system* prepares the body when it is under stress (or when the body perceives that it is under stress). The body has a certain finite amount of energy, thus the body must allow critical functions to receive as much energy as needed, and it will close down those functions that would distract from the other body parts (Greenberg, 1999). Some of the symptoms associated with the sympathetic nervous system described by Guyton in the Rice (1999) text *Stress and Health* (p. 139) are:

1. Increased blood pressure
2. Increased blood flow to support large active muscles, coupled with decreased blood flow to internal (for example, digestive) organs not needed for rapid activity
3. Increased total energy consumption
4. Increased blood glucose concentration
5. Increased energy release in muscles
6. Increased muscle strength
7. Increased mental activity
8. Increased rate of blood coagulation

Interestingly, certain foods and/or chemicals can mimic the sympathetic nervous system and have these same symptoms occur. For example, caffeine and nicotine can activate many of these same symptoms. These are *mimeticsympathetic* agents, that is, they mimic the sympathetic nervous system symptoms. Imagine the incredible effect on the body if an individual is under a great amount of stress and that person aggravates the body's condition by drinking an excessive amount of caffeine and smoking cigarettes! It is no wonder that the body could never "get back to normal." For example, one cigarette increases blood pressure and heart rate for about fifteen minutes. Caffeine speeds up the system and sharpens mental activities (although, ironically, if a person consumes more than two cups of coffee within two hours, the results—in some people—are the opposite; that is, the person might have more difficulty concentrating). If a person smokes a pack of cigarettes (twenty cigarettes) a day, drinks six to eight cups of coffee (or soda) a day, and is also under a lot of stress, that individual's body may not have an opportunity to relax. It could take hours for that person to settle down and fall asleep.

The Parasympathetic Nervous System

The *parasympathetic nervous system* is the system that allows the body to return to normalcy. How long it takes for the parasympathetic nervous system to kick in depends upon the stressor. As discussed earlier, a mean dog starts snarling at a person; the sympathetic nervous system is activated. Either the person is going to run away from the dog or that individual is going to somehow fight it (sometimes referred to as the *flight or fight response*). Whatever the decision, the body's sympathetic nervous system prepares the body. After the danger is dissipated, the parasympathetic nervous system brings the heart rate down and allows more blood flow to those parts of the body that had a reduction during the stressor. The parasympathetic nervous system might be activated within minutes of the initial stressor.

But, what happens when a person experiences chronic stress all day at work? When does the parasympathetic nervous system become activated? It may take hours; in fact, some people keep their stress bottled up inside so that their sympathetic nervous system is chronically activated. People under a great deal of stress need to make sure that they *take time* to let the parasympathetic nervous system bring their body systems back to normal.

The Endocrine System

The *endocrine system* consists of the following glands: pituitary, thyroid, adrenal, parathyroid, pancreas, ovaries, testes, pineal, thymus, and hypothalamus. Each gland has a unique role in helping the body to deal with stress. The glands do, however, have similar functions, and there are a number of reasons for this. First, dealing with stressors is a major function of the body, a function that requires the production of many chemicals and/or hormones. Second, in the event that a person has a physical problem with a specific part of the body (i.e., only one kidney), the body has to rely on other glands to deal with stress.

The Pituitary Gland and the Hypothalamus

Considered the master gland, the *pituitary gland* is a pea-sized gland located behind the eyes. The *hypothalamus,* located at the base of the front part of the brain above the pituitary gland, has a major function in controlling various body functions such as heart rate, blood pressure, temperature, thirst, hunger, and sex drive. The pituitary and the hypothalamus "play off of each other" in directing the endocrine system during stressful times.

The Adrenal Glands

The *adrenal glands* are located on top of the kidneys. The outside of each gland is referred to as the *adrenal cortex*. The adrenal cortex produces aldosterone and cortisol. The inner portion of the adrenal gland is the *adrenal medulla;* it is directly affected by a nerve from the back (posterior) of the hypothalamus, allowing almost instantaneous reaction. When activated, the adrenal medulla releases epinephrine (sometimes referred to as adrenalin) and norepinephrine (sometimes referred to as noradrenalin), which are the hormones that allow for quick energy and strength to handle an emergency—thus, the term *adrenaline rush.* These hormones are critical in helping a person deal with the immediacy of a stressor.

Figure 7.1 shows that the posterior hypothalamus has a direct nerve path to the adrenal medulla, whereas the anterior hypothalamus activates a series of hormones that travel via the bloodstream. Although travel through the bloodstream is relatively quick, it is not as quick as the direct nerve path. When activated by a

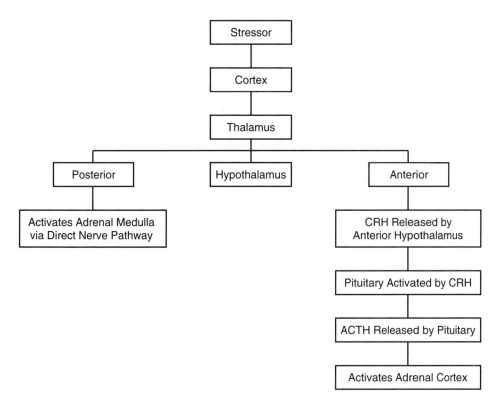

FIGURE 7.1 **Overview of How a Stressor Affects the Adrenal Gland.**

Source: Adapted from *Comprehensive Stress Management* (6th ed.) by J. S. Greenberg, 1999. Columbus, OH: McGraw-Hill.

stressor, the anterior hypothalamus discharges corticotropin-releasing hormone (CRH). This travels a very short distance to stimulate the pituitary gland to release adrenocorticotropic hormone (ACTH). ACTH travels via the bloodstream to activate the adrenal cortex (outside of gland). The adrenal cortex then produces cortisol and aldosterone.

Cortisol provides fuel for battle by increasing blood sugar. In addition, cortisol continues to increase arterial blood pressure and it decreases lymphocytes (white blood cells) from the thymus gland (a very important concept to remember when discussing the immune system—an increase of cortisol decreases the effectiveness of the immune system).

Aldosterone increases blood pressure so that food and oxygen can be transported to active parts of the body. It accomplishes this by increasing blood volume by decreasing urine production and increasing the sodium retention.

Another function of the anterior hypothalamus is to release thyrotropin-releasing hormone (TRH). This hormone also travels to the pituitary gland and allows it to release thyrotropin or thyroid-stimulating hormone (TSH). This activates the thyroid gland to produce thyroxine. Thyroxine

1. Increases basal metabolic rate
2. Increases free fatty acids
3. Increases rate of glucose production
4. Increases gastrointestinal motility (diarrhea)
5. Increases the rate and depth of respiration
6. Increases heart rate
7. Increases blood pressure
8. Increases anxiety
9. Decreases feelings of tiredness

Finally, the anterior hypothalamus (like the posterior hypothalamus) has a direct nerve path to the pituitary gland that allows the pituitary gland to produce oxytocin and vasopressin. Oxytocin constricts blood vessels and contracts smooth muscles. Vasopressin also contracts smooth muscles and constricts blood vessels, but it also increases the permeability of the blood vessels to water, resulting in greater blood volume. Figure 7.2 provides a diagram of these routes.

The Immune System

The emergence of acquired immune deficiency syndrome (AIDS) in the early 1980s really pushed the scientific world to truly understand the role of the immune system. Volumes have been written about it, and some references are identified at the end of this chapter.

Basically, the *immune system* consists of the cells, tissues, and organs that protect the body from disease—the lymphocytes, bone marrow, the thymus gland, the spleen, and other parts. *Immunity* is the state of being resistant to foreign products or substances. It is the body's capacity for identifying, destroying, and disposing of

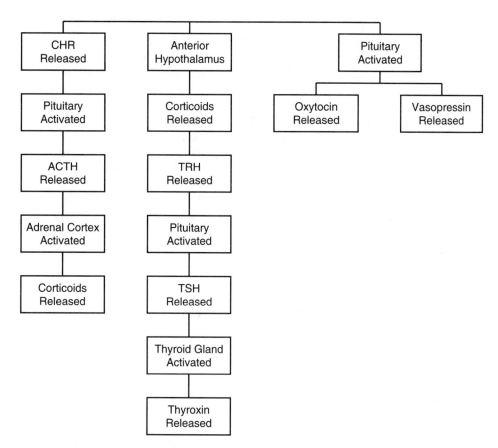

FIGURE 7.2 **Hypothalamus's Role During Stress.**

Source: Adapted from *Comprehensive Stress Management* (6th ed.) by J. S. Greenberg, 1999. Columbus, OH: McGraw-Hill.

disease-causing agents. When such foreign substances enter the body, the body responds by sending out powerful forces to destroy the incoming substances. These incoming substances are referred to as *antigens,* and they trigger the body's immune system. In this situation, white blood cells are the key to the immune system.

Lymphocytes are a class of white blood cells involved in immunity. They are found in the bloodstream, lymph nodes, bone marrow, and certain glands. Two forms of lymphocytes in particular are involved in the immune response. These forms, *T lymphocytes* and *B lymphocytes,* each have their own very specific role in the immune response.

T lymphocytes are produced primarily by the thymus gland (thus, the term *T cell*) and possess the ability to recognize invaders that are dangerous to the body. There are actually three types of T cells. *Helper T cells* are really the leaders of the immune system. These helper T cells identify the enemy (antigen) and then signal to other parts of the body (and to B cells) the need to fight the antigen.

Helper T cells recruit *killer T cells* to fight and kill cells of the body that have been invaded. Killer T cells specialize in killing cells of the body that have been invaded by foreign substances. They also fight and destroy cancerous cells. Finally, *suppressor T cells* are able to slow down and/or stop the attack of B cells and other T cells, which is imperative when the infection has been conquered.

B lymphocytes (so named for the bursa of Fabricius, a part of the intestinal area of birds, where they were first discovered) are produced by the liver and spleen and are the cells that produce the actual antibodies. When an antigen enters the body, antibodies are produced. *Antibodies* are large protein molecules produced in response to the presence of antigens such as viruses. They immobilize the antigens so that *scavenger cells* can devour them. Specific antibodies respond to specific antigens. For example, XYZ flu antibodies respond only to XYZ flu antigen. After the antigens are destroyed, other types of lymphocytes (called *memory cells*) make a memory of the invader so that the system can respond quickly during the next encounter. Many contagious diseases in humans are once-in-a-lifetime diseases because of this system. For example, mumps, measles, and chicken pox produce antibodies that remain in the body for an entire life. Vaccinations are also ways to produce antibodies. Vaccinations produce antigens in a form not to cause disease but to code the memory cells to create immunities. This remarkable system can be illustrated in a four-step procedure:

1. *Recognition of the enemy.* Viruses enter the system, and, during this initial entrance, cells called macrophages destroy a few of the viruses. Helper T cells "read" the antigen and send its messages throughout the body.

2. *Amplification of defenses.* Once activated, helper T cells begin to multiply. Killer T cells and B cells are now called into action.

3. *Conquering the infection.* Some of the viruses have entered the actual body tissue (the only place they are able to replicate). Killer T cells will sacrifice these cells, puncturing the infected cell's membrane and letting the contents spill out. This prevents the virus from multiplying. Antibodies then neutralize the virus.

4. *Slowdown and truce.* As the infection is contained, suppressor T cells halt the entire range of immune responses, preventing them from spiraling out of control. Memory T and B cells are left in the blood and lymphatic system ready for quick response in case an identical virus enters the system.

When a body is stressed, the sympathetic nervous system and the endocrine system are activated. Both of these activations affect the immune system by preventing the release of T cells from the thymus gland, reducing white blood cell production, and allowing the body to more slowly respond to an invading antigen.

The Body's Balance

The body is a marvelous creation that, despite its complexity, runs relatively smoothly. The body always tries to maintain its internal balance. It might be compared to an airline pilot. A passenger on a jumbo jet has a relatively smooth ride most of the time. Granted, there may be times that the ride is rough, but the pilot and the onboard computers are constantly striving to balance any abnormal situations such as wind gusts, turbulence, and weight imbalance. As the plane encounters one set of problems, the pilots adjust their controls to have the plane get back on a steady ride. The body does the same thing; as it encounters "turbulence" along the way, it deals with such unexpected problems, but then it brings itself back to normal, awaiting the next disturbance.

Obviously, the jumbo jet needs occasional maintenance; if this maintenance does not occur, serious problems can develop. The same is true of the body; it needs to "recover" from periodic "disturbances." If it is not allowed to recover, its balance may become so lopsided that drastic steps may be required to get back to normal.

Consider how the endocrine system, the immune system, and the sympathetic and parasympathetic nervous systems work together when a person is exposed to stress. First, consider the role of blood pressure. Blood pressure is the amount of pressure exerted onto the blood vessels and is measured in two components. *Systolic pressure* is the pressure created when the heart contracts. *Diastolic pressure* is the measurement taken when the heart relaxes and refills with blood between contractions. To state what constitutes *high* blood pressure is difficult, since there are so many different concepts on what is considered *abnormal.* For decades, 120/80 mm Hg (120 millimeters of mercury pressure for systolic and 80 for diastolic) was the *norm,* yet most medical guides indicate that this can vary depending upon a number of factors. More recent medical studies have shown that anything about 140/90 mm Hg is something a person and his or her physician need to monitor (Turner, 1994). Note that a onetime high reading does not indicate a problem, but a long-term series of high readings might be of concern. When blood pressure is consistently above 140/90 mm Hg, the term *hypertension* is used. Hypertension is chronic or excessively high blood pressure. Long-term, uncontrolled hypertension could result in some type of cardiovascular accident (i.e., stroke or heart attack) in which the vessels lose their pliability. Uncontrolled hypertension can also lead to kidney problems.

So, how does stress affect blood pressure? When an individual is under stress, the sympathetic nervous system increases the output of the heart, which increases blood pressure. In addition, the release of oxytocin and vasopressin is also increased, which causes contraction of the smooth muscles. This, in turn, allows constriction of the blood vessels. A smaller opening automatically increases blood pressure.

Finally, a discussion of arteriosclerosis can help explain some of the devastating effects of high blood pressure. *Arteriosclerosis* is a term used to describe changes in the walls of the blood vessels. These changes can be caused by such things as cholesterol, fatty plaque, and calcium. The elasticity and the diameter of the vessels are affected (Blonna, 1996).

Imagine a hose that is old and rigid. Turning on the water full tilt may actually cause the hose to burst. This can be compared to a person's blood vessels. Growing old naturally causes arteries to "harden," and this can be accelerated through a variety of factors, including diet and stress. Now, in addition to the hose being rigid, imagine the hose has a deposit lining the entire hose. What was one-half inch in diameter is now, say, one-fourth inch. Again comparing to the blood vessel, there is more pressure put on the blood vessel because the same amount of blood is trying to get through a much smaller space.

The liver produces over three-fourths of the cholesterol that the body needs. The liver then removes excess cholesterol (produced by the liver and through diet). However, the liver can only remove so much cholesterol. Any additional amount of cholesterol circulates around the bloodstream and can eventually attach itself to the blood vessels. When under stress, the liver produces more cholesterol. When under chronic stress, the liver constantly produces cholesterol and the extra amount of cholesterol eventually attaches itself to the walls of the blood vessels (Van Dorner & Orlebeke, 1982).

Prioritization During Stress

When stressed, the body has finite resources, and must conserve energy. Blood flow will be minimized in those parts of the body that do not aid in the "flight or fight." For example, consider the earlier example of the walk in the woods. Physiologically, the critical areas of the body are the brain, the heart and blood vessels, and the muscles. Thus, these are the areas where the blood flow is prioritized when the body is under stress. Those areas that are not prioritized include the skin, the digestive system, and the urinary system. The skin is the largest organ, then the digestive system. Both systems are rich in blood vessels. Yet, when under stress, the body needs as much blood (to obtain oxygen) as possible. The body has a finite amount of blood; thus, when stressed, it will close down the skin and the digestive system to allow extra blood to circulate throughout the body to help the "more essential" organs (i.e., cardiovascular system, brain).

Being under stress occasionally is not a problem; the body can deal with it accordingly. When you are walking in the woods and think you hear a wolf, your eyes sharpen, your breathing intensifies (to get more oxygen into your system), your heart rate increases (to send more blood through the system), and your blood pressure increases (because of the increased blood flow). In addition, your hands will become cold (because the blood is taken from the skin) and your intestinal tract will be affected. As already discussed (and an essential part of this prioritization), aldosterone signals your kidneys to slow down filtering the sodium out of the blood, which allows for an increase in blood volume, which, in turn, raises the blood pressure.

More blood glucose is needed to assist the muscles in maintaining their ready state. Cortisol is produced by the cortex of the adrenal gland to trigger the liver to release more glucose (Blonna, 1996). Also note that when the body produces cortisol, it also minimizes the number of lymphocytes available to fight infection; thus, people who are under stress are more vulnerable to a host of infections, including cancer (Dantzer & Kelley, 1989; Herbert & Cohen, 1993; Cohen & Rabin, 1998).

Techniques/Exercises

1. In small groups, design an analogy to the immune system to more easily teach it to others. For example, you might use the military, sporting teams, or computers to help teach the different functions.

2. Survey fifteen to twenty people on the top five items that cause them stress. In addition, ask them what types of symptoms they have when they are over-stressed.

3. Bring a variety of stress management books (or make this a library research project). In small groups, identify how the following diseases or symptoms are affected by stress:

    a. HIV/AIDS
    b. Heart disease
    c. High blood pressure
    d. TMJ
    e. Loss of sexual desire
    f. Arthritis
    g. Backaches
    h. Asthma
    i. Depression
    j. Acne

4. Do a diet analysis to see how much of your diet might activate the sympathetic nervous system.

5. Find five websites on the Internet that deal with stress. Identify what the purpose is of each website, what (if any) products they are promoting, what training the people have had who are making such claims, and whether the claims might be "acceptable" to the experts in stress management.

Summary

Stress is sneaky in that it reveals itself through many problems that people would not contribute to stress. Stress can affect the body in many ways, and, if allowed to continue, stress allows the body to become more vulnerable to a variety of health-related problems.

The body's ability to function is based on not only the central nervous system but also the sympathetic and parasympathetic nervous systems. The endocrine system also has a strong impact on how the body deals with stress. The endocrine system primarily releases hormones to prepare the body for certain functions. Finally, the immune system is especially influenced by stress. If too much stress is allowed to accumulate it can wreak havoc on the endocrine system and immune system.

DISCUSSION QUESTIONS

1. Describe how the sympathetic and parasympathetic nervous systems differ and how they work together to help maintain homeostasis.

2. Identify how stressors influence the immune system and how long-term exposure to stress can impact a person's health.

3. Explain the difference between psychosomatic illnesses, somatogenic psychosomatic illnesses, psychogenic psychosomatic illnesses, and psychoneuroimmunology.

4. Describe the "common" symptoms of stress. How can a person determine if something is stress induced or if it is due to some other problem?

5. Distinguish between real and perceived stress, and give an example of each.

6. Describe the pathways of the various hormones when the hypothalamus is activated by stress.

RELATED WEBSITES

http://ncptsd.org/West_haven.html—Clinical Neuroscience Division. Studies on stress and brain function as well as treatment for trauma patients. Also included are studies by international researchers and training for the next generation of researchers.

http://www.mcms.dal.ca/danat/anat_res.html—Anatomy and Neurobiology. This site provides research articles and activities regarding the human brain, its function, and responses during stress.

http://www.teachhealth.com—Medical basis of stress, depression, anxiety, sleeping problems, and drug use.

http://www.unl.edu/stress/mgmt/#toc—Stress Management: A Review of Principles. This site presents concepts of stress management education including understanding stressors and responses, sources of stress, physiology of stress, decision making, and more.

http://www.users.cts.com/crash/d/deohair/psychoph.html—Biofeedback: Review, History, and Application. Article by Donald E. O'Hair, Ph.D., explores theories and techniques of biofeedback.

REFERENCES

Blonna, R. (1996). *Coping with Stress in a Changing World.* St. Louis: Mosby.

Cohen, S., Kamarck, T., & Mermelstein, R. (1983). A global measure of perceived stress. *Journal of Health and Social Behavior, 24,* 385–396.

Cohen, S., & Rabin, B. S. (1998). Psychologic Stress, Immunity, and Cancer. *Journal of the National Cancer Institute, 90,* 3–4.

Dantzer, R., & Kelley, K. W. (1989). Stress and Immunity: An Integrated View of Relationships Between the Brain and the Immune System. *Life Sciences, 44,* 1995–2008.

Girdano, D. A., Everly, G. S., & Dusek, D. E. (1997). *Controlling Stress and Tension* (5th Ed.). Boston: Allyn & Bacon.

Greenberg, J. S. (1999). *Comprehensive Stress Management* (6th Ed.). Columbus, OH: McGraw-Hill.

Herbert, T. B., & Cohen, S. (1993). Stress and Immunity in Humans: A Meta-Analytic Review. *Psychosomatic Medicine, 55,* 364–379.

Jermott, J. B. (1985). Psychoneuroimmunology: The New Frontier. *American Behavior Scientist, 28*(4), 497–509.

McQuade, W., & Aikman, A. (1974). *Stress.* New York: Bantam Books.

McGuigan, F. J. (1999). *Encyclopedia of Stress.* Boston: Allyn & Bacon.

Rice, P. L. (1999). *Stress and Health* (3rd Ed.). Boston: Brooks/Cole.

Schafer, W. (1999). *Stress Management for Wellness* (4th Ed.). Ft. Worth, Harcourt College Publishers.

Schafer, W. (1992). *Stress Management for Wellness* (2nd Ed.). Ft. Worth, Harcourt Brace Jovanovich College Publisher.

Seaward, B. L. (1997). *Managing Stress: Principles and Strategies for Health and Well-being.* Boston: Jones and Bartlett.

Turner, J. R. (1994). *Cardiovascular Reactivity and Stress, Patterns of Physiological Response.* New York: Plenum Press.

Van Dorner, C. J. P., & Orlebeke, K. F. (1982). Stress, Personality, and Serum Cholesterol Level. *Journal of Human Stress,* 24–28.

Whitehead, W. E. (1998). Gastrointestinal syndromes and disorders. In E. A. Blechman & K. D. Bownell (Eds.), *Behavioral Medicine and Women: A Comprehensive Handbook* (pp. 646–653). New York: Guilford Press.

CHAPTER

8 Stress Management

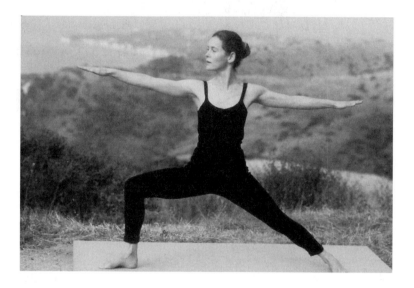

Chapter 7 gave an overview of stress and how it can affect a person's health. This chapter identifies specific strategies to (1) cope with stressors and (2) reduce the effects of unnecessary stress.

In the late 1970s and early 1980s, there was a very effective and memorable television commercial for Framm oil filters. A stern-looking mechanic looked into the camera and said, "You can pay me now, or you can pay me later." His point was that either way he was going to get paid. The customer could choose to pay an extra buck or two during each oil change to use Framm oil filters, which would theoretically extend the life of the engine. If the customer chose not to, that was fine, but eventually the consequence would be a new engine.

Obviously, Framm was trying to get the consumer to purchase its product, but the statement that the mechanic makes is also relevant to stress management: A person can take care of stress now or not worry about it, but eventually that person will "pay" for it. That payment may be in the form of a cold, flu, or exhaustion; but, rest assured, the debt will be paid. Hopefully, only minor problems such as colds result. However, all too often, people deal with the cumulative effects of stress through such serious problems as heart disease, stroke, accidents, or cancer.

The point is that everyone is exposed to an enormous amount of stress every day. People cannot live without a certain amount of stress, and it is perfectly acceptable to be under more stress on some days than others. In fact, as discussed earlier, people are often at their best when they are under stress. Their minds are sharper, they are able to move and respond more quickly, and they experience other benefits. The problems occur when the cumulative effects of stress start showing. It is up to the individual to help the body deal with this stress. Thinking about it is only the beginning. The key to coping with stress is to have a plan of action that includes *multiple* strategies.

Remember that no one strategy is perfect for everybody. It is important to develop a series of strategies to deal with stress, and it is wise to have alternative plans just in case the preferred strategy is not effective or available. For example, imagine a person who utilizes long-distance running to deal with stress. Imagine what would happen if that person suffered an injury that left running out of the question. What would the person do to cope with his/her stressors?

Five Strategies for Dealing with Stress

Consider the following five strategies for dealing with stress: (1) alter your lifestyle; (2) prioritize; (3) use social support; (4) use humor; and (5) structure activities (either active or passive) to reduce stress. Discussion of each of these five areas follows.

Alter Your Lifestyle

Altering—or as some people call it, *avoidance*—is a relatively simple strategy in which you must first assess the events that are causing stress in your life. First, after some contemplation, list the times and/or events at which you are most often stressed. This listing of times and events can be therapeutic in that it provides an opportunity for you to do some deep soul searching as to what leads to stress. Girdano, Everly, and Dusek (1997) call this *social restructuring;* others call it *social engineering* (Seaward, 1997). Instead of using the term *avoidance,* Seaward prefers using the term *path of least resistance.* Whatever you call it, the key is to try to arrange your life so that you can eliminate head-to-head conflict.

Once you have listed all of those events that cause stress, look at which ones can be avoided. You must perceive avoiding not as a bad thing but rather as a negotiation with yourself to save some "wear and tear" on your body. For example, suppose that you often become very irritated at having to wait in line at the grocery store. This might even be exaggerated when you are in the express lane, behind a person who is incredibly slow at writing a check, or behind a coupon-clipping tycoon who has a coupon for every item bought.

A person who is practicing altering (or avoidance) would assess when the best time is to go grocery shopping. For example, if you hate crowds and/or waiting in line, do not shop on the first Friday of the month when Social Security checks arrive (and when many people who receive Social Security buy their groceries). Do not go shopping at the peak times (most grocery stories are open twenty-four hours a day). In some instances, there will be no choice; but, too often, people who are overstressed feel that they do not have a choice when, in fact, they do, indeed, have many choices.

An example often given among college students is campus parking. Granted, parking may present a problem on campus; in fact, many campuses are significantly lacking spaces so that the parking permit is merely a license to *hunt* for a space. Specifically, at the University of Minnesota/Twin Cities, it is difficult to park within one mile of campus (and that is only if the parking gods are in a good mood). Most spaces are between one and a half and two miles from campus. But, it is known and accepted, and those who need to utilize parking facilities plan accordingly.

If you are a student and parking on campus is a stressor for you, identify and brainstorm all possible alternatives. Typically, a list might include carpooling, using mass transit, locating parking a distance away and walking, riding a bicycle, or arriving earlier than usual when spaces are not at such a premium.

After listing all of the options, review and assess which option is most appropriate. For example, there may be a large empty lot across campus that is never full during the day. You could park there, alleviate the stress, and enjoy the walk across campus (the exercise would probably be good for you). There are people who drive around lots looking for an empty space (perhaps even keeping the car running while sitting in the lot's driveway waiting for a car to leave), allowing their stress to become more and more intense. You could drive the extra halfmile, walk, and still get to the classroom before the person waiting for the space nearby.

Another common strategy to avoid parking lot anger is to realize that the lots become incredibly crowded between certain times. Obviously, if you are arriving just a few minutes before class, chances are that you will be caught in this congestion. Of course, this will lead to stress. However, by planning to arrive just fifteen minutes earlier, you might be able to avoid almost all of the stress of finding a parking space. You might even find a space close to your classrooms.

Go through all of your identified stressors and pinpoint those areas that can be altered (or avoided). Obviously, some of the stressors cannot be avoided, but many can. This is also helpful if you share stressors with others; there is something about power in numbers. You will quickly discover that you are not alone in many of the stressors that you face and that in many instances somebody else has figured out some way to avoid or alter a similar situation. The question is, what stressors can you reduce or avoid by merely altering your lifestyle?

Prioritizing

Here is a descriptive example of what is meant by *prioritizing*. Imagine the following scenario. There is a line at the checkout of a grocery store. There are numerous people waiting in line, and the person at the front unloading groceries is having a difficult time going through checkout. Behind this person are several people, many of them expressing dissatisfaction with the person unloading the groceries. Some are anxious and want to get out of the store; some are angry with the person (perhaps he has twelve items in a ten-item line). However, there is one person standing in line who is relaxed and almost oblivious to the situation.

Assuming that nobody in line has a sick child that they have to rush off to, or that nobody is late for an important meeting, why is that one person not upset at having to wait in line? Go inside the minds of some of these people and listen to what they are saying:

> *Person 1:* "I can't believe how slow this person is. People like this should be barred from stores. Now watch, he'll write a check in a cash-only line. Gee, I wish they would hurry up!"
>
> *Person 2:* "Why do I *always* get stuck behind some klutz? It's even worse; they have more than they should have in their cart."
>
> *Person 3:* "This nimrod, why is he even using coupons? What's he saving, about fifty cents?"
>
> *Person 4:* "You know, it's not too often I get to have ten minutes all by myself without the kids, my wife, or my boss bugging me; it's kind of nice."

Persons 1, 2, and 3 are obviously stressed about waiting. Yet, Person 4 has a very different perception. It appears that he is actually enjoying waiting in line. Prioritizing is the process of assessing the importance of certain issues in life. It is hard to do, but it can have some major impact on how you manage stress. Most of the stress people deal with is based on their *perception* of the situation. Thus, the goal is to change your perception of the information you receive (stressor), how it is evaluated, and the meaning attached to it (Girdano et al., 1997).

As already stated, prioritizing is one of the most difficult things to do, but it can be one of the strongest ways to reduce stress. This applies to a person's *values* and changing a person's values is incredibly tough. A value has worth attached to it. Many people consider what people do, versus what they say, as true indicators of their values. For example, people may state that health is a value; yet, if they do activities that harm their health, they would be perceived as having their actions speak louder than their words.

A number of factors—parents, religion, peers, culture, the era in which a person was raised (i.e., the 1930s versus the 1990s), experiences, education, and place of residence —influence a person's values. One person's values are not better or worse than another's but different. To help others prioritize, you must be cognizant of their values and what might influence them and be aware of their lifestyle and what they consider important. Although it is not simply "black or white," many stresses are caused by a person's values being challenged, which can leave the person feeling threatened. For example, since the 1970s, more and more women have become employed in the workforce. Initially, spouses who supported their wives working still expected them to keep the house clean, have meals prepared, and to maintain the household similar to their mothers (who probably did not work outside the home). Men (and women, too) have done a great job of making women feel guilty for working outside the home and not "taking care of" their family. Of course, it is clear that the husband should (and is slowly starting to) do more things about the house, but there is still this haunting feeling among millions of women that if the house is not clean it is their fault.

The bottom line is that there is no way to maintain the house the way that June Cleaver (*Leave it to Beaver*), Carol Brady (*Brady Bunch*), or even one's own grandmother did, not when the majority of women are working outside the home—though that value is strongly supported by those raised in the era in which women stayed at home. The fact that a large percentage of women are single parents exacerbates the stress. The stress that women feel is a value-laden type of stress, that is, the stress is based on a value that many people have.

Since in many instances, altering and prioritizing go hand in hand, what could a person in the preceding situation do to alter or prioritize? First, assess the need and determine who could help. Children old enough to understand can be told to put things away when they finished with them. Children can put their clean, folded clothes away; children can help with basic housework (this is not about violating any child labor laws; it is just about having them help out with the basics).

Second, assess how urgent it is that every dish be cleaned and put away before you go to bed. A dishwasher is a great place to store dirty dishes, and you can be doing the environment a favor by waiting for a full load before running it. Identify those areas that you consider an absolute must and those that can be modified without sacrificing your integrity. Again, altering or prioritizing may come into play.

Consider the wife of the one of the authors. She is very meticulous at keeping the house clean. The children, including the three-year-old, know to put things away when they are through with them and before they get something else out. Another policy is to touch an item once. In other words, whoever gets the mail does not just look at it and put it on the kitchen table. That person looks at it and puts it wherever it belongs (i.e., the garbage, the bill file, the personal file). This technique, in and of itself, helps reduce clutter a great deal.

Another way to prioritize is to assess the importance of getting something done "your way." Many people want it done their way or no way at all. These individuals tend to invite a lot of stress into their lives. For example, consider the man who had a difficult time with his wife over folding towels. When he first got married, he was one of those few men who actually did as much work as (if not more than) his wife around the house. He felt comfortable cooking; dusting; and washing, drying; and folding clothes. Yet, he and his wife would get into the craziest arguments because he folded towels in half instead of into thirds. *OK,* one would think, *no big deal,* but it was very frustrating to both individuals. He was raised in a family in which the towels were folded in half; she was raised in a family in which the towels were folded into thirds. Instead of feeling appreciated for doing the laundry, he felt miserable that he had failed in some aspect of their relationship. She felt that he was folding the towels that way just to *irritate* her. She eventually stopped arguing, but, after the towels were put away, she refolded them. Thus, a simple task now took time for two units of people to do instead of just one. The man now looks back at that marriage and shakes his head, saying that the cause of their divorce was that he folded the towels *wrong*. This marriage probably had more problems than just folded towels, but little things like this cause excessive amounts of stress within people and between relationships. There are so many things around the house that need to get done that, to reduce stress, people need to assess how important it is to do something in a particular way versus whether the activity gets done.

There are also examples of when more drastic steps need to be taken. Consider the woman who was upset that nobody in her family would help with the cleaning of the house. She, like her spouse, worked outside the house full-time. They both came home tired. However, once at the house, he would not do anything to keep it clean. She got home, started dinner (not an easy task because she was cooking for five people), cleaned the kitchen, and then worked on the housecleaning. This did not take into account any work that she might have brought from work. She would be busy from the moment she got home until well past 11:30 p.m. She was up the next morning at 5:30 a.m. to help get the family's day started.

All efforts to obtain assistance went unheeded. The woman got angry; that did not work. She threatened; that did not work. Finally, she made an ultimatum to her family—"From this day on, I am not going to do any more cooking"—and she stopped cooking. The first few days were rough. The husband did not like to cook, did not do a very good job, and did not want to; but, after a few days of peanut butter and jelly dinners, he started to cook.

This woman's rationale was that she could not keep doing all aspects of the housekeeping. The time that she had previously spent cooking was now used to straighten up the house. Thus, when dinner was over, the housework was done and she could spend some time with her children and her husband. She had less stress, and, although it was a tough task to not do something that she felt obligated to do (cook for her family), it had a substantial impact on her stress level.

More recently, she has worked out an agreement with her husband and the children. She does now occasionally cook; while she is doing that, the rest of the family members are cleaning the house. Sometimes, doing something drastic draws the attention of other people. What this woman did reduced the stress in her life. It is not selfish for people to take care of themselves—especially when they are responsible for other people (i.e., parents).

It is important to be flexible. Redesigning a constricted frame of reference can occur over time. The following exercise (Borysenko, 1984) demonstrates how you can take a different perspective on ideas that you might deem to be irreversible. Take a few moments to solve this nine-dot puzzle. The object is to connect all of the dots with four, straight, continuous lines without lifting up your pencil. No curves are permitted. Allow yourself some time before reading further.

•   •   •

•   •   •

•   •   •

If you had any difficulty with this teaser, do not despair. Try the puzzle again; this time, do not restrict yourself to the confines of the box shape. Redesign the pattern to fit your needs.

Good job. Whether you succeeded or not, you realized that the solution lay in going outside of the parameters of the box. Having overcome this obstacle, you understand the need to expand your frame of reference in relation to this puzzle or anything else.

People often limit themselves through thought, much like with the box in the preceding example. These self-imposed limitations function to impede growth and limit success in reaching goals. People's stress response schemata are based on seasoned response modes, or stress boxes. Individuals are accustomed to dealing with situations in this manner without realizing that these ingrained responses are contributing variables in the overall stress equation. The solution remains in recognizing that each person is capable of breaking out of the confines of the box and emerging stronger and more adept at challenging the bounds of even larger boxes. This newfound inner resolve can intensify the person's drive to succeed by reducing the stress created by the "boxed-in" feeling and by fostering self-actualization.

A more personal note on what it takes to prioritize a person's life involves one of the authors who had the very fortunate opportunity to become friends with a colleague who was suffering from cancer. This colleague was dying; he knew; and the people he worked with knew. Although the author did not see his colleague's emotional progression with the disease, this individual seemed to be in the stage of acceptance. One day during a one-on-one conversation, the idea of future planning came up. The colleague chuckled and said that his idea of future planning was vastly different than that of most other people; obviously, he knew that his days were numbered.

Subsequently, it has become apparent to this author that too often people prioritize areas that maybe are not that important. A new philosophy of life has emerged for him that is related to stress: *How important will this be when I am on my deathbed?* Of course, you have probably heard that when you are on your deathbed, you are not going to be thinking, "Gee, I wish I had spent more time at the office"; you are more likely to think, "Gee, I wish I had spent more time with my children (spouse, friends, family)." The point is that if a person thinks, *How important will I think this is when I am on my deathbed?*, that person's priorities might change.

It is also important to talk to your friends about what is important. Sharing your stressors with others may help you to see that many of your stressors are only *perceived* stress. In a classroom setting, when people share with the group their "stress" at not having something completed (i.e., folded towels), the importance of the issue becomes minimized.

An important aspect of prioritizing is determining how much time there is to do something and getting as much done as possible during that time. This is known as *time management*. Time is considered by many to be one the most precious commodities in the world. Though people may attempt to control time, slow time, or even speed time up, the reality is that not one of these notions is possible. The best people can do is simply to *manage* their time. That may seem impossible when there are so many things to do and so little time, but there are methods for managing time that can add valuable moments to a person's life.

Time management is *not* about becoming inflexible with your schedule. Actually, when you manage your time, you have more time for flexibility and spontaneity in your life. Consider the following options for managing your time.

First, draw a horizontal line at the bottom and one at the top of a piece of paper. Then, divide the remaining space into the times of the day that you are awake. For example, your top line may be 5:00 a.m., and your bottom line may be 12:00 midnight. In this example, your space would be divided into nineteen hours. You might be thinking this is too early to wake up and/or too late to go to sleep, but that is why you create your own chart. After dividing your paper into the hours of the day, write within the time slots when you have commitments. For instance, if you have class from 1:00 p.m. to 5:00 p.m., then those hours would be considered *committed hours*. Remaining hours would be considered *discretionary hours*. Certainly, if you are a student, your commitments do not merely revolve around school. Perhaps you are working or need to devote a certain amount of time to study each week; or you must allow time for meals or time to drive to the university and/or work; or you have other commitments that are simply unchangeable. After completing a chart for each day of the week, you will have a better idea of what hours are devoted to necessary tasks and what hours remain for discretionary time. (See Table 8.1 for one day's chart.)

Certainly, this will provide you with a global picture of how you are spending your time. Remember, once time is spent, it cannot be recaptured. Therefore, you must use your time wisely. Consider how this exercise can help you. Instead of simply hanging out between classes, you could use part of this time to study, pay your bills, write a letter, or whatever else is necessary. Although you may enjoy talking with your friends between classes, this may be one of the behaviors that limit your time. This is not to say that you should not talk to your friends; it only suggests that many people are simply unaware of where their time is going.

TABLE 8.1   Sample of Time Management Plan

7:00 A.M.–8:00 A.M.	Get ready for school/Travel to school
8:00 A.M.–9:00 A.M.	Psychology class
9:00 A.M.–10:00 A.M.	Study
10:00 A.M.–11:00 A.M.	Economics class
11:00 A.M.–12:00 noon	Lunch
12:00 noon–1:00 p.m.	Work
1:00 P.M.–2:00 P.M.	Work
2:00 P.M.–3:00 P.M.	Work
3:00 P.M.–4:00 P.M.	Work
4:00 P.M.–5:00 P.M.	Work
5:00 P.M.–6:00 P.M.	Work
6:00 P.M.–7:00 P.M.	Travel home
7:00 P.M.–8:00 P.M.	Dinner
8:00 P.M.–9:00 P.M.	Study
9:00 P.M.–10:00 P.M.	Free time
10:00 P.M.–11:00 P.M.	Free time

Truthfully, one of the most important steps in time management is awareness; only when you are aware of how your time is spent can you make changes that will lead to better time management.

According to Covey (1989), time-management matrix in Table 8.2 illustrates how people choose to use their time. Consider the four quadrants of the illustration, and consider where you are spending your time. For example, going to class, studying, or working would be considered *important, but not urgent* (Q2). These are simply necessary tasks that individuals are committed to. Talking on the telephone, watching television, surfing the net, and similar behaviors would be considered *not urgent, and not important* (Q3). These activities are "of the moment" and feel good but consume large amounts of a person's time. If they are activities that a person enjoys, then they should be placed should be somewhere into the person's schedule. Thus, the person controls the activities rather than these activities controlling the person's schedule.

For the following seven days, complete time-management tables like the one shown in Table 8.1, and examine how it makes you more aware of your time and how it is being spent. Then, throughout the day, check off which quadrant applies to each activity. For example, place a check in Q3 while watching television and so on with your other activities. Then, examine the quadrants to see where you are spending the majority of your time. Again, this is only a tool to help you to become more aware of how you are spending your time. Using this exercise in conjunction with your schedule can enable you to manage your time more efficiently, therefore providing you with additional time to engage in more of the activities that are meaningful to you.

TABLE 8.2 Time Management Matrices

Not Important **Not Urgent**	**Important** **Not Urgent**
Organizing papers, straightening files, and involving oneself in tasks that simply do not make a difference.	This is the quadrant where most effective time managers spend more time.
Not Important **Urgent**	**Important** **Urgent**
Answering telephone and opening mail.	Otherwise known as a crisis or an emergency.

Use Social Support

Over the past two decades, health educators have become more familiar with, supportive of, and accepting of the fact that social support plays a critical role in helping individuals deal with stress. What is social support? *Social support* is the social connection that a person has with other people; it is especially important when a person is under stress (Pierce, Sarson, & Sarason 1996). It is more than just a pool of friends; it extends through a person's work environment, business, and civic efforts. The research is showing that the broader a person's social-support network, the more likely that person will be able to deal with stress. Such a network can increase its members' "self-esteem, a sense of well-being, and support one another in coping with developmental transitions and life stress" (Hartup & Stevens, 1999).

An individual should have a social-support system that consists of a variety of individuals. For example, imagine a group of people between the ages of twenty-three and twenty-six who are all teachers and are all friends. Imagine that one of them loses his or her job. Of course, the friends will be saddened by the loss and they will be supportive, but chances are they may not have any insight into what it takes to get a new job. Chances are they all know the same people or "types of people." They may not even know what they could do with their skills— other than teaching. However, if a person makes an effort to make connections with a variety of individuals from a variety of ages and business interests, that person might be able to get more advice on how to deal with this major stressor (losing the job). People often confuse *social-support network* with *best buddies*; that is not the case. It is important to make connections with all types of people. In fact, people get linked into social-support networks to both give and take.

People can increase their social-support networks by going beyond what they normally do. Volunteering is a great way to expand a social-support system (although this should be considered a benefit of volunteering, not the primary reason to volunteer). Becoming involved with church or other civic groups is another option.

Yet another way to increase social support is to do business locally. It is possible to save some money on items such as car insurance if bought through the mail. However, buying auto insurance from a local agent keeps money in the community, and contacts are made that may extend beyond just car insurance. For instance, a connection with an insurance agent might, in the case of the unemployed teacher, provide an opportunity to use teaching skills to sell insurance.

Research from the late 1970s and later has shown that social support *buffers* one from the effects of stress. Talking out concerns, knowing that somebody is there to help through a rough time, or helping somebody out personally appears to be "good for the soul." However, social-support networks need both give and take. Have you ever been invited to dinner at somebody's house? It is not unusual to ask if you can bring something. How does it feel when you are told "no"? You might feel very awkward coming to somebody's house for dinner without bringing anything. Oftentimes, even if you are told not to bring anything, you do. Typically, you might bring a bottle of wine or some type of dessert.

As already noted, the wife of one of the authors keeps the house immaculate. She is also a great cook and makes exceptional lasagna. When she does make it, she tends to make a lot, so it is no big deal to invite extra people over for dinner. A co-worker of this author has been invited over a number of times for dinner. She graciously accepts, always brings something to contribute (i.e., dessert), and always leaves full, grateful, and commenting that she needs to reciprocate by having the host family over to her house. Well, in reality, she lives alone in a small house that is too small to hold a family with three children. Social support, in this case, does not mean providing the same "services." Whereas the author and his wife provide a dinner, the co-worker colleague provides a social support at work!

People get involved with other people for various reasons. One is obviously to gain from others' talents, but it is also important to be able to *give* to others. The co-worker invited to dinner often brings some dessert (i.e., ice cream). The first few times this occurred, the author's wife insisted that she take the remaining ice cream back home with her. It was clear that the co-worker was very uncomfortable with taking it back home. She *needed* to feel that she contributed to the dinner. The fact that she spent more money on the ice cream than she would have if she had gone to a restaurant for a single dinner is irrelevant.

Social support between people works only if both people can give and take. If one person is taking all the time, they will feel awkward and will stop asking. On the other hand, those that give all the time need to know that it is also acceptable to take.

By taking, a sense of honor is provided to the giver. Taking support also helps to buffer the effects of stressors that are encountered.

Use Humor

The fourth method of dealing with stress is through the use of humor. This is not to say that humor can *eliminate* many of the problems that people may encounter, but it certainly can help people *cope* with awkward and difficult times. In the mid-

1960s, Norman Cousins was diagnosed with a disease that had a very small chance of recovery. After some studying, Cousins discovered that the disease was enhanced by stress. He decided that he would attempt to alleviate his pain through the use of laughter. He spent time watching various movies and shows that allowed him to laugh. He discovered that laughing for ten minutes could reduce his discomfort and pain for up to two hours. He continued this "therapy," and soon his disease went into remission. He has attributed his recovery to his use of humor (Cousins, 1978). Although most people may never use humor to that extreme, it can be used nonetheless to help buffer against the effects of stress.

It is difficult to define how a person can become more *humorous*. Humor is personal, and what one person finds humorous another may find offensive. Rather, it is important for a person to develop the attitude of not taking too many things too seriously. Humor allows people to laugh at themselves in a fun, caring fashion, not in a mean-spirited manner.

Perhaps a way to start is to do what Cousins did, that is, find something that makes you laugh. Cousins found Laurel and Hardy movies exceptionally funny; some people, on the other hand, find little humor in their movies. Some of the current situation comedies are offensive to many people. Humor is unique to each individual; what one person finds funny, another may find boring. Two movies, *Used Cars* and *Animal House,* are considered funny by some people; these movies provide belly laughs and a time to forget about the worries of the day. However, many people may be offended by the "antics" in the movies.

Structure Activities to Reduce Stress

The preceding techniques are very important for helping a person to deal with stress. These alone may be sufficient; on the other hand, as already discussed, they may be part of a multieffort strategy. Structuring activities to reduce stress can include two components—those activities that are considered *chair bound* and those that must be done *out of chair.*

Out-of-chair activities take a certain amount of physical work to do. The following can be considered as physical: (1) exercise; (2) Yoga/stretching; (3) tai chi; and (4) massage. *Chair-bound* activities are those activities that can be done just sitting in a chair or lying down. Three of the key techniques are mental imagery, progressive relaxation, and meditation.

However, a discussion of the role that breathing plays must come first. Perhaps nothing is more at the basis of relaxing than breathing. Some stress-management practices focus solely on breathing to decrease arousal of the body (McGuigan, 1999). In fact, Van Dixhoorn (1999) has worked extensively with cardiac patients teaching them how to use breathing to minimize their stress.

Most people breathe without considering much about it. They inhale and exhale thousands of times a day. But what is it that breathing does to help people with relaxation? First, as the body works (which is all of the time), it manufactures waste products. These waste products are picked up by the blood cells in exchange for oxygen. As the blood is transported through the lungs, the waste products are discarded and oxygen is picked up. Bear in mind that not all blood cells make the exchange in the lungs. One of the keys to relaxation is making sure that fresh oxygen is supplied to parts of the body. Imagine a very crowded marathon with everybody running in the same direction. A runner comes up to a water station to get water, but it is quite possible that because of the crowd that person may not be able to get the water. If by chance the person misses this particular water spot, it is not going to "kill" him or her and in most instances the runner can pick up water at the next stop. However, if obtaining water at several of these water stations fails, chances are that finishing the marathon becomes impossible, or, if it is completed, it is done with great physical discomfort.

The second aspect is more psychological. Breathing can be a relaxing and soothing activity—especially if it is done properly. But what does *breathing properly* mean? How can a person breathe improperly? Please read through this next section, then put the book down and follow the directions:

> First, lie on your back on the floor, the bed, or a couch. Make sure you are comfortable. Breathe for the next two minutes, and pay particular attention to your abdomen and to your chest. Both the abdomen and the chest will rise and they will fall. Pay particular attention to when each (chest and abdomen) rises and falls.
> Now, put the book down and do what was just asked of you to do.

What did you find out? When you breathed in, did your chest or abdomen rise? When you breathed out, did your chest or abdomen fall? Physiologically, the ideal way to breathe is what is sometimes referred to as *diaphragmatic breathing* (Schafer, 1999). When inhaling, the stomach should rise and expand. When exhaling, the stomach should flatten out (Blonna, 1996). The reason for this is that by expanding your stomach you are allowing your diaphragm to pull down and allow more air to enter into your lungs. This allows for greater efficiency of oxygen exchange within the red blood cells. Have you ever had the situation where you took a deep breath and realized how good it felt? This is actually getting more oxygen into your system.

The *external* strategy in breathing is also important. With some exceptions, you should attempt to breathe in through your nose and allow the expiration to take place through the mouth. Think back to a time when you had a cold. Your nose might have been so congested that the only way you could breathe was through your mouth. Typically, you wake up with extreme dryness in the mouth. Breathing in through the nose allows the air to be moisturized, warmed, and cleansed. Breathing out through the mouth is soothing. To help individuals focus on their state of relaxation, stress-management instructors often use the feel and sound of the air rushing through the throat.

You can incorporate using breathing as a relaxation tool into your lifestyle with little or no difficulty. A massage therapist has given one of the authors a card that reminds him to *breathe*. Every time he sees that sign, he is reminded to focus on breathing. Obviously, you need no equipment to do this activity, and you can do this while performing any other tasks. If you are attempting to quit smoking (or to reduce your snack intake), you know that sometimes the cravings can be overwhelming. Simply putting down whatever you are doing and concentrating on your breathing for a minute can help you overcome such cravings.

In many activities, people are often encouraged to start their activity with a deep, cleansing breath. For many, this is the start of their relaxation effort. A deep, cleansing breath is done by inhaling through the nose fully, filling the lungs. You should hold your breath for just a short time period (three to five seconds) and slowly allow the air to be expired out through your throat.

As stated at the beginning of this chapter, there is no perfect stress-management technique. You must choose what you are most comfortable with. Breathing can be all that you need to help you with your relaxation. Ten minutes of focused concentration on your breathing can do wonders. Following is another example and demonstration. As before, please read this next section, then put the book down and do what you have read. Then come back to reading the book. The activity is only two minutes in length, so even if you are pressed for time, this will not take a great amount (and there is a good chance that you will actually be more refreshed afterward):

> Sit in a comfortable chair, and do not have any part of your body pressed against another part (in other words, do not cross your legs or ankles). Do not lean forward with your chin in your hands. Sit comfortably, hands somewhere on your lap. Find a clock with a second hand that you can focus on. Here is your challenge. Starting with two deep cleansing breaths, try to get between fourteen and sixteen breaths within two minutes. A breath is considered an inhalation and an expiration. For this to work, it is imperative that you strive to get fourteen to sixteen breaths for this session. That is about seven to eight breaths per minute, which is about seven to eight seconds per breath cycle.
>
> Now put this book down, find your clock, and do your activity.

Assuming you have indeed done the activity, what are your thoughts? Were you able to achieve the goal of breathing fourteen to sixteen times for these two minutes? Try to remember what you were thinking about while you were doing this. You were probably really concentrating on finding the right *tempo* of breathing. You probably were very conscious of your breathing, each breath in and each breath out.

Now, consider some questions. While you were doing this, did you think of anything else? Were you worried about any upcoming tests or major papers? Were you worried about that relationship that you are in with that special person? Did you think about how you were going to pay some of your bills this month? If you did, chances are that you allowed those thoughts to leave quickly because you were concentrating on your breathing. But, it is quite probable that none of those thoughts came into your mind. Why? Because you were concentrating on your breathing, which is how breathing can serve as an efficient and effective stress-management technique. Remember that breathing has a critical function in all types of stress-management activities.

As you may have noted from this activity, another critical factor in stress management is concentration. By concentrating, you are able to prevent those *negative* thoughts (remember that most stressors are caused by thoughts) from entering your system. Breathing can, in and of itself, be a way to cope with daily stressors. The advantage is that you can do this in almost any location and usually inconspicuously to the outside world.

This breathing discussion illustrates a function of the mind-body relationship. If the mind can be *relaxed* (as in the case of breathing), then the body follows suit. During the preceding activity, if someone could measure your bodily functions (ideally with some type of machine like Dr. McCoy held above a patient's body on the original *Star Trek* series), the person would find that during this two-minute time period the following things happened:

1. Your heart rate was reduced.
2. Your heart output increased.
3. You had better oxygen exchange.
4. Your muscles became more relaxed.
5. Your blood pressure dropped.

These are pretty good things to have happen to your body. However, the preceding two-minute activity is not necessarily the breathing relaxation approach that a person should follow. This activity is to illustrate the power of concentration. Obviously, a peson can go longer than these two minutes (remember, experts recommend somewhere between fifteen to twenty minutes a day of doing something relaxing). You could put on some very relaxing music (two or three songs) that would equal this time period, and you could just sit back, focus on some item (or close your eyes), and just concentrate on your breathing. When the songs are over, the activity is over.

Chair-Bound Activities.   If a person can achieve these physical benefits from a *mind* activity, it only makes sense that a person can achieve a state of mental relaxation by doing a physical activity. Again, in the mind-body relationship, if one becomes relaxed, the other will follow suit. In other words, when the body becomes relaxed, the mind follows suit. If the mind becomes relaxed, the body then follows suit. If focusing on breathing alone is uncomfortable, reverse it and concentrate on the physical body; the mind, in turn, will become relaxed (please note the importance of breathing in this activity).

Progressive Relaxation.   Muscles have two states, a state of contraction and a state of relaxation. Obviously, you can *contract* any muscle on command, but most people do not know that you can also *relax* any muscle on command. It takes training, but it is possible. A researcher named Jacobson (1955) discovered several decades ago that people could heighten their awareness of the tension in their muscles by first contracting and overtensing such muscles. Then, once their focus was on that part of the body, they could concentrate on relaxing that same part. Keep in mind that there are thousands of different strategies and that there are volumes written on Jacobson's writings. Following is a "modified" approach to relaxing your muscles.

First, find a comfortable place to lie down. You may sit in a chair, but comfort is most important. Do not have any pressure points on your body (i.e., no crossing of knees). Since the examples given are based on your lying down, some modifications may be needed if you are sitting in a chair.

Second, loosen up any tight clothing such as shirt collar, belt, and shoelaces. Third, if you find it uncomfortable to lie flat, you can place your head on a small pillow and/or place something (i.e., pillow, rolled towel) under your knees. Take off your glasses and place them in a safe spot. For those individuals who wear contacts, if you cannot keep your eyes closed for a long period of time, consider removing your contacts. Finally, turn off your phone and/or answering machine (or at least turn the volume down) so that your concentration is not disturbed.

Once you are comfortable lying down, take two to three deep cleansing breaths. Close your eyes, and again take two or three breaths. Starting with your head, scan your body, noting any feelings that you have, any particular aches or pains, any sense of heaviness, or any sense of warmth.

Evaluate this experience. You may note that time seemed distorted. You may think of this activity as being much shorter than it was. You may view it as a much longer event. If you are new to these activities, some type of mechanism to alert you to the time may be needed. (It is best to avoid using an alarm clock; the shrill sound of the alarm will probably undo what has just been accomplished. Other options might include using a less obtrusive timer on your computer or asking somebody to gently knock on the office door after a certain period of time.) As you were concentrating on your arms, legs, abdomen, and head, chances are that you were not able to spend a lot of time worrying about the stressors that you face each day.

Mental Imagery.   Simply stated, mental imagery is picturing events in the mind. The mind is a powerful organ that can affect all parts of the body. For example, imagine having a slice of lemon placed on your tongue. Close your eyes and imagine seeing the lemon. Watch it being sliced in half with juice and seeds spilling forth. Then imagine another thin slice being made and having it placed on your tongue. Imagine the tartness, the sourness, the increased saliva flow, and the puckering sensation from *having* that lemon on your tongue. The amazing thing is that there is no lemon on your tongue.

So, use this powerful tool—the brain—to help you relax. Mental imagery, like muscle relaxation, has had thousands of pages written about it. What is written in this chapter is a very brief synopsis of the authors' interpretation of mental imagery. More important are some practical tips that you can incorporate into your lifestyle.

As with muscle-relaxation activities, it is important to be very comfortable sitting or lying down. Make sure all tight and/or restrictive clothing is loosened or removed, and make sure that your shoelaces are untied. Typically, you can do this sitting up, but lying down is also a viable option.

The beauty of any of these strategies is that they can be modified to meet your particular needs. The length of the activity and how you perform it (sitting or lying) can both be modified with no problems. The key point is that you are concentrating on relaxing the mind or the body, with the other following suit. You can just focus on those things that make you happy.

Think of a beautiful scene that you have witnessed. One of the authors lived in Maine in 1978. He would use a mountain path for one of his running routes (it took about forty-five minutes to run to the top). When he would get to the top, he typically would turn around and run back (another thirty-minute trip). As with many people who are into serious running, he was really into training hard and for many weeks after arriving in August he would just concentrate on the run. One day in late September, during the peak of the fall foliage, he stopped when he reached the peak of the mountain. He looked at the valley below. It was like a picture—the foliage with the bright colors, overlooking a small village, a church steeple sticking out above the tree lines, cool crisp air. That picture still remains in this author's mind. When he wants to relax with a visual image, that is what comes to mind. Twenty-five years later, he still remembers it.

Meditation.   Many of the techniques discussed in this section "borrow" from other techniques. Perhaps the only difference in meditation compared to the muscle relaxation, breathing, or mental imagery is the slight difference in focus on why it is being done. Whereas most people say they do mental imagery to try to reduce stress, many people who meditate say they do it to better understand themselves, to communicate with their spiritual side, or to seek answers from God. *Meditate* comes from the Latin word *meditari,* which means to reflect, ponder, or think about (McGuigan, 1999).

Meditation can be categorized into two efforts: transcendental meditation (TM)—or a modification thereof—and prayer. A professor in Czechoslovakia met with one of the authors. This professor taught stress management. He came under increasing amounts of pressure to not "teach" meditation because of the influence of the Catholic Church. Apparently, the church did not like the word *meditation.* He decided to refrain from the word meditation, because most people thought of it (falsely) as having to do with religion—especially Eastern religion. Instead, he referred to the event as *quiet time* or *prayer,* which has received no complaints. The bottom line is that yes, meditation can be spiritual in nature. However, it does not have to be. It is up to individuals to interpret however it is best for them. It works as a coping device regardless of what it is called.

So, how does a person meditate? Again, the key word is concentration. Benson (1975) has taken the complex and often mystical properties of transcendental meditation and has restructured it to be more to the liking of Western society. This approach follows.

First, as with all such activities, you need to find a comfortable position. The lotus position may seem good, but, if you are physically unable to do it comfortably, then it can do more harm than good. Sit in a comfortable chair, undo all restrictive clothing, take off your glasses, and sit comfortably. Take two or three deep cleansing breaths.

Rice (1999) claims that there are four elements to meditation: a quiet environment, an object to focus on mentally, a comfortable position, and a passive attitude. Finally, a major key to meditation is your breathing. Carefully monitor each breath as it enters through your nose and continues down your windpipe and into your lungs. Allow your diaphragm to expand (make sure you breathe properly). After you hold the breath for a few seconds, slowly allow the breath to leave via your throat and mouth. With TM, you are given a certain word or phrase (mantra) to repeat with each breath. However, Benson's research (1975) found that any single-syllable, nonthreatening word could serve the same purpose. Thus, he suggests using a simple word like *one, love,* or God.

The theory behind this approach is that through this repetition of breathing and focusing on one nonthreatening word, the body (and mind) starts to relax. As with most other stress-management strategies, it is suggested that a person practice this strategy around fifteen minutes a day.

Similar to Benson's approach (1975) to meditation, prayer requires the same elements but with a focus on communication with the individual's God. Schafer (1999) indicates that prayer can be used to relieve anxiety. The concern that both Schafer and Seaward (1997) have is that the person becomes dependent upon prayer to answer all of life's problems without taking on responsibility for such problems.

Techniques for prayer can be similar to those already discussed. However, you can substitute a deep thought directed toward God. Seaward (1997) quotes Jackson H. Brown: "Do not pray for things, but rather pray for wisdom and courage" (p. 292).

Out-of-Chair Activities. As already noted, out-of-chair activities take some physical work. The following paragraphs discuss some common out-of-chair techniques.

Exercise. People are quick to think that exercise is the cure-all for all stress problems, but it is not. Exercise can be as much a stressor as it is a stress reliever. As with most issues with stress, much of it goes back to how the activity is perceived.

Consider the following question. Physiologically, what is the major difference between being under stress and exercising? First, both have heart rates that are substantially elevated; blood pressure is also increased along with cardiac output. Muscles are tense; a reduction of blood flow to unnecessary systems takes place (i.e., urinary and digestive tracts). Sweating takes place. So what is the major difference? Do not say that it is because the body can distinguish between good stress and bad stress, because it can not. When your heart is beating faster, it does not matter what caused it; it is beating faster.

The major difference between the two (and this is where exercise is a good stress reducer) is that during exercise your breathing is heavier. Because it is heavier, you are able to obtain fresh oxygen and replace the by-products of stress (and normal body functions) with oxygen. When you are under a lot of stress (say that you are under the clock to get a term paper done by tomorrow a.m.), your heart races, your blood pressure increases, your muscles are tense, and so on. But, you are not sitting there breathing like you have just completed a one-mile run; your breathing is regular. Thus, your body is producing all of the by-products of cell metabolism and it is not able to replace them with fresh air as quickly as if you were exercising. Obviously, there are other benefits to exercise (muscles become stronger, have more tone, are more resilient), which can never take place if you do not exercise.

Basically, any type of exercise can help reduce stress, if you allow it to. Consider this last statement. Perhaps you know a very competitive person who after a game of racquetball (or golf, or tennis, or whatever that person selects) is more stressed than before they started? A very competitive and good racquetball player (national ranking) experienced any game as a life and death event. If he missed a shot, he would swear, get incredibly angry, throw his racquet, and otherwise be miserable. Even if he won, he was always critical of his game. He was more stressed after than he was before. Certainly the physical movement may have helped him with his cardiovascular and muscular systems, but it did nothing to help him relax.

Exercise is not a good event to do to reduce a person's stress if it is a competitive or an ego-loaded activity. In other words, for exercise to help reduce stress, the activity must be noncompetitive and ego-void (Girdano et al., 1997). This is especially true if an individual has had some extensive experience with a particular activity. For example, at one point, one of the authors was a very competitive (and fairly decent) distance runner. During those time periods of his life, running was not relaxing; it was extremely stressful. He noted each workout for his stamina, time, length of distance, and pulse rates. He monitored everything he ate (almost to a point of compulsion). Racing was serious business. It was tough for him to go out and *enjoy* a run. Obviously, it would have been a mistake for him to use running as his coping mechanism. Running was certainly a benefit to his physiological self (and to a lesser extent his mental self), but it was not a stress-reducing activity. He had to use other mechanisms to deal with his stress. Even today, nearly twenty years after his most competitive years, it is still very difficult for him to go out for a run just for fun. It is, however, more of a stress reducer than it once was.

Walking, swimming, running, and biking are all great ideas for reducing stress—assuming that a person backs away from being too competitive. Many people like to exercise with somebody else; others prefer to be by themselves.

As with using exercise to improve fitness, if you use exercise to reduce stress, you need to do it on a regular basis and for a substantial period of time (fifteen to thirty minutes). You can arrange such activity at any time during the day. Some people use their lunch breaks for their walks; others do it first thing in the morning. Some prefer it in the later day or evening. It is probably best to avoid heavy exercising late in the day or evening, as it might make it difficult to relax and fall asleep.

If you are just starting an exercise program, it is wise to start with a walking regimen. Assuming you have no physical problems walking (i.e., knee pains), you should wear a good quality walking shoe, and comfortable clothes (do not overdress) and start a four or five days a week walking routine. Start with fifteen minutes and add two to three minutes each week. Once you have reached forty-five minutes, you will have an excellent foundation to obtain good physical health.

If you have a desire to do any other type of activity, it would be wise to contact somebody at your university's exercise science/physical education department or the university's athletic training program for a personalized plan.

Yoga/Stretching.   Similar to many of the concepts with exercise, Yoga is another active method that can be used to reduce stress. The previous chapter discussed the mind-body relationship. That is, if your mind is relaxed, the body follows suit. On the other hand, if you can relax your body, your mind will then become relaxed. There are numerous types of Yoga, but the specific one discussed in this section is called *Hatha Yoga.* It is a very disciplined activity in which partipants focus their energies on parts of their bodies. Yoga is typically thought of as stretching; in reality it is much more. It is a combination of the mental, physical, social, and spiritual self (Blonna, 1996). By concentrating deeply with each movement, you not only can stretch a particular part of the body, but you can also create and maintain a certain amount of mental discipline. To effectively stretch, you need to concentrate on your breathing, the part of the body where the *pull* is taking place, and proper body alignment while performing the stretch. Throughout this time period, as you focus your attention on the stretch, your mind is allowed to be free of concerns and worries that may otherwise surround you. There is no guarantee that Yoga will prevent stressors from coming into existence. Rather it is a way to allow you to take time each day (hopefully) to not allow those stressors to bother you.

The physical benefits of stretching are also important. Many back and neck problems are the result of poor flexibility. Especially as a person ages, the muscles become less flexible. Thus, it is absolutely essential to take time to stretch.

This section does not necessarily focus on the true dimension of Yoga, but it does provide some basic guidelines. Someone interested in learning more about Yoga can look in the phone directory for any local services regarding Yoga or can check with local YMCAs, a wellness center, or a local health provider.

Following are a few basics regarding Yoga. First, do not think of this stretch as a competition. This is especially true with novices. They will see somebody who is very flexible and will try to *compete* with them. Flexibility is highly personal and is obtained slowly (especially if a person has not stretched on a regular basis before). You should avoid the temptation of comparing your progress to others. Also, some people, no matter how much they stretch, will never be as flexible as some people who never stretch.

You might find differences and irregularities in your flexibility on different sides of your body. For example, you may find that your right hamstring is more flexible than your left; then you should plan to spend a little extra time with your left side.

The trick to stretching is to do it on a regular basis for a sizable amount of time (i.e., twenty minutes). It is also important to do the stretching in slow, non-sudden movements. Forget the high school gym class of calisthenics where you bounced to get loose. Rather, you should slowly reach down to the point of the *burn,* and then hold it for several seconds. (Bouncing to get loose can actually have the opposite effect.) Make sure that you breathe during the stretch–do not hold your breath. In addition, by focusing on your breathing, you are able to concentrate more on your stretch and not go into oxygen deprivation.

Finally, the proper body alignment for the stretch can make a big difference in reaching its maximum effect, which is one reason that taking Yoga or a stretching class is beneficial. The trained instructor can observe body mechanics to allow for maximum stretch. For example, the placement of your head can make an incredible difference on the stretch of your hamstrings.

Following are a few key stretches that can help your flexibility and also help you to develop mental discipline (the real benefit of Yoga). Obviously, derivations exist, and you should make modifications accordingly. The diagrams are courtesy of the webpage The Yoga Site.*

1. The Rib Stretch (Trikonasana—the Triangle)

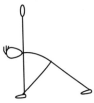

Standing with your feet apart at about shoulder width, turn the left foot away from your body. Point arms out to the side and slowly rotate the trunk so that your left hand starts to point to your left foot and your right arm points in the air. Your head should face toward your right hand. The stretch should be really noticeable in the right ribs, the right hips, and hamstrings. Breathe in and out and hold for ten seconds. Slowly bring your trunk upright. Repeat the procedure the opposite way.

2. Shoulder (or partial shoulder) Stand (Ardha Sarvangasana)

Lie on your back. Slowly slide your feet up to your buttocks with knees bent. Placing your hands on your buttocks for support, raise your legs and point them in the air. You should be resting on your shoulders. Be sure to breathe. When you become more flexible, you can slowly allow gravity to bring your ankles over your head. Again, be sure to breathe.

3. The Sun Stand (Tadasana)

Stand with your feet together, pointed forward with your hands to your side. Take several deep, cleansing breaths. Slowly bring your arms up from your side and point the fingers outward. Continue bringing them up over your head, and place your palms together over your head. Reach high for the sky, point your head up, and look at your hands. This will stretch your arms, back, and neck. Continue breathing. You can even rise to the balls of your feet. Slowly lower your feet, hands, and head back to the starting position. You can do this several times, with each round taking a minute or two.

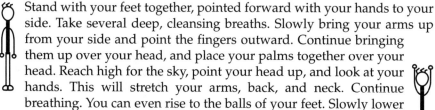

4. Hamstring Stretch (Uttanasana II)

Inhale, and raise your arms overhead. Exhale, bend at the hips, and bring your arms forward and down until you touch the floor. It is OK to bend your knees, especially if you are feeling stiff. Either grasp your ankles or just leave your hands on the floor, and breathe several times. Focus on your breathing. This helps both your hamstrings and your lower back.

5. Lower Back Stretch (Adho Mukha Svanasana)

Start on your hands and knees. Keep your legs about hip width apart and your arms shoulder width apart. Your middle fingers should be parallel, 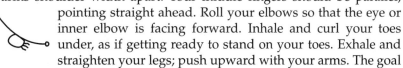 pointing straight ahead. Roll your elbows so that the eye or inner elbow is facing forward. Inhale and curl your toes under, as if getting ready to stand on your toes. Exhale and straighten your legs; push upward with your arms. The goal is to lengthen the spine while keeping your legs straight and your feet flat on the ground.

Again, these are not any substitute for a Yoga class, and, if any Yoga experts are reading this chapter, they are shaking in dismay that *Yoga* and *stretching* are used interchangeably. Just keep in mind that the primary goal of Yoga is to create mental discipline. You can obtain the same type of focus with ordinary stretching.

Tai Chi. Tai chi is an ancient oriental activity that focuses on mind discipline and movement. Whereas Yoga is predominantly stretching, Tai chi has various movements, stretches, and strides. Tai Chi is used to help individuals maintain some control over their physical selves and is sometimes referred to as a *moving meditation.*

According to Chinese tradition, there is a life force that runs throughout each individual. This life force is called *chi* (pronounced *chee*) (Seaward, 1997). Focusing on this life force allows a person to clear the mind of unnecessary stressors (at least while doing the activity).

Proponents of tai chi (and those of Yoga) claim that, by practicing such mind discipline, people will start to prioritize their lifestyles and perhaps the events that would normally cause them stress will somehow not seem to be that big of a problem. Such claims have not been substantiated through scientific research, but there are many people who give testimonials to the value of these activities. There are millions of people of Chinese origin who have used tai chi (and Yoga) who have dramatically changed their lives—not only in their physical presence but also with their minds. When people can practice mind control over their physical movements, the ability to transfer such mastery to emotional aspects is improved.

Massage. Human touch is one of the most critical components of having a healthy life (Van Boven, 1997). Studies of infants who have been denied such touch show them to be more susceptible to illness, more aggressive, and taking longer and having more difficult times maintaining close, intimate relationships. Clearly, humans were meant to be physically close to one another, not just in sexual intimacy but through nonintimate involvement (light kissing, hugging, or just plain physical touch).

Massage is an activity that allows a person to relax physically, which then allows the mind to follow suit. Massage can be something given to somebody through either a professional massage therapist or just through a friend or loved one; it benefits not only those who receive but also those who give massage; or it can even be given in the form of self-massage.

In the history of the United States, massage has somehow gotten a nasty reputation. Perhaps it is because many people have seen or been part of the *massage parlor* agenda. In many instances, such massage parlors were fronts for organized prostitution. However, during the past twenty years, professionals in massage—massage therapists—have worked hard to promote the idea that massage has an incredible soothing power. In many areas in the country, massage therapy is now third-party reimbursable, which means that health insurance will now pay for such services.

Massage can benefit people physically as well as emotionally. As with most aspects of stress management, if a person can relax physically, the mind follows suit. Thus, as a person receives massage, it is unlikely that the person will have worries during that time.

The problem with this is that most people cannot afford to *pay* for a professional massage on a daily basis; thus it may not have the same benefits as other stress-management activities because of its infrequency. However, as stated earlier, massage does not necessarily have to be done by a professional to derive a benefit—massage can come from a caring individual, or a person can participate in self-massage.

Becoming a professional massage therapist requires training of approximately two years in length with approximately 500 hours of coursework and numerous years of practical experience (Seaward, 1997). Although at this time massage therapists are not licensed, many states do certify them. Florida, for example, has an elaborate certification process. Thus, if a person wants to verify that a massage therapist is legitimate, the therapist's academic training and any certifications can be requested. Many states do not have licensure or certification for massage therapists, yet many massage therapists make a point of obtaining their certification in those states that do. Thus, many massage therapists seek Florida certification.

You can expect to pay anywhere from $50 to $100 for a full-body massage. Most massage therapists recommend a full hour for a full-body massage. However, if you are receiving a partial massage for just a targeted part of the body (i.e., legs), then a thirty-minute massage may be sufficient.

Generally speaking, the person entering the therapy room will be asked to disrobe and to drape his or her body with a sheet. A person can choose to be completely undressed or to keep underwear on. For those individuals who desire complete nudity, the massage therapist maintains dignity and privacy by using the sheets to drape the person and only working on the designated area of the body (i.e., the back).

After the client disrobes and covers up with a sheet, the massage therapist enters. It is common for the massage therapist to ask a series of questions
about the client before proceeding with any massage. The therapist needs to
know if the client has a sore back or neck or any other problems. It is very
important for an individual to continuously communicate with the therapist
on how he/she is doing. If a certain part of the body is sensitive, the massage
therapist needs to know. If the person is ticklish, the therapist needs to be told.
These issues are also important to remember if a friend or loved one gives the
massage.

Types of Massage

There are dozens of books available on various types of massage. Two types are presented here: Swedish massage and self-massage or shared massage. Swedish massage is
one of the most popular types of massage approaches in the United States. Self-massage
or shared massage is massage that people can give to themselves or others without a
great deal of training.

Swedish Massage

According to Seaward (1997), there are five progressive steps in a Swedish massage. The
first step is referred to as *effleurage,* which is light stroking of the skin. It is primarily for
preparing the person for the next series of steps. The second step, *petrissage,* is when the
massage therapist "rolls, rings, and squeezes" (p. 379) the tissue. The third stage, *friction,*
includes more deep pressure on the tissue between the massage therapist's thumbs and
forefingers. The fourth step, *tapotement,* resembles soft karate chops to the specific part
of the body. The fifth step, *vibration,* is when the therapist shakes the area to improve circulation.

Self-Massage or Shared Massage

This section is for individuals who would like to provide themselves (or others) with an
amateur massage. This is not to take away from the value of a massage from a trained
therapist, but it is possible for a person to self-massage or provide a massage to others
without any special training. Following are several types of massage that a person can
perform. The important thing to remember if you are giving or receiving a massage is
communication. Let the other person know if you need something softer, more intense,
or whatever. If in doubt, be gentle.

1. *Lifting of the skin.* This is when you gently lift the tissue of the skin and allows it to roll
   back to its original location.
2. *Pinching.* Not the typical idea of pinching, this is when you pull the tissue with the
   fingers and move the tissue when it is lifted.
3. *Rubbing, very simple.* This is when you use the flat of your hand and rub it against the
   surface of the skin. This is sometimes used as a precursor to other types of massage.
   It warms the skin and allows the recipient to get used to having a physical touch take
   place.

(continued)

Types of Massage   continued

4. *Slapping.* Using the palm and fingers of the hand, you slap the tissue. Obviously, this is inappropriate for certain parts of the body. For example, slapping may be good for the bottom of the feet but may not be good for the head.

5. *Pressure points.* You point or insert your finger, thumb, and/or knuckle into various parts of the body to loosen up any nodules or tensions. For example, you can follow the ridge of the back of the skull with your thumbs. Press your thumbs into your skull and hold tight for several seconds, then move them along.

Another example of pressure points would be following the scapula (shoulder bone in the back) around its outer area. Place your finger/thumb into the skin, maintain pressure while slightly rotating, and hold for about ten seconds. Then move the pressure over a few centimeters and repeat. Continue until you have encompassed the entire scapula.

A foot massage can be a very relaxing activity. The foot is one of the most abused body parts. It is often ignored and kept in a closed, tight shoe. Nothing can refresh you more than a good foot massage, either on yourself or on another. You can start with some long deep rubs along the arch. Next, do some light circular rubs on the top of the foot (be careful of the bones). Make sure that you massage the toes and between the toes. Finally, slapping the bottom of the feet can help rejuvenate tired feet. For most people, using lotion makes it easier to provide such a massage. As already indicated, it is important to constantly talk to the partner to be assured that the experience is enjoyable.

Note: Many different types of massages are available. For more information on the specific types of massages available from a massage therapist, visit one of the various websites listed at the end of this chapter.

Techniques/Exercises

1. For the next week, take a daily slow walk along a particular path in your community. Make the walk solitary. Note the area as you walk, and for each day see if you can discover something different about the path.

2. Make a list of everybody who serves in your social-support system. See if you can find areas that you need to improve, and identify a strategy to go about filling such gaps.

3. Give and receive a foot massage with somebody.

4. Identify one major stressor that you are experiencing on a regular basis. Brainstorm on ways to reduce and/or eliminate this stressor. Rank your findings. Then, starting with your first choice, set up a strategy to see if you can eliminate and/or reduce that stressor over the next two weeks. If the first choice does not work, try the second, and so on until you have exhausted your list.

5. Call a massage therapist to determine cost, procedures, and other issues such as certification and third-party reimbursement.

Following is the solution to the nine-dot exercise provided in this chapter. Remember, the trick is not to be bound by the parameters of the box.

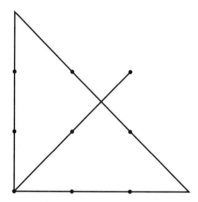

Summary

It's really not that important what is done to combat the stressors of life. However there are two strong strategies that everybody should incorporate. One, work out ways to prevent stress from happening, realizing of course that one cannot alleviate all stress. This can be done by re-prioritizing what is important, re-alter events so that you can avoid those items that cause stress, or rearranging your time to allow for more efficient use of the day.

The second approach in dealing with stress would be to take time every day to refocus and to try to dissipate the stressors that can't be prevented. These are pro-active efforts to attempt to reduce the stress that you are accumulating. Activities such as exercise, Yoga, breathing, and a variety of other "chair-based" activities can help one to dissipate the stress they may be experiencing. Together, both strategies can be used to reduce the potential negative consequences that stress can play on one's mental health and wellness.

DISCUSSION QUESTIONS

1. Identify the pros and cons of the five strategies for reducing or eliminating stressors that are discussed in this chapter.

2. Explain the rationale behind the author's contention that individuals should use a multifaceted approach to reduce stress.

3. Discuss the role that breathing has in stress-reduction activities.

4. Discuss the role that concentration has in the various aspects of stress management.

5. Identify the role that exercise can play in reducing stress. How does exercise tie in with massage, Yoga, or tai chi? What precautions must be kept in mind when using exercise as a stress reducer?

RELATED WEBSITES

http://www.aomc.org/stressreduction.html   Stress: Techniques for Stress Reduction. This site provides exercises and tips for coping with various stressors.

http://oz.sannyas.net/quotes/med03.htm   Exploration of Dynamic Meditation. Includes explanation of its purpose, technique, and instructions on its use.

http://www.shsu.edu/~counsel/shortr.html   Short Relaxation Technique. This site explores various methods of relaxation exercises.

http://www.mbsr.com/   Mindfulness-Based Stress Reduction. This site includes discussion, training, a teacher directory, journal, and book index page.

http://ub-counseling.buffalo.edu/Stress/ Stress and Anxiety. Includes stress and time management, test anxiety, overcoming procrastination, and study skills for students.

http://www.aome.org/stressBC.html   This site discusses the basic concepts of stress, stress reduction, and coping skills.

http://www.stress.org/   American Institute of Stress. Comprehensive site includes job stress, AIS monthly newsletter, information packets, and legal consultation.

http://imt.net/~randolfi/StressPage.html   Stress Management and Emotional Wellness. Includes comprehensive list of links, discussion forum, quotes, bookstore, consultation, and speaker information.

http://www.talamasca.org/avatar/yoga.html   This site explores Yoga, its benefits, and additional techniques. It also provides links to various Yoga technique sites.

http://www.gday-mate.com/   Stress-Management Site. This site provides a definition and description of stress as well as treatment advice and stress links.

http://www.yogasite.com/welcome.html The Yoga Site. An electric collection of Yoga connections.

REFERENCES

Benson, H. (1975). *The Relaxation Response.* New York: Morrow Press.

Blonna, R. (1996). *Coping With Stress in a Changing World.* St. Louis: Mosby.

Borysenko, J. (1984). *Minding the Body, Mending the Mind.* Reading, MA: Addison-Wesley.

Cousins, N. (1978). Anatomy of the Illness (as Perceived by the Patient). *New England Journal of Medicine, 295*(26), 1458–1463.

Covey. S. (1989) *Seven Habits of Highly Effective People.* New York: Simon & Schuster.

Girdano, D. A., Everly, G. S., Dusek, D. E. (1997). *Controlling Stress and Tension,* (5th Ed.). Boston: Allyn & Bacon.

Hartup, W. W., & Stevens, N. (1999). Friends and Adaptation across the Life Span. *Current Directions in Psychological Sciences, 8*(3), 76–79.

Jacobson, E. (1955). Neuromuscular Controls in Man. Methods of Self-Direction in Health and Disease. *American Journal of Psychology 68,* 549–561.

McGuigan, F. J. (1999). *Encyclopedia of Stress.* Boston: Allyn & Bacon.

Pierce, G. R., Sarson, B. R., & Sarason, I. E. (Eds.). (1996). *Handbook of Social Support and the Family.* New York: Plenum Press.

Rice, P. L. (1999). *Stress and Health* (3rd Ed.). Boston: Brooks/Cole.

Schafer, W. (1999). *Stress Management for Wellness* (4th Ed.). Orlando, FL: Harcourt Brace.

Seaward, B. L. (1997). *Managing Stress: Principles and Strategies for Health and Well-Being.* Boston: Jones and Bartlett.

Van Boven, S. (1997). Giving Infants a Helping Hand. *Newsweek* (Special Issue May). In D. Corbin (Ed.) (1999), *Perspectives in Stress Management.* Belluvue, IA: Coursewise.

Van Dixhoorn, J. (1999). Implementation of Relaxation Therapy Within a Cardiac Rehabilitation Setting, in D. Kenny, J. C. Carlson, F. J. McGuigan, & J. L Sheppard (Eds.), *Stress and Health: Research and Clinical Implications.* Boston: Allyn & Bacon.

9

Spiritual Well-Being

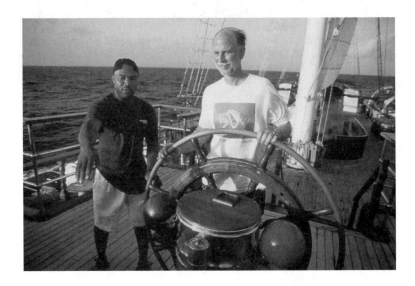

What thoughts first came into your mind when you read the title of this chapter? Did you assume it would be about mysticism or magical and unseen powers? Some may have considered that the chapter would be devoted to church membership and attendance or religious dogma. Perhaps notions of faith and healing first came to mind. Your notions about what spiritual health means likely reflect your previous experiences or attempted experiences of a spiritual nature. These could range from thoughts of a fully organized and structured religious service to a solo walk through a peaceful park at sunrise. Your thoughts may have been of a positive or negative nature and this may reflect the types of experiences you have had in dealing with things that you have assumed to be of a spiritual nature.

There once was a man who had set a life goal for himself to become a "holyman." This individual described a holyman as someone who focuses on the meaning of life and the essence of being and doing well. It seemed like a worthwhile goal. He agonized over the path to follow to prepare himself for his aspired role in life. Since this man did not believe that there were any accredited holyman schools, he set out on a course of self-directed study. He reviewed the methods of Hebrew, Catholic, Muslim, and Buddhist scholars in their strivings for spiritual enlightenment. He devoted much effort to master "shamanic techniques" as a pathway to the all-knowing, all-seeing method of understanding that seemed to continually elude him. His personal library was immense, and what book he could not purchase he would obtain from the library. He seemed to be a kind, accepting, and understanding man with good intentions. But often he became troubled. His search repeatedly left him frustrated, and over time he became impatient with himself, as well as others. His impatience with himself was based on never quite reaching the level of understanding and awareness he set as a personal goal for himself. In addition, he had trouble with others who seemed to be continually falling behind him in his ceaseless quest for learning. Whether or not he ever became a holyman is unclear. That he became increasingly unhappy and ultimately caused unhappiness in others is more clear.

The question here is, Where is the true spiritual nature to be found? Can you become more spiritual solely through the study of sacred writings, through the mastery of dogma, through devotion to the teachings of a spiritual leader, or through repeated enrollment in workshops, retreats, or seminars offering to point the way? Is spiritual well-being a quality that must be offered to us by others, or is it an innate, inherent matter that is waiting for a chance to express itself?

Spirituality Defined

There are many varied, and sometimes conflicting, definitions of spirituality. For the purposes of this textbook, some of the more noteworthy definitions of spirituality will be examined and applied to the promotion of mental health.

Hussein (1994) cites the World Health Assembly's definition of the spiritual dimension of health as being "a phenomenon that is not material in nature but belongs to the realm of ideas, beliefs, values, and ethics that have arisen in the minds and conscience of human beings." Hussein further notes that many of the great thinkers of the past have declared that human beings are composed of a combination of body, mind, and spirit. He uses the analogy of a building and its foundation to describe the spiritual dimension, and suggests that the "invisible and intangible spirit" is like the foundation (unseen beneath the surface) serving as an indispensable support to the more obvious building (the body and the mind). Banks (1980) has offered a thorough and involved description of spirituality that includes something that is known by belief or faith, gives purpose and meaning to life, offers a sense of place in the universe under an influence that is beyond the natural or rational, and acts as a unifying force in integrating other dimensions of human health to create a whole person.

While Banks's description includes several notions of commitment to a supreme being, others disagree and believe that knowledge or acceptance of a Supreme Being is not a critical factor in defining spirituality. Viktor Frankl, in his classic work *Man's Search for Meaning* (1992), suggests that, while religion and spirituality can have much in common, spirituality is a human dimension and it can develop and function in those without a formal belief system. Remen (1988) states that a yearning for the spiritual is found in all humans and that it is an essential human need and something from which humans cannot separate themselves. She further states that it does not involve ethical, moral, or religious factors.

Schafer (1996), on the other hand, views religiosity and spirituality as being more conjoint. He defines *religiosity* as "religious belief, practice, or both" and *spirituality* as "meaning, purpose, and direction." While many regard the spiritual dimension as not material in nature, Chandler, (Holden, and Kolander 1992) contend that "spirituality is a natural part of being human and can be conceptualized in an understandable and practical fashion." They suggest that human beings have an innate capacity to seek experiences of a spiritual nature and that such experiences enable a transcendence or movement beyond a current state to a higher one. Such growth, they claim, enables a greater knowledge and a worldview that promotes a clear perception of life's purpose. They further contend that this growth enhances the development of more effective ethical and value systems.

Morris (1996) describes the spiritual component of health as including the "transcendent and existential features pertaining to an individual's relationship with the self, others, and a higher being (however that may be conceived)." Her point that the higher being may vary in personal conception is an important one in that it allows for a sense of the spiritual in a variety of belief and understanding systems. She further notes that spiritual relationships can provide hope and a sense of meaning to life. It is interesting to note that, like so many other observers of the role of spirituality in health, Morris comments on the important overlapping and interrelationship between spirituality and the other dimensions of human health. Deats (1995) describes spirituality as a belief in a higher power along with a sense of meaning and purpose to life. Ingersoll (1994) describes spirituality as including: a concept of a divine, absolute force greater than the individual self; a sense of meaning; and a systematic force that acts to integrate the dimensions of life.

After considering some of these notions and perceptions, it might be reasonable to suggest that spirituality has dual components. One segment is related to a supreme being or higher power and is usually addressed via a religious orientation. The other portion is more existential in nature and relates to that sense of meaning and purpose in life that so many scholars and philosophers discuss. These portions of spirituality can be complementary or not. Rossi (1998) suggests that spirituality is an essential need of human nature and that people all participate in spirituality even if they are unaware that they are doing so. She further states that all humans are seeking the spiritual dimension, albeit with differing degrees of enthusiasm and need. Rossi has compiled numerous definitions of spirituality, and, like those already cited, they all seem to embrace a common thread that includes

- Providing a sense of meaning and purpose to life
- Serving to coordinate all other dimensions of human health (holism)
- Involving a belief in a power or force greater than the individual

The Search for Spirituality

There are many reasons behind the search by human beings for experiences related to the spiritual dimension. When so many seek and report positively regarding an aspect of their lives, there must be something of noteworthy value involved. The opinions expressed by those who experience a sense of spirituality, that improved the quality of their life help to provide an understanding of this phenomenon. Whether a person is following a transcendental spiritual path, one with a religious orientation, or a combination of the two, a manifest spirituality enables human beings to find meaning and purpose to life. This may include a relationship to God, a supreme being, or a significant force for good in the universe. Further, a well-developed spirituality can offer a sense of unity and direction among people.

This alone would be a great motivator to seek a heightened degree of spirituality. The cry uttered by some politicians in recent years for a "return to family values" implies a loss of some of the characteristics considered to be components of spirituality. Studies such as those conducted by the American Council on Education and cited by Coontz (1992) suggest a reduction in altruistic behavior and a sense of importance to having a meaningful philosophy of life. Whether or not society would be better if it returned to a value system of the past, the fact that many listen to the request for the return to family values suggests that there is a sense among many that those factors in life that relate to the moral, ethical, value, and spiritual could be improved. Seeking a sense of how to connect with the spiritual is a contemporary issue, but it may always have been so.

The impression that a world could exist in which individuals understood their motives and acted in a manner that was in the best interest of others, as well as themselves, allows for the peaceful universe that has been desired for so long. Behaving based on love and understanding of a "big picture" in which all living things were accorded a sacredness and acceptance is a very tempting one indeed. Clinebell (1995) suggests that this search for the spiritual domain entails a desire for such things as a sense of trusting and belonging in a community that supports spiritual growth, a relationship with a loving God, and a functional and reasonable philosophy of life. Stein (1989) believes that one of the sources of appeal in the search for spiritual development is the coping resource that spirituality provides. If individuals have faith in a benevolent supreme being and/or have well-developed notions of the meaning of life, it is quite plausible that they would possess better coping abilities.

An article published in *Time Magazine* (Wallis, 1996) reports that about 80 percent of people in the United States believe that prayer or the power of God can heal sickness. Maugans and Wadland (1991) discovered that seven out of ten physicians surveyed reported that they have inquiries about religious counseling from patients with terminal illnesses. It seems that a spiritual connection or sense of support from spiritual sources is a very important part of coping with illness for people in the United States.

Chapman (1987) suggested that a well-developed sense of spirituality promotes a sense of relationship to fellow human beings. This joining together with others establishes a "connectedness" that is a two-way street allowing people to both give and receive help, joy, and fulfillment. This connection with other people that seems to accompany the development of the spiritual dimension seems to promote the notion that human beings are all one family. Terms like brother, sister, and father used by members of spiritual communities imply a sense of family-like bonding. This desire to connect with others is much more than cultural according to May (1981). He suggests that the spiritual realm of existence is best understood by recognition of the fact that all humans are essentially common to people's deepest sense. Genetic codes passed on from prior generations carry the blueprint or design of the universe. But even more basic to people's oneness is the fact that every human being is both comprised of and sustained by the same basic elements and atmosphere of the earth.

Humans are all a part of the same larger life cycle, and the innate or core goodness that is potential in all humans may owe its presence to this composition of genetics and common elements. The phrase used in many Western burial ceremonies—"dust to dust and ashes to ashes"—implies this. The spiritual notion of an afterlife, reincarnation, or the continuation of the life force following death, has a founding in this principle of commonalty, connectedness, and continuity.

A culture's spiritual goals are often directed toward the young and more actively promoted by the women in a society. Bly (1996) suggests that young women in particular have a longing for the spiritual. This seeking of spirituality, he claims, is evidenced by the types of pilgrimages that take place in virtually all parts of the world and in almost all cultures. He further suggests that the higher rates of church attendance by women may indicate a higher level of spirituality or a seeking of spirituality by that gender. The spiritual needs of men, however, have been made evident by the rise of contemporary men's spiritual organizations. One of the most visible of these was organized by a former football coach and is so well attended that it meets in sports arenas and football stadiums.

The fact that human beings seem to search for a level of spirituality might be explained by the rewards offered by this dimension of mental health. Some of these rewarding and fulfilling notions include the following:

1. There is meaning and purpose to life.
2. Life is worth living.
3. I fit into the grand scheme of things.
4. I have worth.

5. There are important things beyond my own needs.
6. I can make a difference.
7. The world is a good place.
8. The human race is a family.
9. Others care about me.
10. There is a superior power, force, or being that cares about me.

Ponder the following questions and then answer in the spaces provided.

1. In rank order, list the five most important things in life.

   a. _____

   b. _____

   c. _____

   d. _____

   e. _____

2. Compare and contrast indicators that people are generally "good" or "bad."

   good   *bad*

   a.

   b.

   c.

3. Discuss any signs or other forms of evidence that indicate that there is or is not a greater power or supreme life force guiding the universe.

   _____

   _____

   _____

   _____

4. Based on the thoughts generated in this assignment (or any other thoughts you may have), prepare a brief description of what, to you, is the "meaning of life":

   _____

   _____

   _____

   _____

The Benefits of Spirituality

There is evidence of a variety of benefits that seem to accompany a well-developed spiritual dimension in people. Miller (1985) demonstrated a negative relationship between spiritual health and such undesirable characteristics as hopelessness, alienation, and loneliness in chronically ill adults. Hodges (1988) found that among parents who have experienced a death of a child, those with a higher level of spiritual health were likewise more likely to exhibit psychological health. In studies examining the effects of spiritual health on college students, researchers discovered that the existential component of spiritual health (finding meaning and purpose in life) had a positive impact in coping with life changes as well as in promoting hope for the future (Fehring, Brennan, & Keller, 1987; Carson, Soeken, & Grimm, 1988).

While the two aforementioned studies revealed a greater impact by existential spiritual health than religious spiritual health, other studies demonstrate a positive effect on mental health resulting from religiously oriented spirituality or church attendance. An example is the work of Levin (1996), who concludes that spiritual practice promotes a health-related lifestyle as well as providing a social-support system that enhances coping abilities. Some studies have revealed that it does not seem to matter what form or style of religious practice is involved in maintaining health. Using samples of Hindus, Buddhists, Muslims, Jews, Catholics, and Protestants, Levin and Vanderpool (1989) discovered a reduced illness and death rate associated with high blood pressure (hypertension). A study by Ross (1990) revealed that those with the higher levels of religious beliefs experienced lower levels of psychological distress. Dull and Skokan (1995) offer the suggestion that religious beliefs can encompass a sense that life's events happen for a reason and that God is directing a larger plan. He further suggests that those with a strong religious sense might interpret problems in life as part of a plan to strengthen faith.

Chima (1996) suggests that spirituality plays a positive and important role in the recovery from drug and alcohol abuse. Seigel (1986), in discussing the role of religious belief and prayer in the healing process, said. "To me it is the absence of spirituality that leads to difficulties." However, he also suggests that for some people a strong religious belief can interfere with their recovery from illness. He regards such thinking as reflecting an attitude that says, "If God gave me this illness, then who am I to get well?" So Seigel, who is a leading proponent of belief and faith as a key factor in healing, differentiates between those characteristics developed on the basis of spiritual well-being and adherence to a strict religious dogma. He goes so far as to suggest that spiritual life need not be reflected in any commitment to an organized religion and that, for him, spirituality is the acceptance of what is reality. The key benefits of spirituality to mental health seem to involve

1. A common ground for connecting with others
2. A potential to accept (if not understand) differing points of view
3. Support/connection with others who have similar beliefs
4. Acceptance that there is a powerful force or supreme being watching over people, capable of offering help or working with them to solve problems
5. The comfort or peaceful calm that many with well-developed spiritual natures describe

Identifying Spirituality

A spiritual experience involves deep thoughts or feelings about the meaning and purpose of life, the forces that govern the universe, or a person's concept of a creator or Supreme Being. Consider for a minute the prospect of an actualized human being. This is a person who has accomplished all that is possible for himself/herself. Think about all that is possible for you as well as all that you realistically wish to be. Keep in mind that at one point in your life you will achieve your best. Picture just how this will be. How will you look? What will your voice sound like? What will be important to you? What will you be able to accomplish at this point in your life? Of course, the many dimensions of a person might cause a situation where you will be at your absolute best in different things at different times, so it might be wise to consider this actualized person in two ways. The first would involve being actualized in each of the dimensions discussed throughout the book.

What would you be like at your physical best? How would this differ from your characteristics at your mental, social, or emotional best? Can you form a mental image or notion concerning your appearance and manner of speech and dress? What things would you choose to occupy your time when you are at your absolute best? Who would you choose for friends and associates, where would you live, and with whom would you live? What sort of music would you listen to, and how would you choose to spend your recreational time? Create a mental picture of yourself at your absolute best in the various dimensions of the human experience, and record any noteworthy observations in the space that follows.

Dimension	*Characteristics/Attributes*
Physical	
Social	
Mental	
Emotional	
Spiritual	

What did you discover concerning perceptions about yourself from completing the preceding exercise? _____

_____

At what approximate age were you at your best in each dimension? _____

Was there any difference as far as the continuum of your lifeline where you attained this absolute best status? _____

_____

Were any of the dimensions easier or more difficult for you to visualize? _____

_____

Make special note of any of the characteristics you visualized in your actualized spiritual self. _____

_____

_____

In what ways was the actualized spiritual self similar to the actualized physical, mental, social, or emotional selves? _____   _____

_____   _____

In what ways was the actualized spiritual self different from the selves of the other dimensions? _____   _____   _____

_____

To which of the other dimension selves was your actualized spiritual self most similar? _____

Why do you think this was so? _____

Now consider the fact that at some point in your life you will be at your average best when all of the dimensions of human health are considered. Try to gain a mental picture of yourself at your absolute best when all of these dimensions are taken into consideration.

Which of the dimensions is most noticeable? _____

Rank the dimensions in order of apparent importance as seen in your visualization of yourself at the point of highest actualization when all dimensions are considered:
1. _____
2. _____
3. _____
4. _____
5. _____

If you were to compare your spiritual views with those of your parents, in which ways would they be similar? _____

_____

In which ways would your spiritual views differ from those of your parents?

_____

List and describe the four most noteworthy or memorable spiritual lessons in your life:

1. _____

_____

_____

2. _____

_____

_____

_____

3. _____

_____

_____

4. _____

_____

_____

_____

Did each of these experiences have something to do with each other or were they separate and unrelated in nature? _____

_____

At what age(s) did you experience these lessons? _____

Who were/are the main guiding forces in the development of your spirituality?

_____   _____

_____   _____

What about similarities and differences between the spiritual beliefs and nature of the most loved people in your life? Do your beliefs and views run in a parallel, complementary, or contradictory fashion? Are you able to accept any different notions about the spiritual dimension in others with whom you associate? Are they able to tolerate any differences in you?

_____

_____

_____

What major questions do you have regarding your spirituality?

_____

_____

What would you consider to be the best source for answers to these questions?

_____

_____

Developing, Fostering and Maintaining Spirituality

Over the life span, most people will pass through a series of experiences, relationships, and methods of viewing life that will result in changes in their spirituality. Others may remain quite static or at least experience less variance in their spirituality. Keeping in mind some of the earlier definitions of spirituality, do you believe that your personal spiritual nature and its interpretations have changed appreciably or remained more central to the way they are now?

Deep, and perhaps long established, spiritual feelings may change slowly, remain relatively unchanged, or undergo dramatic modifications. Such things as the strength of the feeling, the support or reinforcement of the feeling, or environment or life experiences may cause people to question, challenge, or even discard a component of their spiritual perceptions. This latter situation could either leave space for a new spiritual model to develop or some spiritual notions may displace an earlier one.

An important question that a person must continually ask is, Am I more spiritually mature when my notions about myself and my place in the universe become constant and unchanging or when they are open and seeking new thoughts and ideas? Frequently, people become troubled by transitions in spirituality. But recognition of that, as Kegan (1982) suggests, is, as an individual emerges from the old to the new, that there is not a repudiation of earlier notions but a development and growth from the point the original notion allowed the person to occupy. This new relationship to the universe may create questions in people and others around them regarding who they are and what they are becoming.

Epstein (1983) has noted that when people's experiences become inconsistent with their personal view of reality they may distort or deny these experiences in order to maintain harmony with their beliefs. A good goal would be to always define beliefs in terms of reality rather than attempting to define reality in terms of beliefs. The person undergoing spiritual development is capable of viewing these inconsistencies as indicators of growth and will attempt to understand and even incorporate these new notions into her/his spiritual insight.

If modification of a person's spirituality occurs, it is not necessarily for the better or worse; it may simply be a response to prior life experiences, personal needs, and current factors in the person's life. A reassessment of life, a new set of experiences, or a new way of viewing the universe and the person's place in it may all be involved. This need not be viewed as a breakdown or disintegration of spirituality, but rather a means of maintaining balance and harmony between the person, the universe, and the new experiences and perceptions. Circumstances change, new demands are placed upon people, and new questions that require a spiritual answer about life may arise.

Personal circumstances, skills, knowledge, and discernment can and often do change. These changes may require different answers or methods of seeking answers. Hopefully, these changes yield results that are more rewarding and bring even greater meaning and understanding to human beings through enhanced spiritual well-being.

It is important to regularly consider the meaning and purpose of life. Viktor Frankl (1997) refers to this as *pondering* or *self contemplation.* Frankl's approach entails spending some time in bed each morning thinking for several minutes about the meaning of the coming day and, in particular, the meaning it has for you personally. Frankl's method of self-contemplation or pondering is a method that could enable anyone to develop a mental picture in which that person fits into the grand scheme of life. To get to this point, the person would ideally be able to keep selfish, envious, angry, fearful, vengeful, and other such notions out of the mix.

An important, perhaps even essential, step to the development of spiritual health would be to free yourself of these nonproductive patterns of thinking prior to pondering the meaning of life. How can you ever empty your mind of such thoughts? Is it realistic to attempt to do so? Do such thoughts originate from a means of survival? Would it ever be in your best interest to eliminate such thoughts completely? Since these are human patterns, would you be less human if you totally eliminated them? These questions may be purely academic, since it is unlikely that you could ever totally eliminate all negative thoughts or emotions. Some stress management techniques, however, involve "freeing the mind" and working to temporarily cleanse yourself of negative thoughts to make room for the unimpeded positive. In order to contemplate the meaning of your existence and to determine if it is worthwhile, it is important to do so free of negative distractions. Is it better to free your mind of all thoughts and thus be open to more spiritual infusion or to keep your mind in tune with your past experiences and the current realities of your life as you seek to gain a notion about yourself and the "grand scheme"?

Observations of the individual, described at the beginning of this chapter, who sought to be a "holyman" certainly indicate that study and thought alone may not be the best path to spiritual health. But what of the person who releases all thoughts and emotional responses to the world in which she/he resides? Can lessons concerning spirituality ever be applied in a realistic sense? When considering opening yourself to spiritual growth, it might be of value to balance the following:

Free and empty the mind to gain spiritual enlightenment.	Develop spiritual health within the framework of everyday life.
Abandon or radically change daily life to accept new modes of thinking.	Attempt spiritual development within the established lifestyle.
If friends and associates cannot comprehend the changes move and/or establish new social networks	Modify life to balance new spiritual insights with associates.

A leader in the spiritual health movement, Deepak Chopra (1998) describes the Sanskrit term *prakriti* as the true self. This prakriti, or true self, enables each person to express himself/herself in light of his/her unique strengths and weaknesses. He claims that people are born understanding this but may forget or somehow lose contact with this primal comprehension. In order to recapture the wonder of life, Chopra suggests that you

1. Walk barefoot on grass to connect with and absorb energy from the earth.
2. Walk beside a natural body of water to allow it to infuse your being.
3. Feel the light and warmth of the sun and its energy-giving power.
4. Walk near abundant vegetation and inhale the healing breath of the plants.
5. Gaze at the night stars, allowing your awareness to extend through the universe.

Summary

Whether spiritual health means a strict religious commitment or a simple recognition of nature's beauty, the spirit that touches a person's soul is another guiding force that completes a holistically healthy person. Spiritual health encompasses many things, such as writings religious doctrine, sermons, workshops, retreats, or seminars offering answers to worldly questions. Who am I?, Why am I here?, and other such plaguing inquiries often define the search for self. This search can sometimes overtake people's lives.

Recall the concepts of interconnectedness from Chapter 1. When it is understood that each aspect of holistic health is driven and affected by the others, the importance of spiritual health is more clear. Assume that the aforementioned questions are left unanswered. Without a definition of self, a person might feel lost and fall into a bottomless cycle of self-doubt and wonder. This could lead to depression, drug addiction, or even suicide attempts. Chapter 10 focuses on the happiness a person can find in answering these questions and moving into a spiritual acceptance.

DISCUSSION QUESTIONS

1. What steps could be taken to comprehend the meaning of life for yourself?

2. What key stages of your life have fostered the greatest amount of spiritual growth?

3. How can you balance a seeking for spiritual values with the realities and demands of day-to-day living?

4. How can you avoid using transcendence as an excuse to avoid the challenges and rigors of *real* life?

5. Is it possible to attain a state of detachment while maintaining a sense of identification with the needs and purpose of others?

6. Would avoiding some of life's challenges through escape into the world of mindfulness and meditation be contrary to positive mental health?

7. Is there such a thing as unhealthy spirituality?

RELATED WEBSITES

http://www.geocities.com/RodeoDrive/1415/indexb.html Spirituality Defined. The concept is broken into subcategories to further explain spirituality. Also included are Yoga, quotes, and poems.

http://www.womanspiritrising.nu/index.htm This site is dedicated to the spirituality of women and women's needs.

http://www.academicinfo.net/nrms.html Academic information regarding religious movements and alternative spirituality. Provides a source for educational links to various topics including many religions, anthropology, and sociology.

http://www.saintmarys.edu/~incandel/spirituality.html Spirituality. Offers insight to everything from New Age practices and therapies to overcoming addictions.

http://www.spirithealth.montana.edu Spirituality and Health Home Page. A guide to existing organizations, research, funding, and upcoming events. Conferences and seminars.

http://www.kun.nl/tbi/sis.html Studies in Spirituality. An international scientific forum for spirituality. *Studies in Spirituality* is a journal, which is published annually.

http://www.owlnet.rice.edu/~ezenker/spirituality.html Spirituality. Love. Baha'u'llah. Environment. Spirituality and the Arts. Relating to Others. Baha'i Links. Main Page. Spirituality and the Arts.

REFERENCES

Banks, R. (1980). Health and the Spiritual Dimension: Relationships and Implications for Professional Preparation Programs. *Journal of School Health, 50,* 196.

Bly, R. (1996). *The Sibling Society (p. 177).* New York: Random House.

Carson, V., Soeken, K. & Grimm, P. (1988). Hope and Its Relationship to Spiritual Well-Being. *Journal of Psychology and Theology, 16,* 159–167.

Chandler, C., Holden, J. & Kolander, C. (1992). Counseling for Spiritual Wellness: Theory and Practice. *Journal of Counseling & Development, 71,* 168–169.

Chapman, L. (1987, Fall). Developing a Useful Perspective on Spiritual Health: Love, Joy, Peace, and Fulfillment. *American Journal of Health Promotion,* 13.

Chima, F. (1996). Assessment in Employee Assistance: Integrating Treatment and Prevention Objectives. *Employee Assistance Quarterly, 12,* (2), 47–66.

Chopra, D. (1998). *Healing the Heart (p. 1407).* New York: Harmony Books.

Clinebell, H. (1995). *Counseling for Spiritually Empowered Wholeness: A Hope-Centered Approach* (pp. 81–828). New York: The Hawthorne Pastoral Press.

Coontz, S. (1992). *The Way We Never Were.* New York: Basic Books/Harper Collins.

Deats, F. (1995, May/June). The Dilemma of Making Referrals, Clinical Judgment, Personal Bias, and Pragmatic Reality. *EAP Digest, 15* (4), 33–35.

Dull, V., & Skokan, L. (1995). A Cognitive Model of Religion's Influence on Health. *Journal of Social Issues, 51,* (2), 145–160.

Epstein, S. (1983). The Unconscious, the Preconscious and the Self-Concept. *Psychological Perspectives on the Self, 2,* 219–274.

Fehring, R., Brennan, P., & Keller, M. (1987). Psychological and Spiritual Well-Being in College Students. *Research in Nursing and Health, 10,* 391–398.

Frankl, V. (1992). *Man's Search for Meaning* (4th ed.). Boston: Beacon Press.

Frankl, V. (1997). *Viktor Frankl Recollections (p. 32)*. New York: Insight Books.

Hodges, M. (1988). *Relationship of Spiritual Well-Being to Emotional Well-Being in Bereaved Parents.* Unpublished master's thesis, Mississippi University for Women, Columbus, MS.

Hussein, A. (1994). Exploring the Mind and Spirit. *World Health, 47* (2), 8.

Ingersoll, R. (1994). Integrating Spiritual Experiences in Counseling. *Counseling and Values, 38,* 11–23.

Kegan, R. (1982). *The Evolving Self: Problems and Process in Human Development (p. 82)*. Cambridge, MA: Harvard University Press.

Levin, J. (1996). How Religion Influences Morbidity and Health: Reflections on Natural History, Salutogenesis, and Host Resistance. *Social Science & Medicine, 43,* 849–864.

Levin, J., & Vanderpool, H. (1989). Is Religion Therapeutically Significant for Hypertension? *Social Science & Medicine, 29,* 69–78.

Maugans, T., & Wadland, W. (1991). Religion and Family Medicine: A Survey of Physicians and Patients. *Journal of Family Practice, 32,* 210–213.

May, R. (1981). *Freedom and Destiny (p. 9010)*. New York: Norton.

Miller, J. (1985). Assessment of Loneliness and Spiritual Well-Being in Chronically Ill and Healthy Adults. *Journal of Professional Nursing, I,* 79–85.

Morris, E. (1996). A Spiritual Well-Being Model. *Issues in Mental Health Nursing, 17,* 440.

Remen, R. (1988). On Defining Spirit. *Noetic Sciences Review, 63.*

Ross, C. (1990). Religion and Psychological Distress. *Journal for the Scientific Study of Religion, 29,* (2), 236–245.

Rossi, D. (1998). *Spiritual Health Education.* Paper presented at the national convention of the American Alliance for Health, Physical Education, Recreation, and Dance, Reno, NV.

Schafer, W. (1996). *Stress Management for Wellness* (3rd ed.). Fort Worth: Harcourt Brace.

Seigel, B. (1986). *Love, Medicine, & Miracles (p. 179)*. New York: Harper & Row.

Stein, K. (1989). *Conceptual Models of Nursing:Analysis and Application* (2nd ed., pp. 331–346). Norwalk: Appleton & Lange.

Wallis, C. (1996, June 24). Faith and Healing. *Time,* 58–63.

CHAPTER

10 Life's Goals and Happiness

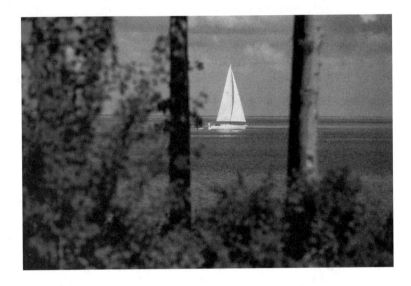

There are three main concepts that contribute to a person's ability to achieve his/her dreams. The first is achieving self-acceptance. People need to have an understanding of themselves and have a degree of confidence in their abilities. Self-esteem is an important factor in determining how a person will *behave* and, as a result of these behaviors, the degree to which that person will *succeed* or not succeed in life. If people do not believe they have the ability to create a better life for themselves, then the second concept is obsolete. This second concept maintains that people need to be goal-oriented. People need to set goals for themselves that will help them move closer to happiness. This is not an easy process, nor is it one that will ever be finished. The key is for a person to maximize his or her ability to establish, monitor, and revise goals. How do people set appropriate goals for themselves and achieve success in those goals? The answer to this question lies within the principles of cognitive and behavioral psychology.

People need to have an understanding of what drives their behavior to be able to successfully change it in a way that will help them move toward their goals. The integration of being self-accepted and goal-oriented, along with having the knowledge of how to change behavior to maximize potential, can lead to a mental balance of fulfillment and personal satisfaction. This chapter serves to teach people the general concepts of what goals are and the different ways of framing goals to promote success. Further, it goes beyond the basic concepts to provide readers with practical knowledge in setting, moving toward, and keeping a positive attitude toward their goals. First, some of the basic theories of personality that are particularly relevant in the area of having a positive attitude and happiness are presented. Then, because it is important to have a basic understanding of the theoretical aspects of goals, the basic foundations and, finally, the applications and implications are discussed.

Personality Construct

First and foremost, people need to have an understanding of their personality construct. Their personality construct is one indication of people's capacity to manage the myriad of situations that they encounter on a daily basis. According to Table 10.1, each person reflects certain qualities from each of the four quadrants with some characteristics emerging as predominant traits (Dawson, 1989). Analyzing which area people fit into can help them understand how they respond to stressful situations.

The top left corner of the table indicates the *analyticals*, individuals that are logical or linear in nature. They prefer the independence of working alone to that of a team effort and often have difficulty interacting in social settings. The stress levels for analyticals are mainly a result of perfectionism in getting the job done. The time it takes to complete the task might in fact take longer than anticipated because of this self-imposed demand for exactness, which in turn leads to higher degrees of stress.

The top right corner accommodates the *drivers*, the decisive individuals who enjoy their degree of authority and exhibit a tendency for noncompromise. Drivers possess a well-developed internal locus of control, an indication of their desire to seek out and succeed in high-profile positions and activities. They attract amiables who acquiesce to their authoritarian manner and ability to delegate. The drivers'

TABLE 10.1   Personality Matrices

	Passivity	Assertiveness
Goal-Oriented	Analytical	Driver
People-Oriented	Amiable	Socializer

need for control over all aspects of their lives leads to high levels of stress, especially when things do not go according to plan.

The lower left corner shows the *amiables*, the passive, socially oriented individuals whose stress emerges when their unspoken needs are not met. Although they are very people-oriented, amiables lack the degree of assertiveness that is required in many situations to voice their opinions and their demands to those around them. Career ambitions are limited to positions of nonauthority due to this subservient orientation. Stress surfaces when the inner conflict of desiring a change in the amiable's environment is not met with appropriate action, resulting in feelings of inadequacy and frustration.

The *socializers* are described as motivators because they understand and implement the concept of interpersonal motivation. They demonstrate their ability to communicate well with others by completing tasks with minimal stress and misunderstanding. Due to their charisma, socializers are able to exact a quality performance from those with whom they work. Socializers strike a balance between passivity and assertiveness in their approach to solving problems and creating solutions.

Bear in mind that each of these styles has positive and negative qualities. For example, analyticals might deal very well with facts and logic but have difficulty developing interpersonal skills that come naturally for amiables. There is no *right* or *wrong* style for anyone; perhaps the best approach is maintaining the flexibility to combine them when they are best suited to the task at hand.

Still referring to Table 10.1, locate which qualities fit your ideas of yourself. The horizontal scale indicates the two opposite poles of passivity and assertiveness. The vertical scale shows the range of orientation from goals to people. Place an X along the horizontal axis of the passive-assertive scale at a point that best describes your personality. Place another X along the vertical axis on the goal-oriented–people-oriented scale at a point that corresponds to your personality. Connect the two Xs with a line to provide a clearer visualization of where your primary qualities are distributed. Remember that the attributes you derived from the table only emphasize how certain traits correspond to different levels of stress.

This exercise serves as an aid in understanding how stress impacts individuals and their corresponding actions in relation to others. It is important to know that perception if an individual is dealing with stress in order to make changes in his or her life. At times, anxiety and uncertainty can create stress. When individuals have goals, they are more directed and focused and, thus, are more organized and more efficient in terms of time management. This supports the notion that there is an inverse relationship between an individual's amount of stress and whether or not he or she has set goals. This is true if an individual does not become obsessed with his or her goals, by which stress is created.

Another way of looking at personality is to assess what drives behavior. Behavior is not random; it happens for specific reasons. Because achieving goals depends on demonstrating certain behaviors, knowledge of the four different forces that drive human behavior is needed. Roger Dawson (1992) developed this model, called *ACDC*.

The *A* stands for *accept*. In this force, it is most important to earn the acceptance of others and a person's behavior is meant to achieve this acceptance. All people are driven by this force during childhood and usually outgrow it as they move toward adulthood. If a person does not outgrow this, then the need to be liked persists and the person will strive for acceptance throughout his or her life.

The first *C* stands for *control*. These people need to have control over all aspects of their lives and over other people. They spend their lives trying to achieve and maintain this control. This need for control can be a benefit as in a salesperson's ability to close a deal; however, it can also be very negative as in the actions brought by Hitler. Often, people with this control force grew up in very secure environments but did not have a great deal of love.

The *D* stands for *direction*. People with this force need to see their ideas and beliefs prevail. They often have stubborn philosophies and seem to think that being right is better than being loved and accepted. These people are typically raised in an insecure environment with a lot of love. Political debates may reveal examples of this force.

The second *C* is for *competence*. These people have a very strong desire to be excellent at whatever they do. They can often fall into this force by prior achievements. For example, students who get all *A*s will fall into patterns in which they have to get an *A* on everything.

Think about these four forces. Which one best describes you? Identifying which force best fits, you will have an understanding of why you are where you are and how you can get to where you want to be (Dawson, 1992). Each one of the forces has positive and negative sides. For example, people who best fit with *accept* are most likely very likable people who can resolve conflict and keep peace. These same people, however, are not very good at taking a stand and fighting for what they want. Thus, these people have qualities that can be helpful or not so helpful. Your job is to be aware of what drives your behavior and use that information to develop ways that will motivate you to work toward your goals.

Personality also involves the interpretation of what happens in the world. Sometimes motivation is not enough. How does a person keep going and keep working toward something with the onset of tragedies or negative events? Dawson (1992) suggests that what matters is how a person reacts and not what actually happens. This reaction will determine in part how that person behaves in the future. It follows, therefore, that a person's behavior depends on his or her interpretation of what happened. If individuals' interpretations lead to behaviors that take them away from their goals, then they need to change their interpretations. Reactions are dependent on three main perceptions. The first is *permanence versus impermanence*. How particular events are perceived, either as a permanent condition or an impermanent one, carries a strong impact. To be optimistic, a person should be encouraged to view good events as permanent in that they will always happen and bad events as things that are due to chance or a fluke.

The second perception is *personal versus impersonal*. This speaks to issues of internal versus external locus of control. A person with an internal locus of control sees events as happening because of something he or she did or something internal.

A person with an external locus of control, on the other hand, sees events as happening due to some external force. It was not that person's doing but something in the environment that caused the event. As with the first idea, people need to view good events as to their credit and bad events to someone else's fault in order to think positively. This does not mean neglecting responsibility for taken actions, but it does mean developing a positive attitude that will foster mental well-being. In other words, it is okay to see bad events as an owned fault as long as it is not taken to an unnecessary extreme.

The final perception is *pervasive versus isolated.* People need to view good events as indications that good things are happening all over instead of being isolated events. For example, a person should view finding a job as an indication that the job market is doing well instead of thinking, "I was just lucky."

Together, these make up a blueprint for healthy, optimistic behavior. Look at the different sides of each idea. Which side represents your personality? If you tend to be optimistic, great! If you see yourself as being pessimistic according to these ideas, then you need to change your thinking to be more positive. A positive attitude is essential for achieving ultimate happiness and satisfaction. Remember that just because you act one way in a situation does not mean you will always act that way in future situations. Applying labels to yourself is dangerous in that it limits your abilities to achieve further, lowers your self-esteem, or, at the other extreme, can cause depression if you expect too much of yourself.

All of the issues presented in this section are valuable. You need to have an understanding of your personality makeup to understand your behavior and to be able to think positively. Consider the following story:

One day there was a man who was overwhelmed with worry, and, after exploring many alternatives, he decided to visit his physician. He felt no sense for living and could concentrate on nothing but his worries. He could only concentrate on all of the problems, and he was unable to experience the beauty that was clearly evident before his very eyes.

When he explained his feelings to the physician, the doctor thought for a moment and quietly wrote the man a prescription. He asked the man what he enjoyed most as a boy. Without hesitation, the man responded, "Going to the beach." The doctor paused and proceeded to write something else on his prescription pad. The doctor inquired whether the man would be willing to take one day away from work. In a despondent voice, the man responded that he would. The doctor handed the man his prescriptions and carefully dispensed the directions.

He said, "Drive to the beach, and do not read the first of four prescriptions until 9:00 a.m. Then, open the second prescription at 12:00 noon, the third at 3:00 p.m., and the fourth and final prescription at 6:00 p.m. Once you have experienced these prescriptions, we will meet again."

The man thought the idea strange but drove to the beach and obeyed the directions of the doctor. He found a secluded spot at the end of the beach and slowly opened the first prescription at 9:00 a.m. The first of the four prescriptions simply read, "Listen." For three hours, the man did nothing but listen to the seagulls, seashore, and children playing in the distance. This time seemed to take forever, but soon enough it was 12:00 noon. The man more anxiously opened the second prescription that read, "Reflect." For three hours, the man reflected on aspects of his life. Some of these brought back good memories, and others were painful. These hours seemed to go by much more quickly. When 3:00 p.m. arrived, he slowly folded the second prescription, placed it in his front pocket, and opened the third envelope. This prescription read, "Reexamine reason for living." This prescription brought much thought and consumed three hours without warning. Somehow, he was beginning to understand the meaning of his day. When 6:00 p.m. arrived, he unraveled the fourth prescription, which instructed the man to locate a stick and write his worries in the sand. After the man did so, he slowly walked toward his car. However, before he drove away, he looked back and noticed that the water had washed away all of his worries.

This story demonstrates that, to create a feeling of satisfaction in their lives, people need to go through a process of assessing and revising the way they approach success and deal with stress. It also shows how important a positive attitude really is.

This connection between goals and happiness is an important one. There are always stories about individuals who struggle to overcome great odds to succeed in situations that most would consider intolerable. These people often explain that their goals kept them happy and motivated. On the other hand, it is important to not allow goals to overtake day-to-day life. As the old adage goes, "Life is what is happening while people make other plans." According to Jerry Braza (1997), in his book *Moment by Moment: The Art and Practice of Mindfulness,* joy and happiness are by-products of the practice of mindfulness. To be mindful is to live fully in the present moment. How often are opportunities for happiness missed because of "mindlessness?" "In an attempt to hurry, we frequently miss the opportunity to enjoy the little pleasures that are happening moment by moment" (Braza, 1997). How many sunsets, smiles, and small adventures have you missed?

Main Concepts in Goal Setting and Goal Pursuit

A discussion on the basic concepts of personality that are essential in achieving dreams should be followed by the main concepts in setting and pursuing these dreams. The notion of goals is one that is intertwined with the constructs of values and motivation. Elliot, Sheldon, and Church (1997) offer a definition of personal goals. They state that *personal goals* are conscious, personally important objectives that an individual pursues in his or her daily life. They exist to provide individuals with a purpose, structure, and sense of identity. Another similar definition of personal goals is that they are an individual's cognitive representation of his or her personal motivations (Jolibert and Baumgartner, 1997). They are related to values in that both establish a desirable objective. The difference, however, lies in the idea that values constitute what a person must do whereas personal goals constitute what a person wishes to do.

This intermingling of goals, motivations, and values forces a consideration of the concept of the self. Jolibert and Baumgartner (1997) discuss the different dimensions of the self, such as ideal self versus self as perceived by others, and offer that these are extremely important concepts when examining motivation and personal goals.

An insightful resource for examining how people perceive themselves and how they are perceived by others is the *Johari Window* (Figure 10.1).

Psychologists Joe Luft and Harry Ingham devised this diagram for people to see the different ways in which they communicate their aspirations and themselves. To productively implement goals, individuals must know their personal agendas and the place where they fall. In realizing this, more efficiency in means, modes, and methods of goal execution can be created.

Types of Goals and Goal Framing

There is wealth of research in the area of goal types. Researchers have studied different types of goal orientations and their consequences. *Goal orientation theory* is a conception of motivation that focuses on goals that are perceived for achievement behavior (Middleton & Midgley, 1997). This orientation is important because it provides an individual with a framework within which events are interpreted. Reactions are based on the interpretation and can result in many different cognitive, behavioral, and affective patterns. This may explain, in part, why students tend to set short-term goals with the hope that they will lead to success in long-term goals. This is consistent with Bandura's idea that short-term goals provide a feeling of self-satisfaction that reinforces and sustains an individual's efforts and motivation (Howe & Poole, 1992). Learning about the different types of goal orientations can help a person choose effective goals.

There are two main types of goals that are seen throughout the research. They are based on their direction toward an outcome. *Approach goals* are goals in which the individual is trying to move toward a desired outcome. *Avoidance goals*, on the other hand, are goals in which the individual is trying to move away from an undesired outcome. These two goals are based on the motivational orientation of approaching success and avoiding failure, respectively (Coats, Janoff-Bulman, & Alpert 1996; Elliot & Sheldon, 1997). Therefore, the type of thinking a person

	Behavior known to self	Behavior unknown to self
Behavior known to others	**Open**	**Blind**
Behavior unknown to others	**Hidden**	**Unknown**

FIGURE 10.1   Johari Window

engages in, positive or negative, helps determine the type of goal orientation. For example, suppose a college student has an upcoming midterm examination. This student can have one of two main goals. On the one side, the student could want to *not fail* the exam, which would create an avoidance goal. On the contrary, the student may want to obtain an *A* on the test, which would create an approach goal.

Coats and his colleagues (1996) explored the effect that approach and avoidance goals have on self-satisfaction. They found that the greater the number of avoidance goals, the greater the depression, lower self-esteem, and lower optimism. Conversely, they found that the greater the number of approach goals, the lower the depression. Follow-up self-evaluations revealed that avoidance goals are more difficult to accomplish, are less likely to be accomplished in the future, and were viewed as less important. It was also reported that there was less happiness when avoidance goals were accomplished as opposed to approach goals. This research supports the concept that framing approach goals can produce more favorable self-evaluation and are associated with greater psychological well-being. The authors suggest that avoidance goals may have a "circle of negativity." In other words, people form avoidance goals because of past failures and a desire to avoid future failures; however, at the same time it may decrease their perception of success.

Elliot and Sheldon (1997) offer support for this idea as well. In their research, they describe four basic levels of goal representation. The first is *task-specific*, in which guidelines for performance are set. *Situation-specific*—orientations that represent the purpose of achievement activity—is the second. The third level is *personal*. These represent ideographic, personalized achievement pursuits that often transcend particular situations. Finally there are *self-standards* and images of the self in the future.

This study (Elliot & Sheldon, 1997) focused on the nature of avoidance achievement motivation at the personal goal level. They found that high fear-of-failure scores were associated with a greater number of avoidance goals, and the greater the number of avoidance goals, the less enjoyable and fulfilling the experience. They further suggest that experiencing a feeling of competence with respect to a person's goals is a psychological necessity for well-being. Having avoidance goals, therefore, may be incongruent with psychological well-being. This may suggest that framing approach goals can be an effective strategy in working toward fulfillment and happiness.

The idea that approach and avoidance goals elicit different emotions is further supported in research done by Higgins, Shah, and Friedman (1997). They used the terms *promotion goals* and *prevention goals*, which are synonymous with approach goals and avoidance goals, respectively. They found that utilizing promotion goals created *cheerfulness-related emotions* such as happy and satisfied when a goal was attained and *dejection-related emotions* such as disappointed or discouraged when a goal was not attained. Prevention goals were found to create *tranquility-related emotions* such as calm and relaxed when a goal was attained and *agitation-related* emotions such as tense and uneasy when a goal was not attained.

Another distinction in goals is related to competency. *Performance goals* are goals in which an individual is focused on demonstrating his or her competence relevant to others. People who adopt this type of goal can focus on obtaining positive judgments (approach) or on avoiding negative judgments (avoidance). *Learning* or *mastery goals* focus on the development of competency and task mastery. In this type of goal, people are trying to improve and increase their abilities (approach) (Elliot & Sheldon, 1997; Erdley, Cain, Loomis, Dumas-Hines & Dweck, 1997).

Erdley and his colleagues (1997) used performance and learning goals to examine *social goals*. They also looked at the effect of different personality types. Specifically, they looked at students with an *entity theory of personality,* in which a person believes personality is a fixed quantity, and *incremental theory of personality,* in which a person believes personality is malleable and increasable. The research found that children's goal orientation was predicted by their theory of personality, which in turn influenced their responses to social rejection. It was indicated that children who enter a challenging social situation with a focus on performance goals are more likely to react to failure helplessly and defensively. In addition, they found that despite the type of goal orientation, entity theorists were more likely than incremental theorists to blame their failure on their inability. Further, entity theorists were more concerned with attempting to minimize risk and avoid a negative judgment of themselves. This evidence can help explain some of the maladaptive behaviors—such as withdrawal and aggression—seen in children, because these findings indicate that goals play an important role in the interpretation of social cues and behavior patterns.

Most of the research looks at performance and learning goals as achievement goals that are approach oriented. Middleton and Midgley (1997) examined performance and task (learning) goals from both an approach and an avoidance orientation. They used sixth grade, middle school students in mathematics classrooms. Findings suggest that a distinction between task and performance goals is more influential than a distinction between approach and avoidance goals. Task goals were found to facilitate task engagement through affective and cognitive processes, whereas performance-approach goals were unrelated to academic efficacy and positively related to avoidance behaviors in the classroom and test anxiety. For self-regulated learning and academic self-efficacy a task goal orientation was the strongest predictor for self-efficacy and self-regulation. Further, performance-avoidance goals were the strongest predictors to avoid seeking help in difficult subject areas.

The issue of *goal framing* is an important concept that is related to success and life satisfaction. It has been demonstrated that mastery or learning goals produce more positive outcomes than performance goals (Elliot & Sheldon, 1997; Erdley et al., 1997). Roney, Higgins, and Shah (1995) examined whether the way a performance goal is framed impacts motivation and emotions. They found that people in the negative-outcome-focus condition (failure threatened) showed an increase in agitation-related emotions more than dejection-related emotions. Persistence was also greater in the positive-outcome-focus condition (success oriented). In a subsequent study, it was found that performance feedback framed in terms of positive-outcome focus led to better performance on a task and greater persistence with a more difficult task. These studies indicate that framing a goal in different ways can affect the emotions produced by either attaining or failing to attain that goal and that it can also influence motivation. This suggests that failure feedback has a different impact on a person depending on how it is framed.

Take a moment to look back over the goals you consider most important and answer the following questions:

How did you phrase them?
Are they approach oriented or avoidance oriented?
Are they performance goals or learning/mastery goals?

This type of reflection, although it sounds very technical, is necessary to succeed and achieve self-satisfaction. Based on what you have learned about the different types of goal orientation, how do you feel about your goals? People need to evaluate their goals on an ongoing basis and be able to make decisions about revising them. By going through this process of revision or *reframing* of your goals, it becomes easier to focus on the behaviors needed to attain them.

Factors That Affect Goal Pursuit

Theories of motivation are at the core of goal orientation. Elliot and Church (1997) examined a hierarchical model of approach and avoidance achievement motivation in which goal concepts are portrayed as concrete representations of more abstract motivational dispositions. They tested and gained support for antecedents and consequences of achievement goals. Under the antecedents, Elliot and Church found that people who believed they could attain competence in an achievement situation would orient toward the possibility of success and adopt approach goals. Intrinsic motivation is a consequence that is facilitated through the adoption of mastery goals. The authors attribute this finding to the fact that mastery goals are *grounded* in an approach form of motivation. This, in their opinion, elicits responses that challenge and excite people, as well as create feelings of interest and enjoyment.

Within these theories, other concepts such as self-concept, self-esteem, and self-efficacy are involved. It is important to discuss at this point the differences between these three concepts. Although these three terms are often used interchangeably, they each represent a different idea. *Self-concept* can be defined as the perceptions people have about themselves in terms of personal attributes and roles they fulfill (King, 1997). This does not include value judgments or attitudes toward the self. Instead, it is more of a description of what actually exists. *Self-esteem*, on the other hand, is the evaluation people make of their self-concept description and the extent to which they experience satisfaction or dissatisfaction with it (King, 1997). This refers more to people's feelings about themselves and their attributes. Self-esteem is usually thought of as being either positive or negative, whereas self-concept is a relatively neutral concept. For example, a person may describe himself/herself as overweight, which is that person's perception or self-concept. This is different, however, from having negative feelings about being overweight, which is related to self-esteem.

The third concept, *self-efficacy*, differs from self-esteem in that it refers more specifically to the degree to which an individual possesses confidence in his or her ability to achieve a goal (Greene & Miller, 1996). It is similar to self-esteem in that there is a value judgment being made; however, this judgment is specifically related to ability to achieve a goal. Therefore, it follows that self-esteem is a more general and global concept whereas self-efficacy is more domain-specific.

For example, a person may have a generally high self-esteem in which he or she has positive attitudes toward himself or herself as a person. However, this person can have both high and low self-efficacies. The person might feel very competent in the area of math, thus creating a high self-efficacy in this area. On the other hand, this person may have more trouble with writing, creating a low self-efficacy within this area. The distinction between these three terms is an important one to make. Given this information, it is easy to understand how self-efficacy is more directly related to the process of goal setting and goal attainment.

Although there is evidence that self-esteem has an effect on the types of goals people choose (Adler & Weiss, 1988), examination of self-efficacy may make more sense. Greene and Miller (1996) support this concept. They found that perceived ability, or self-efficacy, relates to goal orientation. Both of these affect cognitive engagement during a task and are linked together. People who adopt learning goals engage in more self-regulation and use more cognitive learning strategies. It has also been supported that students with a high self-efficacy will use more cognitive strategies and have a higher level of cognitive engagement in a task. General self-esteem may also be an important predictor of goal-setting behavior (Adler & Weiss, 1988). Together, these concepts are essential in creating happiness and fulfillment. A person needs to have both a positive self-esteem and a feeling of self-efficacy in certain areas to feel competent and to gain self-acceptance.

It has been mentioned that having a certain type of goal orientation can have cognitive and affective results that are specific to that orientation (Coats et al., 1996; Higgins et al., 1997). Many researchers look at the pursuit of goals and its role in psychological well-being. There have been numerous studies that look at subjective well-being and how this is related to goals. *Subjective well-being* (SWB) can be defined as an aggregate of positive affectivity, negative affectivity, and life satisfaction (Elliot et al., 1997).

Brunstein (1993) also makes this connection, and his research looks at the interaction between goal commitment and goal attainability and its ability to predict SWB. He examined three dimensions that underlie personal goals: commitment to pursue personal goals, evaluation of the attainability of personal goals, and perceived progress in goal achievement. His results found that these three dimensions all play an important role in the development of change in SWB. College students who both had a high level of goal commitment and experienced favorable conditions to attain personal goals displayed positive changes in well-being over time. On the contrary, students who had a high level of goal commitment but experienced poor conditions had impaired well-being. An interaction was also found that indicates that progress in goal achievement may somewhat mediate the influence of goal commitment and goal attainability on SWB. Brunstein (1993) speculates that past experiences of progress may provide a level of comparison for future progress. Therefore, deviations in future progress can be linked to positive or negative changes in SWB. This suggests that keeping an optimistic attitude toward the future might prevent feelings of anguish and might prevent a person from giving up goal-directed efforts while coping with stress.

Research suggests that the use of avoidance goals is negatively related to SWB constructs. Knowing this, Elliot and his colleagues (1997) take this a step further and identify antecedents that may lead to the adoption of avoidance goals. They look at two specific antecedents, neuroticism and perceptions of life skills and competencies. *Neuroticism* is defined as "a general propensity toward emotional instability and overreactivity," and *life skills* are defined as "the competencies and abilities necessary for effective negotiation of daily life" (Elliot et al., 1997). They found support for the belief that neuroticism and life skills are both antecedents to the adoption of avoidance goals. This study suggests that approach and avoidance goals emerge from general emotional predisposition and presumable stable self-perceptions. This finding contradicts Elliot and Sheldon (1997), who suggested that simply reframing goals could be an effective strategy. If goal framing is based more on emotional predisposition, then reframing personal goals in positive terms rather than negative terms will have limited effectiveness.

Once again, look at your four most important goals. Now that they are framed in a way that will promote attainment, think about what the implementation intentions could be. What are some of the problems that you may face in pursuing these goals? How would you deal with this? Think of specific strategies you will use to keep yourself on task and motivated. This process will help you stick with your goals and will increase the rate of completion.

The Goal Process

It is not enough to simply think about a goal that you want to achieve. To increase your chances of attaining that goal, you need to follow a process that will move you in the right direction. Austin and Vancouver (1996) discuss one framework for the goal process. *Establishing goals* is the first step in the process. A person must select a goal and goal content, which may involve many dimensions. This is when the person assesses where he or she is in life and determines where he or she wants to be. The second step is the *planning stage*. This is when specific behavioral paths are developed by which a goal can be attained. It is the *strategy* through which a person will move closer to the goal. In this step, a person needs to specifically link goals to a behavioral script and tactics. These strategies facilitate prioritization of goals. Once a plan is developed, the next step is *striving and monitoring*. The action a person takes can be automatic, unconscious, or elicited from immediate feedback from the environment. A *self-monitoring process* will need to be set up. This aids in the final step of the process, *decisions*. Once a plan is developed and actions are carried out, there are several outcomes. The goal may be attained.

On the other hand, the goal may still be far from achieved. In this case, it is necessary to reassess the goal plan and actions that have taken place. Revisions may be needed to stimulate further growth. The entire goal process is interrelated, with each step depending in some way on the other steps. To begin to achieve lifestyle, social, or career goals, a person needs to learn this process and become goal oriented.

The big question is, What motivates someone? This is an essential part of goal setting. People need to spend time evaluating their lives and determining what they want to improve or change. To achieve a better understanding of this process, write the heading *Long-Range Goals* on a sheet of paper. Your task is to answer the question, What do I want within the next one to ten years? The key to doing this exercise effectively is to take as little time as possible to write down as many items as possible. To help you get started, consider the following half-dozen questions as guidelines (Rohn, 1991):

1. What do I want to do?
2. What do I want to be?
3. What do I want to see?
4. What do I want to have?
5. Where do I want to go?
6. What would I like to share?

Without many and varied types of goals, you could fall prey to the same thing that happened to some of the early Apollo astronauts. Some of them, upon returning from the moon, experienced deep emotional problems. The reason? Once you have been to the moon, where else do you go? After years of training, visualizing, and anticipation, the lunar flight, that moment glorious as it was, was gone. All of a sudden, there seemed to be an end to their life's work, and depression set in. As a result of this experience, later astronauts were trained to have other major projects "on the fire" after their space work was done. This emphasizes the need to constantly push yourself to work harder and achieve more. It is always possible to go further. If it were not possible, life would not have as much meaning.

Now that you have reviewed and balanced your list, choose the four goals from each of four time categories (one year, three years, five years, and ten years) that you consider the most important to you. Doing this assignment is causing you to select a goal, which is the first step to achieving a satisfying life.

Another concept that relates to the goal process is creating *implementation intentions*. These can be defined as anticipated future situations that are linked to certain goal-directed behaviors (Gollwitzer & Brandstatter, 1997). In establishing implementation intentions, people consider what they will do if certain situations come up during goal pursuit. Gollwitzer and Brandstatter examined this concept in their research. They believe that holding such intentions commits a person to perform certain goal-directed behaviors when a critical situation is actually encountered. The results indicate that creating implementation intentions increases the action initiation, completion, and rate of completion of a task. The research also showed that these benefits were only seen with people who reported a high interest in the issue. This suggests that people have an increased chance of goal attainment if they are personally invested in the task.

Time management is another issue that is related to the goal process. Often, people feel as if there is not enough time to get everything done. It is not uncommon to hear people say, "If only I had a couple more hours in the day." These time pressures certainly affect people's ability to pursue and achieve their goals. Because of this, time management is crucial. It is important to make the most of the time you have. The matrix in Table 10.2 depicts four different categories of time management (Covey, 1989).

The top left box reflects the *important/urgent* category. This is otherwise known as a crisis or emergency situation where all efforts are focused on the immediate situation. The top right, or *important/not urgent* category, is where the most effective time managers often find themselves. Here, time is spent on important matters only. The *urgent/not important* category, on the other hand, is where the least effective time managers spend a significant amount of time. In this category, matters are not important, but major time is spent on trivial matters—for example, answering telephones and opening mail. Finally, the lower right corner reflects the *not important/not urgent* category. This corner is otherwise referred to as wasting time—organizing papers, straightening files, and involving yourself in tasks that simply do not make a difference.

These different categories give you an idea of how people can organize their time. Of course, time management is not always within one of these categories. Sometimes, a crisis occurs and you need to devote all of your attention to the emergency at hand. It is important to notice how time is spent and if it is spent productively. Here are some questions to ask: How did you spend most of your day yesterday? What were you doing? How can your time-management skills be improved? These are valuable questions. People need to become aware of how they spend their time in order to come up with ways to maximize the time they have. Maximizing time helps keep people directed and focused. It allows people to be organized, which leads to healthy thinking. When this is achieved, people can successfully work on achieving their dreams.

Dawson (1992) emphasizes another point: that people need to remain enthusiastic throughout the process, even when they hit bumps along the way. Remember that positive attitude that was discussed earlier? Well, it is essential for this process to work. In addition, Dawson (1992) offers guidelines for the goal process.

First, once goals are established, it is important to write them on a piece of paper and carry the paper at all times. This serves as a visual reminder and refo-

TABLE 10.2 **Time Management Matrices**

Important/Urgent	**Important/Not Urgent**
Not Important/Urgent	Not Important/Not Urgent

cuses attention onto the goal. It is also important to have a time deadline on the goal. If there is not a deadline for completion, then what motivation is there? Another step is defining the steps that will lead to the goal. Having a general goal is not specific enough. A person needs to identify what steps he or she can take along the way to get closer to that goal. With this in mind, it is helpful to visualize achievement of the goal. What does it feel like to accomplish it? This visualization will help maintain motivation. Finally, it is essential that a person treat adversities as a learning experience. There will always be setbacks along the way. People are not perfect, and at times they make mistakes. The important thing to remember is that there is always a new day. Remember the discussion about interpreting events that happen to you? A reaction to situations is what really matters. You need to control your behavior even when tragic events happen. So, take setbacks as a learning experience and move on.

Behavior in Goal Pursuit

So far, several issues that affect a person's ability to set up and work toward identified goals have been presented. The information previously discussed is certainly important knowledge to have. There is a very important idea, however, that has not yet been addressed. Identifying goals and working to achieve goals is grounded in one essential need, the need to change behavior. Accomplishing any goal will mean changing some aspect of a person's behavior. For example, suppose a person wants to lose weight. Accomplishing this goal means changing eating behaviors and adding an exercise regime. Any goal you can think of will have certain behaviors that are necessary to have and certain behaviors that are harmful. You need to think about what you want out of life in terms of the behaviors you need to increase or decrease to achieve your goal. Behavior shapers typically define *success* as nothing more than the interaction between what you do, where you do it, and how you reinforce the behavior (Dawson, 1992).

With all of this in mind, it is necessary to recall behavior modification. Changing behavior is not an easy thing to do. If it was, then people would be able to accomplish any goal they wanted, easily. Think about something that you tried to change recently. Maybe you tried to stop smoking or lose a couple of pounds. Do you remember your New Year's resolution? What success did you have with it? It probably was not easy, and you probably became frustrated along the way. How is behavioral change successfully completed? The following section discusses the basic concepts in behavior modification that are essential for change to occur.

The first thing to realize is that behavior does not happen in a vacuum, beginning to end. Rather, behavior is a function of the events that happen before and after the behavior occurs. In behavioral psychology, this is called the *A-B-C model.* The *A* stands for *antecedents.* These include anything that happens before a behavior occurs. What was going on in the environment? Who was there? What where they doing? What were you doing? These are all part of this category. People have a tendency to think that it is the antecedents that cause their behavior, but, while they do have an impact on behavior, they are not the main component.

In the middle, *B* is the behavior that occurs. This is followed by *C*, consequences. *Consequences* are defined as anything that happens after the behavior.

Behavior is a function of the consequences that occur, and people behave in certain ways because of the consequences they have learned to expect. All you need to do to understand this fact is to think about your job. For most people, the major driving force for going to work everyday is that they will be rewarded with paychecks. Receiving paychecks is a consequence that motivates people to keep going to work. Of course, there are other reasons for having a job besides the paychecks. However, if your job suddenly became volunteer work without pay, would you stay? Along these same lines, people are less motivated when they are unsure of what the consequences will be. For example, people would probably not mind putting in lots of extra hours at work if they were sure it would help them get a promotion.

Exploring consequences requires a look at the principle of reinforcement. In behavioral psychology, the *principle of reinforcement* holds that if behavior is reinforced it will be repeated. Think again about your job. You can expect that every two weeks you will receive a paycheck. Thus, the consequence that happens (paycheck) is reinforcing your behavior (working). Reinforcement is a very strong tool and is the best way to change behavior. It helps provide people with the necessary motivation.

There are two basic types of reinforcement, positive and negative. In *positive reinforcement,* something is added to the situation that will increase the likelihood that it will happen again. Receiving a paycheck is one example of positive reinforcement. Another example would be a teacher who gives class members an extra five bonus points on a test if they have good behavior in the classroom. In both of these examples, something is added to the situation that makes the appropriate behavior more desirable. The added item is called a reinforcer. A *reinforcer* can be anything that is motivating and has meaning to an individual. One category of reinforcers is *extrinsic.* Extrinsic reinforcers are often more concrete, materialistic items such as already mentioned.

Another category of reinforcers is *intrinsic reinforcers,* which are more abstract. These types of reinforcers contain things such as a smile, a good feeling, or things people value in life. Often, these types of reinforcers are harder to identify and explain. It is important to think about what motivates you. The concept of reinforcement will always work if you have identified an appropriate reinforcer. A key is to create goals that manifest your own rewards. In other words, try to set them up so that they will be intrinsically reinforced. Using this in combination with an extrinsic reinforcer will help increase success.

The second type of reinforcement is *negative reinforcement.* Be careful not to confuse the word *negative* with something bad. This simply means that something is taken away from a situation that will increase the likelihood that a behavior will happen again. For example, a teacher could say there would be no homework if the students finished their assignment in class. Another example would be a mother who tells her young child he does not have to wash the dishes if he completes his homework. In both these situations something aversive (homework and washing dishes) is taken away if a desired behavior occurs.

Another category of consequences related to behavioral psychology is *punishment.* Whereas reinforcement works on increasing an appropriate behavior, punishment works on decreasing an inappropriate behavior. Both positive and negative exist here as well. Positive punishment is adding something to a situation that will decrease the probability that the behavior will occur again. The added stimulus is something aversive such as having to do extra chores or an extra assignment or being spanked. Typically, this type of consequence is not as effective and should only be used as a last resort. Negative punishment is taking something away to decrease the probability that a behavior will occur again. Examples of this type of punishment would be not being able to go out Friday night or not being able to eat dessert. In general, the research shows that punishment, as a whole, is a far less effective strategy for changing behavior than reinforcement. Punishment does not reinforce *good* behavior, instead, *bad* behavior is identified.

Still, sometimes work needs to be done about decreasing those *bad* behaviors. The best way to do this is to combine reinforcement with punishment. When using punishment, the goal should always be to use it as a temporary strategy until it can be switched to a reinforcement system. It is also helpful when using negative punishment to take away something positive as opposed to adding something negative. This is the more effective of the two strategies.

Since reinforcement is the best approach to learning and maintaining a new behavior, discussion follows on how to set up such a system and apply it to yourself. After selecting a goal, the next step should be to ask yourself, What behaviors do I need to have in order to accomplish this goal? As mentioned earlier, it is not enough to have one complete goal. This goal needs to be broken down into steps and essential parts. From this, you can set smaller behavioral goals that will help you move toward your final goal. For example, a person working toward running in a marathon could start by running every day. This person might need to establish the discipline of running every day before working on behaviors such as distance or speed of running. Once specific behaviors that are needed are identified, the person can set up a reinforcement system to help change his or her behavior. This can include giving a reward for engaging in the appropriate behaviors.

Another related idea is the concept of behavior shaping. *Behavior shaping* is defined as reinforcing successive approximations of a desired behavior. It holds that tasks can be broken down into more specific behaviors and a person can be reinforced for reaching each new level. This, in turn, shapes the behavior into the ultimate goal. This is seen in young infants first learning to talk. When babies speak their first words, everybody makes a big fuss and reinforces it through social acceptance, hugs, kisses, and cheerful noises. After a while, hearing one word from a child is not a big deal anymore and the reinforcement slows down until the point that a two-word utterance is spoken. This is seen as a big step, and, as a result, parents and family once again make a big deal and reinforce the child. This process continues, reinforcing the child each time he or she achieves a new level until speech and language is completely developed. This is a good example to emphasize that shaping is a natural process. It is related to how many developmental milestones and academic abilities are learned. This is a good way to help a person slowly change behavior.

Another method of changing behavior is to reinforce an action that is *incompatible* with the target behavior you want change. The thought here is that it would be impossible for these two behaviors to occur at the same time. Suppose you have a person who has a problem screaming at people when he or she gets mad. This person can use anger-management techniques such as taking a deep breath and counting to ten to calm down. It is physically impossible for a person to be screaming and taking a deep breath at the same time; thus, these behaviors are incompatible. By teaching the new *incompatible behavior,* the person learns an alternate way of dealing with a situation that is more appropriate than the current method. This method of reinforcement is beneficial because it replaces the old behavior with a new behavior, which is often the challenge being faced.

The use of reinforcement is essential for modifying behavior and reaching goals. People need to be aware of their behavior and know a way they can successfully align themselves with their goals. Positive reinforcement is a strong, successful method to facilitate a change in behavior, which is crucial in the exploration of the goal process. The behavioral techniques presented can lead to reinforcement that can perpetuate a person's aspirations and goals.

Nine Steps to a Self-Directed Life

The focus of this chapter has been on how to get what you want out of life and achieve true happiness. Dawson (1992) identifies nine steps necessary for a person to have a more self-directed life:

1. *Select a goal.* This goal needs to be specific, obtainable by your efforts, measurable, and given a time frame.

2. *Determine the chain of events that must precede the successful completion of the goal.* This will depend on personal styles and personality constructs. The key here is to start out slow and make a goal out of specific behaviors required.

3. *Establish a course.* What behaviors must you change in order to get to the goal?

4. *Establish target behaviors and develop a plan that gradually increases your success.*

5. *Develop a reinforcement system.* Select a reinforcer that is motivating to you, and reward yourself when you achieve a step.

6. *Avoid pitfalls.* Try not to make commitments when you are tired or discouraged. Look for willpower, and plan for plateaus along the way. Recognize that reaching a plateau where you feel *stuck* is common, and ride it out. Do not cheat. It is easy to just give yourself the reward even though you did not earn it.

7. *Study role models.* Observe someone who is achieving goals. Imitation is the basis for many learning experiences.

8. *Visualize yourself accomplishing your behavioral goal.* This is far more powerful than visualizing the whole goal. Using visualization will draw you toward the behavior.

9. *Reevaluate your behavioral goals continuously.* Once again, focus on the behavior. Did you over or underestimate yourself? If you did, then you need to lower or raise the criteria for the behavior. Keep in mind, you and your environment are constantly changing. It is important to continually ask, What is the behavior I should be aiming for and what technique should I be using?

Self-Assessment

Following are eight different areas in which you can assess your current strengths and weaknesses. For each area, think about your life and where you are in relation to where you would like to be. Rate yourself on a scale of one to ten, with *one* being *totally dissatisfied* and *ten* being *totally satisfied*. Then, for each area, write a goal for yourself in the space provided for three months, six months, twelve months, three years, and five years from now. Think about where you want to be and which goals can help you get there.

Career
Three Months

_____

_____

_____

Six Months

_____

_____

_____

Twelve Months

_____

_____

_____

Three Years

_____

_____

_____

Five Years

_____

_____

_____

Family
Three Months

_____

_____

_____

Six Months

_____

_____

_____

Twelve Months

_____

_____

_____

Three Years

_____

_____

_____

Five Years

_____

_____

_____

Financial
Three Months

_____

_____

_____

Six Months

_____

_____

_____

Twelve Months

_____

_____

_____

Three Years

_____

_____

_____

Five Years

_____

_____

_____

Health
Three Months

_____

_____

_____

Six Months

_____

_____

_____

Twelve Months

_____

_____

_____

Three Years

_____

_____

_____

Five Years

_____

_____

_____

Relationships
Three Months

_____

_____

_____

Six Months

_____

_____

_____

Twelve Months

_____

_____

_____

Three Years

_____

_____

_____

Five Years

_____

_____

_____

School
Three Months

_____

_____

_____

Six Months

_____

_____

_____

Twelve Months

_____

_____

_____

Three Years

_____

_____

_____

Five Years

_____

_____

_____

Spiritual
Three Months

_____

_____

_____

Six Months

_____

_____

_____

Twelve Months

_____

_____

_____

Three Years

_____

_____

_____

Five Years

_____

_____

_____

Social
Three Months

_____

_____

_____

Six Months

_____

_____

_____

Twelve Months

_____

_____

_____

Three Years

_____

_____

_____

Five Years

_____

_____

_____

Summary

Personal goals are related to achieving good mental health. Goals help a person to become more directed and focused, which leads to less stress and increased self-satisfaction. A person who is mentally healthy needs to be goal-oriented and have knowledge of the techniques that promote goal pursuit. To proceed through this process, a person must, first and foremost, have an understanding of his or her own personality. People are motivated in different ways and have different philosophies. In addition, people need to be aware of how they deal with stress. Knowing this information can aid in developing individualized plans for working toward goals and achieving good mental health.

People can frame their goals in many ways, including approach, avoidance, mastery, and performance. Generally, approach and mastery goals have been shown to promote increased well-being, unlike avoidance and performance goals. The way that people phrase their goals, positively or negatively, can have a great impact on the success and feelings of satisfaction they experience. Self-esteem and motivation are additional factors that are crucial in achieving and maintaining good mental health.

The process through which a person attempts to achieve happiness is another important factor. People need to have knowledge of the goal process in order to learn how to set up, monitor, and assess their progress. Time-management skills are an important part of being organized and focused. A positive attitude is an essential component in this process. People need to be optimistic and remain positive when pitfalls occur, thereby learning from their experiences and continuing to move forward.

Finally, behavior is the mechanism by which people achieve their goals. To get where you want to be, you need to assess your behaviors and determine what behavior you need to change to move forward. Setting behavioral goals is the best way to achieve self-satisfaction. Knowledge of and use of behavior modification techniques will help you create a reinforcing environment in which change can occur. When this happens, you will move closer to your goals and, more importantly, closer to achieving life satisfaction and good mental health.

DISCUSSION QUESTIONS

1. Which of the following best describes your personality: analytical, driver, amiable, or socializer? Based on the type you selected, discuss how this affects how you deal with stress.

2. Name and describe the four forces that drive human behavior according to Roger Dawson.

3. Discuss the three main factors that help a person establish a healthy, optimistic attitude. Why are they important?

4. What is the difference between approach and avoidance goals? Give an example of each, and discuss why one is more effective than the other.

5. According to the research, in what ways can goal framing affect a person's mental health?

6. Compare and contrast self-concept, self-esteem, and self-efficacy. Why are these important for achieving self-satisfaction?

7. According to Roger Dawson, what are the key components in the goal process?

8. Discuss the *A-B-C* model of behavior.

9. Name the two types of reinforcement, and give an example of each. What is the benefit of using reinforcement?

10. Suppose one of your goals is to get better grades in college. Name one behavioral goal that will help you move toward better grades. What steps will you take to achieve this behavioral goal?

11. Braza (1997) in his book *Moment by Moment,* asks the reader to reflect on the following questions:
    a. What am I missing while I am making other plans?
    b. How would I complete the following statements?
       I'll be happy when. . . .
       If only. . . .
    c. What pleasures have I failed to enjoy?
    d. Who are the happiest people I know?
    e. What is their secret of happiness?
    Responses to these questions often illustrate what is really important in one's life. Happiness does not come from getting more or comparing; nor is it found in the future. Look at happy people, study their secrets, and live more fully in the present. According to Braza (1997), "There is no way to happiness, happiness is the way."

REFERENCES

Adler, S., & Weiss, H. M. (1988). Criterion Aggregation in Personality Research: A Demonstration Looking at Self-Esteem and Goal Setting. *Human Performance, 1*(2), 99–109.

Austin, J. T., & Vancouver, J. B. (1996). Goal Constructs in Psychology: Structure, Process, and Content. *Psychological Bulletin, 120*(3), 338–375.

Braza, J. (1997). *Moment by Moment: the Art and Practice of Mindfulness.* Boston: Charles Tuttle.

Brunstein, J. C. (1993). Personal Goals and Subjective Well-Being: A Longitudinal Study. *Journal of Personality and Social Psychology, 65*(5), 1061–1070.

Coats, E. J., Janoff-Bulman, R., & Alpert, N. (1996). Approach Versus Avoidance Goals: Differences in Self-Evaluation and Well-Being. *Personality and Social Psychology Bulletin, 22*(10), 1057–1067.

Covey, S. (1989). *Seven Habits of Highly Effective People.* Simon & Schuster.

Dawson, R. (1989). *The Power of Persuasion.* Niles: Nightingale-Connant.

Dawson, R. (1992). *Beyond Goals.* Niles: Nightingale-Connant.

Elliot, A. J. & Church, M. A. (1997). A Hierarchical Model of Approach and Avoidance Achievement Motivation. *Journal of Personality and Social Psychology, 72*(1), 218–232.

Elliot, A. J. & Sheldon, K. M. (1997). Avoidance Achievement Motivation: A Personal Goals Analysis. *Journal of Personality and Social Psychology, 73*(1), 171–185.

Elliot, A. J., Sheldon, K. M., & Church, M.A. (1997). Avoidance, Personal Goals, and Subjective Well-Being. *Personality and Social Psychology Bulletin, 23*(9), 915–927.

Erdley, C. A., Cain, K. M., Loomis, C. C., Dumas-Hines, F., & Dweck, C. S. (1997). Relations Among Children's Social Goals, Implicit Personality Theories, and Responses to Social Failure. *Developmental Psychology, 33*(2), 263–272.

Gollwitzer, P. M. & Brandstatter, V. (1997). Implementation Intentions and Effective Goal Pursuit. *Journal of Personality and Social Psychology, 73*(1), 186–199.

Greene, B., & Miller, R. (1996). Influences on achievement: Goals, Perceived Ability, and Cognitive Engagement. *Contemporary Educational Psychology, 21,* 181–192.

Higgins, E. T., Shah, J., & Friedman, R. (1997). Emotional Responses to Goal Attainment: Strength of Regulatory Focus as Moderator. *Journal of Personality and Social Psychology, 72*(3), 515–525.

Howe., B., & Poole, R. (1992). Goal Proximity and Achievement Motivation of High School Boys in a Basketball Shooting Task. *Journal of Teaching in Physical Education, 11,* 248–255.

Jolibert, A., & Baumgartner, G. (1997). Values, Motivations, and Personal Goals: Revisited. *Psychology & Marketing, 14*(7), 675–688.

King, K. A. (1997). Self-Concept and Self-Esteem: A Clarification of Terms. *Journal of School Health, 67*(2), 68–70.

Middleton, M. J., & Midgley, C. (1997). Avoiding the Demonstration of Lack of Ability: An Underexplored Aspect of Goal Theory. *Journal of Educational Psychology, 89*(4), 710–718.

Rohn, J. (1991). *Seven Keys to Wealth and Happiness.* Niles: Nightingale-Connant.

Roney, C. J. R., Higgins, E. T., & Shah, J. (1995). Goals and Framing: How Outcome Focus Influences Motivation and Emotion. *Personality and Social Psychology Bulletin, 21*(11), 1151–1160.

11 Mental Health Resources and Helping Professions

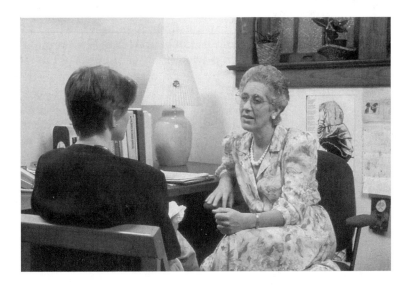

Achieving good mental health is not easy, especially with the multitude of stresses in everyday life. Often, people have difficulty overcoming problems and dealing with stress. There are many psychological problems that can result when a person does not have adequate coping strategies. Every person has difficulty in some areas, and there is a continuum of reactions that people can have. With this in mind, most people can benefit from utilizing resources in the mental health field. "Psychologists are for people who are having bigger problems that I have," and "I can solve my problems on my own" are common misconceptions among the general public. The fact is that everybody needs support and assistance at times. Knowing about the vast array of services offered within the mental health field creates an atmosphere in which people can recognize when they need assistance and how to get it. This is important for students who wish to become mental health counselors along with readers who may someday decide to access help.

This chapter offers an overview of mental health services on a clinical and community level. Different professions within the field are discussed along with information about the process and what to expect in different settings.

Knowing When to Access Help

A key part in achieving good mental health is knowing when to access help. People seek out mental health services for various reasons, ranging from stress in the workplace to major depression with suicidal thoughts. Whatever the presenting problem, the fact remains that the person needs to gain insight into the problem and develop effective coping strategies. Most professionals would agree that the time to access help is when the symptoms begin to interfere with an individual's functioning. For example, people who experience stress at their jobs may be able to deal with it through their own successful coping mechanisms and perform at the expected level. On the other hand, people with this same stress may blow up in the office, screaming at people or becoming violent. This behavior is most definitely going to interfere with job performance and may even cause them to lose their jobs. Another scenario could include the person who performs at the expected level but keeps the stress inside and cannot resolve it. This person may be performing at work; however, he or she may develop chronic headaches that interfere with his or her life. Everyone has problems to a certain degree. It is when these problems interfere with a person's life or goal pursuit that assistance may be needed. In reality, any person can make the decision that he or she needs help. It is also appropriate for certain people (family, managers, teachers, or close friends) to refer a person to access help.

College: A Special Case

In recent years, there has been a focus on college students and their involvement in counseling. The analogy "college is an emotional pressure cooker" depicts the idea that students become vulnerable to a host of problems when they enter college (Hesse-Biber & Marino, 1991). College is a time of transition and new challenges. Often a person is moving to a new place and is forced to start new relationships and adjust to new types of environmental pressures. Because of this, college students are vulnerable to the negative effects of stress. It is suggested that the sophomore year of college is one of the most vulnerable years. Hesse-Biber and Marino's results indicate that sophomores have a higher level of anxiety than both freshmen and juniors. They offer that this may be due to the fact that freshmen have orientations and special programs to help them; however, sophomores do not have a strong social support network and have not yet developed effective coping mechanisms to deal with college stress.

Self-concept is one area that is affected by the adjustment to college. Harrison, Maples, Testa, and Jones (1993) found that students generally reported confidence in their academic abilities; however, they were less secure when comparing themselves to classmates. At first, it appeared as if the students were fairly confident. Through further examination, it was found that problems related to assertiveness, interacting with others in an academic setting, and test anxiety were present. The authors contend that although students may indeed feel confident and achieve success, they concurrently experience a fear of failure that creates interpersonal tension.

The issue of self-concept has also been studied in relation to females and the development of eating disorders. Research suggests that the transition from high school to college may leave females particularly vulnerable (Hesse-Biber & Marino, 1991). It was found that there is a downward shift in self-concept in females during these years. A poor self-confidence, along with lack of assertiveness and academic pressures, may contribute to disturbing eating patterns.

Researchers have investigated the number of college students who access help and the types of problems they report. Pledge, Lapan, Heppner, Kavlighan, and Roehlke (1998) conducted a six-year analysis of presenting problems and found that they became "more serious"—including more emotional and behavioral problems—during the 1980s. They found that this increased severity leveled off and became stable in the 1990s. This implies that the problems of college students seeking help today continue to remain at a more severe level than those from earlier decades. The problems presented included: interpersonal concerns (i.e., feelings of jealousy and guilt and concerns about sexual relationships); vegetative symptoms (i.e., sleep problems, weight change); depressive symptoms (i.e., mood changes, feelings of hopelessness, and suicidal ideation); and behavioral concerns (i.e., substance abuse).

Additional studies looked at the perceived benefit of seeking counseling at the college level. Holzman, Searight, and Hughes (1996) found that clinical psychology graduate students reported positive experiences from initiating psychotherapy. Although many of the students (65 percent) entered therapy to learn the process and improve their abilities as therapists, other reasons were noted. Some of these reasons included personal growth, adjustment or developmental issues, and depression. Survey results indicated that 25 percent of all the respondents stated they had been or were currently depressed during their training. It is possible that being in psychotherapy offers the support needed to adjust and succeed in the college setting. Another interesting note is the finding that the number one reason for students not seeking therapy was finances. It may be that more college students would access help if it were cost-effective.

The example of college students is helpful in making the point that there are hosts of environmental pressures that are inflicted on people as part of everyday life. At times, these pressures become too intense and an individual does not have an effective way of dealing with stress. Often, people tend to wait until they feel the problem is more serious to seek help. This results in a buildup of symptoms, which creates a more complex problem. On the other hand, people can access help at the start of a problem or when there are few symptoms present. Seeking help from mental health resources at these times can be beneficial in preventing a problem, understanding a problem, and developing coping mechanisms.

Intervention: Primary, Secondary, and Tertiary

Generally, there are three levels of intervention. The first is *primary intervention,* in which education and giving appropriate information is the main goal. The purpose here is to give people the ability to recognize problems and resources available so they can make informed decisions. The second level is *secondary intervention,* which involves early detection of problems. Crisis intervention and counseling intervention are often used in this level. The idea here is to catch the problem in its early stages and intervene to prevent the problem from escalating. The final level, *tertiary intervention,* involves more intense therapy and treatments. This is the place where most people access help. It is important to realize, however, that accessing help at the primary or secondary level is very useful in gaining information and preventing more serious problems from occurring.

Clinical Assessment

When a person accesses help from a professional in the mental health field, a process of clinical assessment usually is initiated. A clinical assessment is a process in which the clinician attempts to understand the nature and extent of the presented problem. It is the forerunner for counseling or developing interventions and is usually an ongoing process. In the mental health field, a clinical assessment is not as straightforward as it is in the medical field. A psychologist or mental health counselor is faced with the challenge of discovering the personality characteristics of an individual along with the social environments that individual is embedded in. Since people are not isolated entities, it is essential to gather as much information as possible about a person to conduct a thorough assessment.

Clinical Interview

The *clinical interview* is one of the first ways a mental health worker attempts to collect information. Interviewing techniques vary, with some being very structured and others being more open-ended. The main goal of the clinician is to talk with the client to get basic information on the presented problem, background, personality characteristics, and social/emotional functioning. Basically, the clinician wants to get information on all areas of the client's life. A clinician is rarely going to get all of the desired data during the initial interview. Rather, he/she will talk with the client regarding all areas of the assessment, collecting information as the process unfolds. At times it may be helpful for clinicians to talk with significant people in the client's life for further insight. Counseling settings such as colleges or community programs often utilize this assessment format.

Aside from interviewing, clinicians may need to gather more specific information. This will vary depending on the type of problem and the clinician. There are two main areas of testing that are widely used to gather information: intelligence testing and personality testing.

Intelligence Tests

Intelligence tests provide a more structured and standardized type of clinical assessment. The trained clinician administers a test battery, which gives both sub-test scores and an overall IQ score. Some common intelligence tests used today are: the Wechsler Intelligence Scale for Children, Third Edition (WISC-III); the Wechsler Adult Intelligence Scale, Third Edition (WAIS-III); the Stanford-Binet Intelligence Scale; and the Differential Ability Scales (DAS). A typical intelligence test takes approximately three hours to administer, score, and interpret. It gives a clinician an understanding of the present level of the cognitive functioning of an individual as well as specific strengths and weaknesses. This can provide a clinician with clues as to the resources an individual has to solve problems.

Intelligence tests are used primarily when brain damage or intellectual impairment is suspected to be at the core of an individual's problems. Schools are one place where this pertains. Usually, schools use intelligence tests as one way to help understand a student's learning problems. Because of the nature of this type of testing, it is less critical in many clinical cases and therefore not used as much.

Personality Tests

Personality tests are used to measure many personal characteristics other than intelligence. There are two different types of personality tests: *objective* and *projective*. *Objective personality tests* are more structured and usually include various questionnaires or rating scales. The structure of these types of tests allows them to be more controlled and objective in interpretation. They include such instruments as behavior rating scales, adaptive behavior scales, personality scales, and scales to assess specific disorders (i.e., depression inventory). They give clinicians specific information about how a person is functioning in a particular area. One of the most famous is the Minnesota Multiphasic Personality Inventory (MMPI). This is a self-report tool, which consists of items in various categories (such as social attitudes, moral attitudes, psychological states, and physical conditions) that the client has to answer true or false. The combination of certain questions provides a measure of different clinical scales such as depression or paranoia and of special scales such as anxiety and ego strength. Aside from being used in a therapeutic setting, this test is frequently used for research or selection of people for specific jobs.

Projective personality tests are unstructured tasks in which the client has to respond to pictures or ambiguous stimuli instead of verbal questions or rating scales. The main assumption underlying all projective techniques is that when individuals are presented with an ambiguous stimuli they will project their own characteristics, problems, motives, and wishes onto that situation. They are based largely on a psychoanalytic perspective, thus tap into the individual's unconscious needs and motivations. Interpretation of these tests, therefore, has the potential to reveal very valuable information about a client. A clinician is able to examine how individuals perceive the world, what their current coping mechanisms are, and what issues they may be struggling with. Some of the most widely used projective tests are the Thematic Apperception Test (TAT), the Rorschach Test, and sentence-completion tests. Projective techniques are often used not only for assessment purposes but also as a tool in therapy. The administration of such techniques is seen as analogous to the psychotherapeutic process and can aid in the client gaining insight and increasing self-awareness. In addition, they can enhance the counseling relationship, help a clinician understand a client, and aid in the development of a treatment plan (Clark, 1995; Waiswol, 1995).

Common Practice

Together, these assessment tools allow a clinician to obtain an evaluation in different domains. Research shows that clinicians generally use around nine assessment techniques when conducting an evaluation (Watkins, Campbell, Nieberding, & Hallmark, 1995). Watkins and his colleagues found that, indeed, almost all clinicians surveyed used the clinical interview as a main assessment technique. Further, they reported that the standard assessment tools—the Wechsler scales, the MMPI-2, and the more popular projective techniques (including the Rorschach, TAT, sentence completion, and drawings)—tend to be used most often and most consistently by clinicians regardless of the work setting.

The information gathered throughout a clinical assessment is used in many ways. In schools, it is used to determine if a student needs special education and, if so, what type of program would be appropriate. In the workplace, it is used for selection of employees for a specific job or to find out what type of career is best for a person. In a more clinical setting, the clinical assessment is used to gain an understanding of a person's problem and develop ways to treat the problem. This may include therapy as well as behavioral and environmental interventions.

Psychologically Based Interventions

Psychologists offer a range of services, including testing, assessment, diagnosis, short-term counseling, and long-term therapy. They are usually trained at the doctoral level to conduct thorough assessments and have effective communication skills. Aside from psychologists, there are also certified counselors and social workers that have advanced training in counseling and assessment. More often than not, professionals in a clinical setting spend the majority of their time treating patients with either short-term counseling or long-term therapy. It is important for students to have an understanding of the process of counseling and therapy so they will feel comfortable seeking out help.

To understand the basic process and goals of therapy, it is useful to have an understanding of the different types of orientations therapists have. Therapists often identify with and use a particular theory as the basis for their treatment. Some therapists choose to use combinations of different models that take on a more *eclectic* style. Following is a brief overview of the broad categories of therapies that exist and an explanation of a couple of specific types of therapies within each category.

Psychodynamic Therapy

Psychodynamic therapy focuses on individual personality dynamics from a psycho-analytic perspective. Therapists who identify with this type of therapy are often called *psychoanalysts* or *analysts*. Treatment in this type of therapy is often based on classical psychoanalysis or more modern types of psychoanalysis. The main idea in psychodynamic therapy is that the individual has repressed materials from child-hood that channel energy into the use of defense mechanisms. The goal in this type of therapy, therefore, is for clients to gain insight into their inner motivations and desires in order to turn their energies toward integrating their personality.

Freudian or Classical Psychoanalysis. To have a basic understanding of psy-chodynamic therapy, it is necessary to become familiar with the "father" of psy-choanalysis. The backbone of psychology's understanding of human behavior is Sigmund Freud's *psychoanalytic theory* (Freud, 1935). Classical psychoanalysis is the stereotypical picture of *therapy*, with an impersonal analyst who does not share per-sonal information and a client on a couch discussing his or her childhood. While many people feel that classical psychoanalytic theory has some serious drawbacks, it is the basis for most modern theories and is still widely used in practice.

Psychoanalysis is based on the idea that humans are in constant internal con-flict to resolve aggressive and sexual impulses that occur during daily life. Freud believed that everything occurring in a person's life was a direct result of some prior experience, a concept called *determinism*. According to Freud, free will is sim-ply an illusion that humans have developed, and the effects of internal conflicts about sexual and aggressive impulses are the only determining factors of their behavior (Carson, Butcher, & Mineka 1996; Freud, 1935; Wallace, 1986).

Freud believed that the *psyche* (or soul) was divided into three levels: the unconscious, conscious, and preconscious. *Conscious* information is available by simple recall, for example, your name or home phone number. *Preconscious* infor-mation is only available through concentration. An example might be the infor-mation learned last week in chemistry class. *Unconscious* information is unavail-able to the individual and can only be accessed through psychoanalysis.

To understand human behavior, Freud divided the personality into three structures: the id, the ego, and the superego. Behavior is a result of the struggle between these three structures; and the goal of psychoanalytic therapy is to assist the client to recognize, understand, and resolve the intrapsychic conflict.

The *id* is believed to be present at birth. It is part of the unconscious and does not deal with reality. The id only seeks pleasure and is not tolerant of discomfort. The *ego* develops when a child begins to display socialization skills. The ego is controlled by reality and exists to mediate between the id and the superego. The *superego* devel-ops when a young person internalizes rules and social values. Like the id, it is pre-dominantly an unconscious force and passes judgment on whether an act is "right" or "wrong." Freud believed that humans only have a certain amount of psychic energy, or *libido*. This energy must be divided between the id, ego, and superego in a way that resolves psychosexual conflicts (Carson et al., 1996; Sue, Sue, & Sue, 1994).

Freud believed that many of these conflicts were brought on by the challenges characteristic of psychosexual stages of development. Freud felt these stages were universal, biological, and predictable. Children follow these stages in sequence and must resolve the conflicts that arise at each stage. Inability to resolve these conflicts can result in *fixation,* or lasting preoccupation with the pleasures and issues of that stage as an adult (Carson et al., 1996; Sue et al., 1994; Wallace, 1986).

The first stage of psychosexual development is the *oral stage.* It begins at birth and lasts approximately until the age of one and one-half years. Babies derive pleasure from sucking on a bottle, satisfying their hunger through oral stimulation. An infant who experiences a deprivation of these sensations, such as extreme hunger, can develop a *fixation* on this stage in later life. Freud believed that adults who develop needy personality types are fixated on the oral stage.

The next stage is the *anal stage.* During this stage, elimination of bodily wastes becomes the source of pleasure. The main task of this stage is toilet training. The child learns that in order to gain social acceptance, he or she must delay bodily urges. If the child experiences this as an anxiety-provoking event, he or she may grow up to become an adult who is overly sensitive about others' views (Carson et al., 1996; Sue et al., 1994).

The *phallic stage* is Freud's next level in psychosexual development. During this stage, there is an unconscious incestuous desire for the parent of the opposite sex. Freud called the resulting conflict the *Oedipus complex* in males and the *Electra complex* in females. The Oedipus complex is the male child's sexual desire for his mother and subsequent resentment of his father. The Electra complex is the female child's sexual desire for her father and resentment for her mother. These resentments create a conflict, which is resolved, according to Freud, through the identification of children of both sexes with their same sex parent. Freud felt that inability to resolve these complexes could result in homosexual feelings as an adult.

Freud called the next stage in psychosexual development the *latency stage,* noting that it was a respite from the highly sexual conflicts that occurred in the phallic stage. During this phase, children further develop their personality but do not experience any overtly sexual drives. Freud described this stage as lasting from ages six to twelve (Carson et al., 1996; Sue et al., 1994).

The last stage of Freud's psychosexual development is the *genital stage,* in which adolescents typically develop a desire for the opposite sex. This phase lasts for the rest of adult life, according to Freud.

Psychoanalysts often use the technique of *free association,* in which the client is instructed to say anything that comes to mind. The client free associates, while the analyst take extensive notes or records the session. Dream analysis is also applied. Analysts are also aware of *resistance,* the unconscious reluctance of the client to discuss the matters that are truly important to the therapy (Carson et al., 1996; Freud, 1935).

Although Freud's theory has had a profound impact on the field of psychology, there are many critics who tend to disagree with his emphasis on sexual instincts as the main determinant of human behavior. Because of this, a number of people branched out to create new models of their own. Some of these people include: Alfred Adler, Carl Jung, Erik Erikson, Karen Horney, and Margaret Mahler. All of these people are considered *neo-Freudians* and have made significant contributions to psychodynamic theory.

Adlerian Therapy. Alfred Adler's theory is a good example of a model that was developed as a reaction to Freud's theory. Like many psychological theorists, Adler was originally a Freudian analyst but broke with Freud early because he rejected the sexual basis of crisis that Freud favored. Adler is the founder of *individual psychology*. Individual psychology has a strong cerebral emphasis and is often called *cognitive therapy*. Although Adler believed that certain modifying factors—such as genetics, environment, and early childhood experiences—influence personality and actions, he believed that an individual's conscious thoughts and logic and beliefs are the basis of human behavior (Adler, 1963; Ansbacher & Ansbacher, 1956; Dinkmeyer, Pew, & Dinkmeyer 1979).

Adler further believed that in early life each person chooses a life goal or life script and uses this to fulfill individuality and compensate for inferiority. Individuals consistently make choices that allow them to live up to their life's goals, and these choices result in characteristic ways of reacting to situations. The choice of a life goal is, according to Adler, partly genetic and partly environmental. The behavior of the individual is based on a constant, goal-oriented motivation and can be understood by examining *lifestyle choice*. Lifestyle choice is influenced by four factors: early childhood experiences, place and perceived function in the family, a need for social connectedness, and a human drive for superiority (Adler, 1963).

Adlerian therapists believe that some general conclusions can be reached regarding an individual based on *birth order*. For instance, the first child tends to become a leader and often has conservative attitudes. If a second child is born immediately after the first child and is of the same gender, there is likely to be strong competition between the children. The second child becomes extroverted, seeks approval and attention from others, and often chooses a lifestyle as opposite as possible from the first child. Adlerian therapists believe that, in many cases, interaction between siblings has an even stronger influence on children than the interaction between child and parent (Dinkmeyer et al., 1979).

Social connectedness is also important to Adlerian therapists, who believe that people are primarily social beings and have a strong need to be recognized as valuable to society. Doing things for others, according to Adlerians, gives meaning to life. Social connectedness is also believed to be essential for human survival. If people did not believe they needed one another, there would be no reason to cooperate and the human race would decline (Ansbacher & Ansbacher, 1956).

Adlerians also believe that the *drive for superiority* is a shared part of human nature. As all individuals are compelled by this drive to master their environment, they establish a perception of their uniqueness as individuals. A person must recognize that part of human nature is inferiority and that persons who are healthy work to rid themselves of this inferiority. Rejecting the notion of universal inferiority can lead to exaggerated beliefs in ability, pathology, dysfunctional behavior, and general dissatisfaction with life. On the other hand, Adler believed that individuals are self-determined and can consciously choose to be unproductive (Ansbacher & Ansbacher, 1956). This behavior can lead to fantasy, projection, and neurosis due to faulty beliefs and irrational goals.

Adlerians believe that misbehavior is consciously chosen to further goals and has a payoff when attention is gained, power is sought, revenge is taken, and defeat or deficiency is admitted. This thinking has been applied by parents and teachers in educational situations.

In Adlerian therapy, an understanding regarding the client's lifestyle, goals, and early memories is the focus of early sessions. Adler also placed great emphasis on the client's perceptions of family and the way his or her family interacts. Adlerian therapy is also known for engaging any technique necessary to attract the attention of and arouse the client's thoughts. In cognitive therapy, counselors form a relaxed relationship with their clients, facing them and encouraging trust, acceptance, and respect. The role of the therapist is to help clients understand why they behave the way they do and to explain mistakes in a way that is satisfactory to the clients. Adler described successful therapy as an *"aha"* experience (Adler 1963; Ansbacher & Ansbacher, 1956; Dinkmeyer & et al., 1979).

Adlerians are known for the belief that any technique that attracts attention and arouses the client can pave the way to change faulty logic and to correct personal mistakes and fictional goals. Adler began the use of *paradoxical directives,* a technique that exaggerates undesirable behavior to increase awareness. This technique is often used in marital and family counseling.

Adler's techniques and beliefs appeal to many because they allow the individual to hold the power: individuals are masters of their own fate (Dinkmeyer et al., 1979). Adler's ideas have been used by humanists, existentialists, cognitive therapists, and behaviorists in group, family, and individual counseling.

Behavior Therapy

Behavior therapy is based on the principles of classical and operant conditioning. Unlike psychodynamic therapy, the focus in behavior therapy is on modifying maladaptive behaviors. Behavioral therapists do not put a focus on exploring inner conflicts or childhood events. Rather, they see a maladjusted person who has developed faulty coping strategies that are maintained through reinforcement and who has failed to obtain successful coping strategies for life. With this is mind, the main goal of behavior therapy is to both modify maladaptive behaviors and learn adaptive behaviors while establishing control and self-monitoring.

A behavioral therapist works toward these goals by using the concepts of *reinforcement* and *extinction* (Carson et al., 1996; Sue et al., 1994). *Reinforcement* is the concept that the presence of a reward (pleasant stimulus) or escape from an aversive event will increase the probability that a particular behavior will occur in the future. Reinforcement provides help with teaching a new behavior. It is often, however, the reason a person engages in maladaptive behaviors. *Extinction* is the idea that specific behavior patterns will weaken when they are not reinforced. Thus, removing the identified reinforcement of a specific behavior will help eliminate the maladaptive pattern. Discussion of two different types of behavioral treatments follows.

Token economies operate on the basic principles of operant conditioning. In this technique, a client is able to earn *tokens* or reinforcers that can later be traded in for a more desired reward. The tokens may be tickets, chips, or any other tangible item that can be used as a reinforcer. For example, a child who is constantly calling out in class may receive a plastic chip each time he or she raises his or her hand and waits to be called on. Once the child collects twenty chips, they can be traded in for extra free time to play (Sue et al., 1994).

Token economies are used often in classrooms, as well as with psychiatric patients trying to earn privileges and with clients with developmental disabilities. They can also be used effectively with adults in therapy who are trying to learn a more adaptive behavior or skill. The main goal in this type of technique is for the client to get to the point where the behavior becomes reinforcing in itself, thus allowing natural reinforcers to maintain the behavior. For the child who is constantly calling out in class, the hope is that after a while he or she will experience the positive consequences of raising his or her hand (i.e., being praised and picked by the teacher to answer a question) and that giving a concrete reinforcer such as a toy will no longer be necessary.

Systematic desensitization, developed by Joseph Wolpe, is a different type of behavioral therapy that relies on the basic principle of classical conditioning. Wolpe's approach is used to help reduce anxiety, which is a response to an aversive stimulus. It is a way of extinguishing this anxiety, which is often a reinforced behavior. This type of therapy is very useful in treating anxiety disorders such as phobic disorders and panic disorders.

Systematic desensitization attempts to teach a client an incompatible behavior to anxiety. Specifically, a therapist teaches a client to feel relaxed. Because it is difficult for a person to feel both relaxed and anxious at the same time, the goal is for the client to be able to feel relaxed in the presence of the anxiety-provoking stimulus (Carson et al., 1996; Sue et al., 1994).

The first step in this process is for the therapist to train the client in relaxation. Although there are several types of relaxation techniques, two are more frequently used. The first is *progressive muscle relaxation.* In this type, the client learns to relax by recognizing when body muscles are tense and then relaxing them (Sue et al., 1994). This is accomplished by having the client tighten each muscle group as hard as possible and then slowly letting go. Usually, clients are asked to sit in chairs with their feet flat on the floor, hands on their laps and eyes closed. The therapist prompts the client on which body part to focus on and gives verbal directions. For example, a therapist might say, "Now I want you to focus on your right arm. Tighten your right arm as hard as you can. Feel the pressure and tension building up in your arm. Hold it, keep tightening. Now I want you to slowly release the tension in your right arm. Feel the pressure flowing out of your arm a little at a time. Notice the difference in how your arm feels loose and relaxed." Deep, diaphragmatic breathing is also used at the beginning and end, as well as between the exercises. This is another way to physically calm down the body. The

goal is for clients to be able to recognize when their muscles are tense and immediately release the tension in order to feel relaxed.

Another type of relaxation exercise is *guided imagery*. In this type, the client
is asked to imagine a place that is peaceful and relaxing. With eyes closed, the
client is guided on a "tour" of that peaceful place, which includes smelling, listening, and feeling things about the place (Carson et al., 1996). One common
example of a peaceful place for people is the beach. For example, the therapist
might say, "Now close your eyes and imagine you are at the beach. Look around
and see all the things that are there—the sand, the ocean, seagulls. Now focus on
the ocean. Listen to the waves crashing on the beach. Smell the saltwater in the air.
Now focus on the sand. Feel the softness of it as you walk with your bare feet
down to the water." The goal in guided imagery is for clients to be able to relax
themselves by imagining their peaceful picture.

The second step in systematic desensitization is *creating a fear hierarchy*. The
client is asked to make a list of the least to most anxiety-provoking situations with
respect to his or her fear. For example, when dealing with phobias, a common fear
is flying. This client may make a list in which watching planes take off on television may be the least anxiety provoking. As the list goes on, making airline reser-
vations, taking a taxi to the airport, and boarding the plane are increasingly anxiety provoking. Taking off and flying thousands of feet in the air would probably
involve the most anxiety (Carson et al., 1996).

Once the hierarchy is completed, the client is asked to use his or her relaxation techniques to reduce anxiety. First, the client is asked to imagine the lowest-
anxiety-provoking scene, watching a plane take off on television. The client
relaxes at the same time, using the technique he or she has learned. The client then
moves up the list imagining each scene in order. If one scene is too anxiety provoking, the client returns to a less stressful scene. The therapist and client work on
this until the client can imagine the entire list without any anxiety. This procedure
helps the client learn to relax in anxiety-provoking situations and helps increase
success with real-life situations (Carson et al., 1996).

Cognitive-Behavioral Therapy

One criticism of strict behavior therapy is the fact that it focuses only on observable
behavior and is "mechanistic." It does not focus on cognitive processes. *Cognitive-
behavioral therapy* operates on the idea that psychopathology stems from irrational,
faulty, and distorted thinking a person engages in. It is thought that these negative
thoughts mediate the effects of a stimulus condition and contribute to behavior and
emotions. The main goal of cognitive-behavioral therapy, therefore, is to replace
faulty thinking and negative self-statements with more positive thoughts and self-
statements for the purpose of changing or correcting maladaptive behaviors and
emotions. This change in thinking is often termed *cognitive restructuring*.

Ellis: Rational Emotive Therapy.   Albert Ellis (1967) created one of the first
cognitive-behavioral therapies, *rational-emotive therapy (RET)*. The basic premise of
RET is the belief that cognition produces self-talk that can lead to individuals

being either healthy or maladjusted. Self-talk is merely an individual's internal thought processes that influence how a situation is interpreted. Because it is thought that words provide a tool for interpretation of information and cause both emotional and behavioral consequences, misguided self-talk can produce cognitive errors, which Ellis termed *irrational beliefs*. With time, these irrational beliefs become a habitual pattern (Carson et al., 1996; Ellis, 1967; Wallace, 1986).

An RET therapist uses many different types of cognitive-restructuring techniques for the purpose of challenging the client's irrational beliefs. Because of this, the therapist is thought to be a teacher. Typically, the therapist is very direct and confrontational and is not concerned with developing a close relationship with the client as in other more psychodynamic therapies. Rational-emotive therapy is meant to be a short-term therapy that ends rather quickly.

The first stage in RET is for the client and therapist to agree on the specific goals to be addressed and what specific actions are needed to obtain these goals. During this stage, the therapist encourages the client to describe the self-defeating emotions and behaviors that are present. Then the client needs to explore these statements and resolve whether they stem from a rational or irrational base (Carson et al., 1996).

The second stage involves the therapist forcefully challenging the client to recognize the self-sabotaging statements. The goal is to get the client to realize that he or she is responsible for maintaining the negative consequences. In this respect, this type of therapy is seen as hard work and the therapist often needs to attack and wear down any resistance to change. One way of doing this is to use the *ABCDE* method developed by Ellis. This is a schema used by the therapist to depict how cognition plays a role in developing and maintaining emotions and behaviors. The *ABC* part involves some *activating* event that through some stimulus evokes some response. At first, it is thought that this activating event caused some consequence; however, it is found that, instead, the consequence is the result of self-talk that is initiated by thoughts and beliefs. Once this part is realized, the therapist moves on to *D* and *E* where the client is taught to dispute or challenge the faulty belief and then note the effect it has. After this is accomplished, the client can replace irrational statements for rational ones. It is during this stage that the therapist often gives homework assignments to practice this process. Another homework assignment given is to have the client throw away any exaggerations or overgeneralizations that create a feeling that the situation is hopeless (Ellis, 1967; Wallace, 1986).

The overall goal of RET is to teach clients to take responsibility for emotions and behavior and stop negative self-statements. With this, a client develops a sense of satisfaction with the self. The idea that people have the internal power to create their own happiness or unhappiness is heavily enforced. This type of therapy can be beneficial for adults, although it is often viewed as harsh. Due to the nature of this therapy, it is not recommended for children or people with low cognitive functioning. In addition, it should not be used with people who may not be in contact with reality, as is seen with schizophrenia or mania (Carson et al., 1996).

Berne: Transactional Analysis. Another type of cognitive-behavioral therapy is transactional analysis, developed by Eric Berne (1972). *Transactional analysis (TA)* is a type of therapy that focuses on the interactions and transactions between individuals. Various concepts of ego psychology have been included to stress that individuals have the ability to think, express feelings, and make decisions that result in self-fulfillment.

According to TA, a child learns a way of transacting with others and a *life script* or plan develops as a result. This life script causes the individual to react to others in a customary manner. The purpose or main goal of having transactions with others is to receive recognition, which is termed *strokes*. Every person requires and, in fact, seeks out strokes from other people. It is this chain of events, which includes learning and reinforcement, that helps the formation of personality and how people view the world (Corey, 1986).

In TA, individuals are seen as rational cognitive beings that consciously and deliberately interpret and organize their environment to receive recognition. The strokes received can be positive or negative, and this further reinforces a belief system for continuation of transactional patterns. According to Berne, this explains part of the existence of both functional and dysfunctional behaviors. The main goal of the therapist, therefore, is to teach clients how their actions, feelings, and cognitions contribute to repetitive behaviors and emotions. In addition, clients are taught to challenge and change early script messages in order to learn more functional transactions (Corey, 1986).

As already mentioned, TA includes concepts from ego psychology. In his theory, Berne identified three *ego states,* which he defines as coherent systems of thoughts and feelings that manifest themselves in patterns of behavior. To some extent, the three ego states resemble the three personality structures of Freud: the id, the ego, and the super ego (Berne, 1972).

The first ego state is the *parent ego* or *exteropsyche.* This contains attitudes and behaviors that are learned from parents and other authority figures. There are two substates within the parent ego. The *critical parent* is the part where the rules are located. A person behaves based on moral inferences that are created through the values, judgments, and actions learned from parents. The *nurturing parent* is the part that offers support and encouragement, thus softening the nature of the parent. The second ego state is the *adult ego* or *neopsyche.* This is considered the center of thinking. It contains the rational and unemotional part of an individual. Decisions are based on intellect, and facts are more important than feelings. The third ego state is the *child ego* or *archaeopsyche.* This is the *id* part of the person. It contains impulses that are spontaneous and more playful. It is thought that this state is the most important in examining the personality and underlying self-concept. As in the parent ego, there are two substates to the child ego. The *natural child* experiences total freedom and is completely inhibited, whereas the *adapted child* is influenced by parental beliefs of right versus wrong (Berne, 1972; Corey, 1986).

Together, these three ego states reside within the individual. An individual selects one ego state over another when conducting transactions. The selected state depends upon the interpretation of the situation and past experiences. An individual who is healthy, therefore, is one who can choose the appropriate ego state for a given situation. This balance is necessary for transactions with others to be smooth.

If two people communicate with nonparallel ego states, then the transaction becomes crossed, and *games*, as Berne termed them, are played in which needs are not expressed adequately. Thus, one goal of the therapist is to help the client learn how to state his or her needs and avoid these *games*. Although some more overt games are not that hurtful, covert games in which there is an ulterior motive in the message can be very hurtful and create dysfunctional roles (Berne, 1972).

Humanistic-Experiential Therapy

Much in the same way that cognitive-behavioral therapies evolved as a reaction to strict behavioral techniques, *humanistic-experiential therapies* evolved as a reaction to psychodynamic and behavioral therapies. Many people felt that the focus on childhood memories/events and changing behaviors left out an important concept of *humanness*. Humanistic-experiential theorists believe that people need to examine responsibility, self-concept, free will, and self-actualization. In other words, people need to look at the full potentials of human beings. These theorists see psychopathology as a result of alienation, depersonalization, loneliness, and a failure to find meaning. Professionals in this school of thought believe the client should be responsible for the success and direction of therapy through the guidance or facilitation of the therapist. The client needs to become more aware of his or her uniqueness and *wholeness* as a person. Two essential forms of humanistic-experiential therapy are client-centered therapy and existential therapy.

Rogers: Client-Centered Therapy.   Carl Rogers developed *client-centered* or *person-centered therapy*. Rogers did not believe that the therapist was supposed to be a prober, interpreter, or director; nor did he believe that individuals have an irrational instinct. Instead, he believed that individuals have the power to heal themselves. People have the capacity to be rational, social, and self-directed. In fact, Rogers believed that humankind is basically good and rational. Individuals use emotions to communicate and express their positive and negative experiences. If communication is blocked, an individual experiences frustration, which leads to an incongruency in feelings and behaviors. It is this incongruency, Rogers believes, that causes maladjustment (Carson et al., 1996; Patterson, 1980; Sue et al., 1994).

The process of client-centered therapy is meant to help an individual discover deep levels of self-awareness and insight. The main goal is *self-actualization*, in which the person evolves to feel a sense of achievement or self-fulfillment. This concept of self-actualization is a universal need according to Rogers. To accomplish this, the client must be given a warm and caring relationship that permits growth and acceptance. The main job of the therapist, therefore, is facilitator, and no interpretations are offered (Carson et al., 1996).

Because of the nature of this therapy, the therapist's attitude is more important than specific techniques. Rogers believed that the client and counselor should engage in a *psychological contact*. This means that the client, coming in with incongruence and vulnerability, is met by a counselor who is both congruent and invested in the relationship. The relationship between the two is essential in this type of therapy. There must be authentic feelings present, a focus on saying what is felt at the present moment, and concreteness (Carson et al., 1996).

In the interest of establishing a warm, nonjudgmental relationship between the client and therapist, Rogers identified three conditions that are essential. The first is *unconditional positive regard (UPR)*. This means that the therapist needs to communicate a genuine caring and recognition of human value to the client. The therapist is then able to share in the feelings of the client, and the client is engaged in the therapy process, which will lead to personality change (Carson et al., 1996; Sue et al., 1994).

The second condition is *genuineness* or *congruence.* It means that the therapist "drops the facade" and is in touch with who he or she is and how he or she acts. The therapist needs to be aware of what he or she is experiencing and be able to communicate it. This helps bring down barriers between the client and therapist. In addition, it helps in the development of trust and respect. This means that the therapist has a responsibility to share honestly, which promotes growth, maturity, and improved functioning (Patterson, 1980).

The final condition is *empathic understanding.* This is a form of "emotional knowing" where the therapist can sense what the client is experiencing at the moment. It is as if the therapist is able to be in the client's shoes and experience that individual's inner world. This empathy is essential, because it encourages the client to continue to become fully involved in his or her own situations. The best way for the therapist to convey empathy is through reflection or paraphrasing of the client's feelings. By doing this, the therapist shows that he or she understands what is being said and shares in the experience with the client (Carson et al., 1996; Corey, 1986).

Together, these three conditions make up the heart of client-centered therapy and are all essential for the therapist to facilitate therapeutic change. Experiencing all of these creates an environment for the client in which he or she can gain insight into personal experiences and challenge dysfunctional ways of living.

Existential Therapy.   Closely related to client-centered therapy is *existential therapy.* As in client-centered therapy, the existential therapist sees people as basically good and rational. Further, existentialism is grounded in the notion of individuals being free. Thus, people are free to decide how they live and give meaning to their lives. They cannot blame others for their unhappiness. They must create their own happiness internally. This concept of freedom was developed in part by Viktor Frankl (1979) through his approach called *logotherapy.* Frankl believed that although external freedom may not always be possible, internal freedom can never be taken away. He used his own personal experiences as a Nazi prisoner to illustrate this. He felt that death gives life meaning and that people who believe they have control over their destiny choose life. This meaning in life is what motivates people to live, love, and work toward self-actualization.

Existential aloneness is a concept that suggests each person is ultimately alone in the respect that no one can fully experience another person's exact feelings. Each individual has the power to interpret aloneness as either a freeing or enslaving experience. Therefore, one thing existential therapy attempts is to have people realize their uniqueness, accept themselves, and accept responsibility for their own actions. Self-awareness is essential for an individual to promote freedom and discover his or her identity. If this does not occur, then meaningful relationships cannot be formed (Carson et al., 1996; May & Yalom, 1984).

Existentialism holds that the *idea actions* individually chosen may create internal anxiety. This anxiety is a result of living and is universally experienced. In fact, this anxiety is seen as necessary for growth and change to occur. Rollo May, who first introduced existentialism in the United States, believed that anxiety enhances intelligence, creativity, and positive change. One of his goals in therapy was to reduce anxiety to fear, which could be objectively dealt with. May holds that human creativity enables people to become self-actualized (Corey, 1986).

One way people experience anxiety is through their awareness of death. People realize that they do not have infinite time; this can create a form of guilt in which individuals fail to accept responsibility for thoughts, actions, and behaviors. This guilt can have a negative or positive effect on the individual. On the negative side, this guilt can allow an individual to rationalize that he or she is a victim and that life and happiness is outside of his or her control. Contrary to that thinking, guilt can also have a positive effect in which it causes individuals to use their full potentials (May & Yalom, 1984).

Knowing the importance of anxiety in existential therapy, it follows that the main goal of the therapy is to help the client conform anxiety as much as possible. The counselor or therapist is there to help the client recognize that his or her life plan is under his or her own determination. Achieving such self-awareness promotes freedom, responsibility, and a commitment to discover a person's identity. This permits the establishment of meaningful relationships with others (Carson et al., 1996; Corey, 1986; May & Yalom, 1984).

Based on the preceding information, it is easy to understand that existentialism is more of an attitude than an actual therapy. There are no specific techniques; in fact, existential therapists use any techniques they feel will help the client. As in client-centered therapy, empathy, genuineness, and unconditional positive regard are key components. The focus is on the here and now, and the therapy does not have a predetermined route. The therapist must put all of his or her own needs aside, rise above them, and concentrate on being with the client. The existential therapist requires this self-transcendence.

The preceding is a brief overview of some of the therapies used in practice today. While it is not exhaustive by any means, it gives the reader an idea of the main goals and processes of therapy and counseling. This information can be useful when a person decides to seek out help. A therapist or counselor can have many different philosophies and styles. In addition, many therapists combine parts of different theories to find a treatment style they feel is appropriate. Some therapies are more or less appropriate for a particular problem than others. If and when a person does decide to access help, it can be overwhelming at best to choose a therapist. Knowing the importance of the therapeutic relationship can help in seeking a good match between a client and therapist. One thing a potential client can do is to ask the therapist what his or her orientation is. This will give a person a feel for the philosophy of the therapist and a means of anticipating how the therapist might conduct therapy. A person may feel more comfortable, for example, with a warm and nurturing orientation of a client-centered therapist than with the direct and confrontational orientation of a rational-emotive therapist.

Additional Types of Mental Health Resources

Aside from choosing a therapist and initiating therapy or counseling, there are many other mental health resources a person can utilize. Remember that a person does not have to wait until the problem builds to access help. As was previously discussed, college students often experience a great deal of stress and related psychological problems. One resource for college students is *university counseling centers*. Each university offers a counseling center, which exists to offer services to its students. The main goal in these programs is to help students maximize their ability to achieve in an academic environment. Counselors assist students in career choices, obtaining academic goals, and developing a positive self-concept (Harrison et al., 1993). These services can help college students enhance their comfort level both socially and emotionally.

In addition, many *community mental health centers* have been set up over the years to provide a multitude of services, including short-term inpatient and outpatient care, emergency services, community consultation, and education. One category of services offered is prevention programs, which attempt to lower the incidence of psychological disorders by adding or strengthening resources to promote mental health. Some prevention programs focus on helping deprived children develop necessary skills, providing support for people who divorce, and helping prevent teenage pregnancy and sexually transmitted diseases (Sue et al., 1994).

Support groups and *self-help groups* exist for a multitude of problems, including alcohol abuse, parenting skills, stress management, bereavement, and dealing with divorce. Group counseling is often helpful in that it helps a person to realize that there are many people out there who experience similar problems. Group facilitators try to help people develop or enhance the skills needed to promote mental health.

Psychiatrists are another group of professionals who offer mental health services. A psychiatrist is trained at the doctoral level in the assessment, diagnosis, and treatment of psychological disorders. They differ from psychologists in that they are medical doctors and therefore have the ability to prescribe medication, which is one form of intervention in dealing with problems such as depression and anxiety. Typically, clients of psychiatrists are on the more severe end of the spectrum and are in need of several interventions. A psychiatrist must have a solid foundation as a general physician and an understanding of general medical conditions, as well as a solid understanding of the use of different types of medications, drug interactions, and side effects; this is essential for diagnosing and monitoring progress with medication. In addition to all the aforementioned, psychiatrists also need a knowledge base in psychodynamics, an understanding of the group process in counseling, and crisis-intervention skills (Birecree & Cutler, 1998; Stein, 1998).

Psychologists, on the other hand, possess Ph.D.-level training. They do not have the ability to prescribe drugs, as they are not medical doctors. Social workers are professionals who can be licensed at both the Bachelor and Master's level. Requirements vary from state to state. However, there are some states that have reciprocity agreements allowing an individual licensed in one state to receive licensure in another state with no additional training. Check with your local State Board of Social Work Examiners for requirements. Third-party reimbursement from insurance companies is usually available for psychiatrists, psychologists, and social workers. *Counselors* are individuals with a master's degree (usually approximately thirty hours of postbaccalaureate education) and fewer internship hours than social workers. Criteria for their licensure varies widely from state to state, and, as such, third-party reimbursement for counselors is often not available unless they are supervised by a psychiatrist, psychologist, or social worker. *Therapist* is a term with no generally recognized meaning; in most states, any individual can call himself/herself a therapist regardless of training or education. Clients must understand the training and abilities of the mental health professional they intend to see.

Summary

Achieving and maintaining good mental health can be a challenging task given all the interpersonal and environmental pressures of everyday life. At times, people need to seek out help in order to work through problems, hopefully before the problem is able to escalate. Through community mental health centers and the various mental health professionals including psychologists, psychiatrists, and social workers, a person can find an appropriate treatment for his or her problem. Professionals use such techniques as clinical interviews, intelligence tests, and personality tests to assess an individual and determine a type of treatment plan that will be beneficial. Short-term counseling and long-term therapy are available for people who need to understand and cope with various psychological problems. There are many different central theories for conducting counseling and psychotherapy, including psychodynamic, behavior, cognitive-behavioral, and humanistic-experiential. Within each of these are specific therapies that have specified goals and techniques for therapy. Therapists can choose to orient themselves according to one of these therapies, or they can borrow different ideas from several of them to create a more eclectic approach. It is helpful for people to have an understanding of the basic concepts and processes of some of the main therapies used today. In addition, it is helpful to know of community resources that are available, including support groups, prevention programs, or university counseling centers. All of the information presented in this chapter is meant to give the reader a broad understanding of the types of resources available in the field of mental health and what to expect from them. There is help out there, and anybody can make the choice to access it in an attempt to achieve good mental health.

DISCUSSION QUESTIONS

1. Explain why some people choose to access mental health resources, and develop guidelines for people to realize when they may need help.

2. Based on the research, what are some psychological problems that an individual may experience during the college years?

3. Name and describe the three main components of a clinical assessment, and explain how a professional uses information gathered in an assessment.

4. List the four categories of psychologically based therapies, and explain the central idea of each with respect to cause of psychological disorders and goals of therapy.

5. Name and describe the three personality structures in Freud's psychoanalytic theory. How does Freud use these to explain human behavior?

6. Explain the main criticism of Freud's psychoanalytic theory, and give an example of a theory that evolved as a result of this criticism.

7. What is the main difference between behavior and cognitive-behavioral therapies? Give an example of a specific therapy within each to illustrate a point.

8. According to Carl Rogers, what are the three main characteristics a therapist must have? Why are these important for therapy to be effective?

9. Discuss the idea of "freedom" as it relates to existential therapy and self-actualization.

10. What is the main purpose of prevention programs? Why is it better to access help at this level?

11. Describe the main role of psychiatrists, and state how they are different from psychologists.

12. Explain the differences in training and education among social workers, counselors and therapists.

RELATED WEBSITES

http://mentalhelp.net   Mental Health Net. A large and comprehensive website that nicely organizes mental health information, aimed mostly at mental health consumers.
http://www.nmha.org/infoctr/index.cfm   The National Mental Health Information Center. A variety of fact sheets and pamphlets are available.

http://mentalhealth.about.com About.com's Mental Health Resources page. A constantly updated, incredibly comprehensive resource with nearly everything related to mental health.

http://www.who.org/msa/mnh The World Health Organization's Mental Health Department website with links to their mission, mental health issues in developing and industrialized countries, and their periodical bulletin on mental health.

http://www.ukppg.co.uk/links.html The Psychiatric Pharmacy Group of the United Kingdom. Very comprehensive page of mental health links, with information for consumers, journals and medical information, governmental reports from the United States and the United Kingdom, and other information.

http://www.nimh.nih.gov National Institute of Mental Health. Current mental health news, information for consumers, clinicians, researchers, and students.

http://hometown.aol.com/jimhofw/jimho.htm Justice in Mental Health Organization. Interesting page on the social issues related to mental illness and advocacy for those with a diagnosed mental illness.

http://www.counseling.org American Counseling Association. Information about therapy and other counseling issues, including career information for students interested in counseling.

http://uhs.bsd.uchicago.edu/~bhsiung/mental.html Dr. Bob's Mental Health Link. Dr. Robert Hsiung's comprehensive page of mental health links.

http://www.mhsource.com/ Mental Health Info Source. Comprehensive page with resources related to treatment, interactive quizzes and assessments, recent articles, and other information.

REFERENCES

Adler, A. (1963) *The Practice and Theory of Individual Psychology.* Paterson: Littlefield.

Ansbacher, H. L., & Ansbacher, R. (Eds.). (1956). *The Individual Psychology of Alfred Adler.* New York: Basic Books.

Berne, E. (1972). *What Do You Do After You Say Hello?* New York: Grove Press.

Birecree, E., & Cutler, D. L. (1998). What Makes a Community Psychiatrist? *Community Mental Health Journal, 34*(4), 433–435.

Carson, R. C., Butcher, J. N., & Mineka, S. (1996). *Abnormal Psychology and Normal Life* (10th ed.). New York: HarperCollins.

Clark, A. J. (1995). Projective Techniques in the Counseling Process. *Journal of Counseling & Development, 73,* 311–315.

Corey, G. (1986). *Theory and Practice of Counseling and Psychotherapy.* Montrey: Brookes Cole.

Dinkmeyer, D. C., Pew, W. L., & Dinkmeyer, D. C. Jr. (1979). *Adlerian Counseling and Psychotherapy.* Monterey: Brookes Cole.

Ellis, A. (1967). Rational Emotive Psychotherapy. In D. Arbuckle (Ed.), *Counseling and Psychotherapy.* New York: McGraw Hill.

Frankl, V. (1979). The Will to Meaning. In *Foundations and Application of Logotherapy.* New York: Simon & Schuster.

Freud, S. (1935). *A General Introduction to Psychoanalysis.* New York: Liveright.

Harrison, T. C., Maples, M. F., Testa, A. M., & Jones, P. (1993). Academic Self-Concept of University Students: Implications for Counseling. *Journal of Humanistic Education and Development, 32,* 69–75.

Hesse-Biber, S., & Marino, M. (1991). From High School to College: Changes in Women's Self-Concept and Its Relationship to Eating Problems. *The Journal of Psychology, 125*(2), 199–216.

Holzman, L. A., Searight, H. R., & Hughes, H. M. (1996). Clinical Psychology Graduate Students and Personal Psychotherapy: Results of an Exploratory Survey. *Professional Psychology: Research and Practice, 27*(1), 98–101.

May, R., & Yalom, I. (1984). Existential Psychotherapy. In R. J. Corsini, (Ed.), *Current Psychotherapies.* Itasca, IL: F. E. Peacock.

Patterson, E. H. (1980). *Theories of Counseling and Psychotherapy* (3rd Ed.). New York: Harper & Row.

Pledge, D. S., Lapan, R. T., Heppner, P. P., Kivlighan, D., & Roehlke, H. J. (1998). Stability and Severity of Presenting Problems at a University Counseling Center: A 6-Year Analysis. *Professional Psychology: Research and Practice, 29*(4), 386–389.

Stein, L. I. (1998). The Community Psychiatrist: Skills and Personal Characteristics. *Community Mental Health Journal, 34*(4), 437–445.

Sue, D., Sue, D., & Sue, S. (1994). *Understanding Abnormal Behavior.* Boston: Houghton Mifflin.

Waiswol, N. (1995). Projective Techniques as Psychotherapy. *American Journal of Psychotherapy, 73*(3), 311–316.

Wallace, W. A. (1986) *Theories of Counseling and Psychotherapy: A Basic Issues Approach.* Boston: Allyn & Bacon.

Watkins, C. E., Campbell, B. L., Nieberding, R., & Hallmark, R. (1995). Contemporary Practice of Psychological Assessment by Clinical Psychologists. *Professional Psychology: Research and Practice, 26*(1), 54–60.

CHAPTER

12 Associated Mental Health Issues

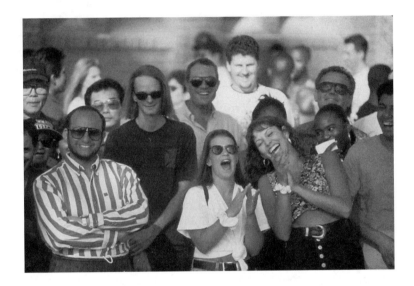

In 1970, the World Health Organization redefined *health* to encompass emotional, mental, physical, social, and spiritual aspects. These different aspects of health interact with one another equally and produce the overall health of the individual (see Figure 12.1). If a person has poor health in a single aspect, it becomes very difficult to develop good health in the other aspects.

For example, much information has been discovered recently about the interplay between physical health and mental health. People with optimistic outlooks often have better immune response, thereby recovering more quickly from illness, as well as being less likely to get sick in the first place.

Mental health also is linked in obvious ways to emotional health. People who have a healthy mental state are more capable of dealing with setbacks and everyday stresses of life. They do not become severely depressed whenever something bad happens, and they do not develop intense anxiety in response to daily occurrences.

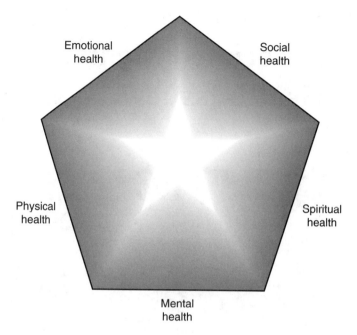

FIGURE 12.1

Mental health also influences social health. Individuals that do not have good mental health often neglect their social health, preferring instead to spend time alone. They can quickly become isolated. On the other hand, some people with poor mental health feel more comfortable in relationships with people, but these relationships are rarely those that increase their social health. They are instead likely to be unhealthy.

Spiritual health is another aspect of overall health and one that mental health also influences. Persons with poor mental health are often uncomfortable with spirituality in any aspect, whereas those with positive mental health are accepting of the beliefs of others and open to experiencing spiritual aspects of life.

Certainly, the World Health Organization definition is a much-expanded version from the previous definition, which defined health as "absence of disease or infirmity." The purpose of this chapter is to fully integrate these important areas of health to understand how mental health affects all aspects of life. Distinguishing areas of importance from those areas that can be considered superfluous will assist in providing clearer perspective on each of these topics and how they interrelate.

Holistic Mental Health

The following is a concept that solidifies this perspective. The philosophy refers to that of a sculptor. Simply said, a sculptor does not simply add more and more clay to the form but strips away the inessentials until the essence is revealed. This same principle applies to the area of mental health. It is simply not possible to be an expert on all the concepts of this book just by taking a course or reading the text cover to cover. Adding concepts in this way results in a weak understanding of the material. One of the most important lessons to learn from this text is to develop the ability to balance strengths and weaknesses in order to experience holistic mental health. In this way, a deeper understanding of the material can be developed.

This focus on developing your own understanding and constructing a holistic view of mental health is a theme common to many areas. For example, there is a story about a young college student who asked a stress-management specialist about whether a particular form of meditation was good. Wisely, the specialist responded by saying, "It's not the form of meditation that is good but the discipline and willingness of the practitioner." The example that was shared with this college student follows:

> One day there was a young child who was convinced that if he took his shovel and dug in his backyard that he would reach water. After digging for several hours and not reaching water, this child began digging in another area of the yard and another and another. This process continued until there were several small holes throughout the yard. Unfortunately, this child grew tired and despondent and never located water.

This story is analogous to individuals who experiment with various forms of meditation, spirituality, and other areas of mental health thinking that one day they will *at last* experience holistic well-being. Simply adding one technique after another cannot do this; it is accomplished, rather, through the careful integration and development of those techniques that are most meaningful to the individual. This chapter, *Associated Mental Health Issues*, provides a form of mental *synergism*. This term applies within the area of mental health because there is not one element that allows a person to be mentally healthy but several areas that, when combined, allow a person to be emotionally healthy and happy. Certainly, some people will relate more to some of the first eleven chapters in this text than others; that is OK, because this simply demonstrates their individuality and reinforces who they are.

Choices Affect Lives

A broad range of qualities defines individuality. For example, consider some qualities that individuals possess and how their strengths and/or deficiencies allow their self-perceptions to be mentally healthy or unhealthy. This perception is important to their self-esteem, as is the manner in which their families, friends, and society as a whole perceive them.

Because of this, it is extremely important to surround yourself with those who are willing to support you in a positive way. Remember that everyone is supporting you for something. There are those who support you for mediocrity, those who support your negative outcomes, and those who support you for success. With whom are you interested in associating? Once again, attitudes are infectious. The larger question is whether or not your attitude is worth catching.

Furthermore, those with whom you surround yourself either energize you or de-energize you. Again, your choices affect your day-to-day experiences. This is not to say that you should dislike negative people, but do yourself a favor and like them from a distance. Your family and friends do make a difference in your overall mental health. Remember that you have a choice as to whom you associate with and how much time you spend with these people.

Often times, individuals get into a habit of complaining about things and not doing anything to change the outcome. One simple saying is: "A person who complains and does not attempt to change the circumstance loses all complaining rights." Certainly, this reinforces the importance of taking an active role within your mental health. Your choices can greatly affect what you experience and the state of your mental health as well as the mental health of those around you.

Treatment of Mental Health

Treatment of mental health issues is an extremely private matter. So, when someone is encouraged to go for help they need to be aware of not only their options but also the methods of treatment that are involved. "Americans are often unaware of the choices they have for effective mental health treatments" (*Mental Health*, 1999). Some of the decisions involved with this process include deciding between basic counseling, psychotherapy, medication therapy, rehabilitation, psychiatric therapy, community-based services, and many more. This confusion often leads people to begin a more comfortable self-assessment. Some people do not seek professional treatment because they are fearful of being forced to accept treatments not of their choice or of being treated involuntarily for prolonged period of times *(Mental Health)*. Again, these fears are associated with the mistrust for the mental health professionals.

There is much misperception regarding the nature of the mental health professions and the effectiveness and nature of commonplace treatments. Many people are deterred from seeking treatment because of the stigma associated with mental health problems. According to recent reports on the state of mental health treatment in the United States, this stigma can take the form of prejudice, discrimination, fear, distrust, and stereotyping. This stigma has led to many people having a reluctance to admit their mental health problems even to themselves, let alone accept treatment for them. Further, the public is largely unaware of the effectiveness of recent innovations in mental health treatment. Patients are offered highly effective treatment options with very few side effects. Even patients with mild depression now have access to a wide range of drug therapies that are very effective. Scientists understand brain chemistry and neurophysiology in ways that were not imagined ten years ago. The public is largely unaware of state-of-the-art treatment delivery systems; recent trends in tailoring treatments to age, gender, race, and culture; and the support that is in place in the area of helping individuals overcome any financial barriers to treatment *(Mental Health*, 1999). Because of this, the first link in the chain of mental health care is more client-centered than in most physical health care systems. Careful and clear self-assessment then becomes more important in this field than in others so that the client can clearly convey his or her concerns to the mental health professionals.

Self-Assessment

People can *self assess* to survey their strengths and weaknesses. Over the years, the authors have collected, experienced, and shared the followings lists of qualities. Because mental health is so broad, A to Z ranges of words that connote both positive and negative qualities are presented here:

> Adaptation, balance, communication, courage, determination, discipline, empathy, empowerment, energy, enlightenment, friendships, group support, happiness, insight, interaction, justice, kindness, laughter, love, meditation, mindfulness, neighborly, optimism, purpose, quiet time, relaxation, self-esteem, spiritual well-being, stress management, trustworthiness, uniqueness, virtue, warmth, excellence, yes, and zeal encompass those qualities that are positive.
> Anger, bitterness, cunning, despair, egotism, fear, glutton, hate, ignorance, jealousy, kibosh, lethargic, malicious, negative, obsession, pessimism, quibble, racist, suspicious, tempestuous, unorganized, vindictive, weak, xenophobic, yell, and zealot are inclusive of those qualities that are negative.

Assessing their traits, both self-perceived and as others see them, can go a long way to helping people determine how they feel about their own mental health.

Effective Communication

How we communicate with others makes a big difference, not only for their own mental health but also for the mental well-being of those with whom they interact. What they say is important, but *how* they communicate that message is also important. It has been said that 55 percent of a message is conveyed through body language, 38 percent through inflection/intonation, and merely 7 percent through the actual words (Helmstetter, 1986). While this does not suggest that choice of words is unimportant, it does reinforce the importance of communicating with the entire body. Being especially aware of their nonverbal communication can help people to work through many aspects of their lives that are difficult because of their relationships with other people.

Positive Mental Attitude

Since Norman Vincent Peale wrote the book *The Power of Positive Thinking* in 1952, there has been much talk about *positive mental attitude (PMA)*. The real question is, Can people control their mental attitudes? Considering the effects that a *negative mental attitude (NMA)* can have, it is doubtful that many people would intentionally possess a negative mental attitude. Somehow, this concept seems absurd when expressed this way, but many people do have NMAs. The question is, Why? Excluding chemical imbalances, who controls your thoughts? Without question, you do. This being the case, it seems obvious that many people possess NMAs because they do not realize that they alone have the ability to change to more positive mental attitudes.

Emerson once said, "The ancestor of every action is a thought." This means that people's thoughts have a profound effect on their behavior. Thus, change the thoughts and behavioral change is soon to follow. The converse of this is the notion of the behaviorist—that changing the behavior will lead to a change in thoughts. However, the cause and effect of this is not important; what is important is to accept that attitude in some way influences behavior.

With this in mind, assume that most individuals with PMAs are optimistic, while those possessing NMAs are pessimistic. Certainly, this is not *always* the case, but it does serve as a general rule. In addition, attitudes are dynamic; that is, they change from thought to thought. However, most individuals have attitudes that are more pronounced and produce what can be refered to as *personality patterns.*

Maybe you are thinking that changing thoughts changes only *words,* but these words form your attitude and behaviors. One of the authors heard someone say several years ago that the average person assimilates fifty thousand thoughts per day. To say that you can control all of these thoughts would be ridiculous. However, to say that you can control the flow of your thoughts is within the realm of reality. With this awareness of the magnitude of your thoughts, consider one additional aspect of how your thoughts produce a pattern or programmed way of thinking.

The fact that you assimilate fifty thousand thoughts per day may not be overly amazing to you, but the fact that it has been estimated that 90 percent to 95 percent of today's thoughts are the same as those thoughts of yesterday is somewhat amazing. If you doubt this statement, reflect on your thoughts of today, yesterday, and last week. Are you considering some of the same worries, and having some of the same positive thoughts, negative thoughts, and daily distractions? It would be extreme to think that you could control or change all of your thoughts, but just imagine how much different your life would be if you were to make a 10 percent attitudinal shift.

For a moment, close your eyes and envision someone you admire or consider to be a mentor. Maybe you know this person well, or perhaps you have only admired him or her from afar. Nonetheless, consider that individual's qualities, especially his or her attitude. Is he or she, calm, insightful, peaceful, and willing to help others? Or, does the person you have in mind possess qualities of selfishness, low self-esteem, and a negative attitude? It is likely that your mentor possesses a helpful demeanor and a PMA because those are the traits that most people admire.

Attitude Adjustment

Consider trying a twenty-one day experiment that is sure to *adjust* your attitude and provide you with a rewarding experience. Beginning this moment, discontinue all criticism for the next twenty-one days. Although this may sound easy, try it, and see how you do. If or when you catch yourself criticizing others or yourself, simply replace this statement or thought with something positive. This is an exercise in training yourself to be aware of your thoughts and to form more positive thoughts. The goal is to learn throughout the process; however, whenever you catch yourself being negative, you must start over at the first day of this twenty-one–day exercise. That is right. Even if you are successful for the initial ten days, you must start over and retrain yourself to compose positive statements and thoughts. While this may seem daunting, many individuals train themselves *physically* several times a week in order to experience good physical health. Why would it be any less necessary to train yourself psychologically?

The Importance of Optimism

Three elements that exist within individuals who are either optimistic or pessimistic reflect situations in which individuals find themselves at either end of a continuum (Seligman, 1995):

1. Personalization
2. Permanence
3. Pervasiveness

With the *three Ps* in mind, think about some situations in your life that brought you happiness or sadness. The following may help you to determine how the three Ps relate to your experiences.

The first element, *personalization,* simply means personalizing a situation. This is otherwise known as *attitudinal personalization.* The second element, *permanence,* simply means allowing that situation to appear permanent; that is, what you are experiencing seems to be long-term and may include such words as *always* or *never.* The third element, *pervasiveness,* simply means going beyond that one isolated situation. That is, one bad or good situation may overflow into other experiences or situations. This is often referred to as *perceptual pervasiveness* (Seligman, 1990).

Now, link these three elements together within optimistic and pessimistic situations and see how they look. Using the following examples, assess whether or not you commonly use language like that presented here. For example, someone might say, "I'm a big loser and I'll never win." First, the person immediately personalizes the situation by using the pronoun *I.* Then, the word *never* is used, adding permanence to the inability to win. Finally, referring to himself/herself as a *big loser* implies that that person does not simply experience a limitation, but experiences negativity that mentally pervades other elements of his or her life. Now, consider an optimistic view. Imagine someone saying, "I'm the luckiest person in the world; I'm always finding money." It was fortunate that this person found a few dollars, but it is unlikely that he or she is *always* finding money. However, this permanent attitude pervades his or her life.

Optimism makes people more likely to identify the *good* experiences over the *bad*. Optimistic people tend to perceive the good things that happen as a result of some merit they possess and the bad things that happen as a result of chance. Pessimistic people, on the other hand, tend to perceive bad things that happen as global things that they *deserve* and good things as chance events that are unlikely to reoccur.

Following is an E-mail that is representative of the aforementioned theory on PMAs/NMAs and optimistic/pessimistic perceptions:

Jeff was the kind of guy you love to hate. He was always in a good mood and always had something positive to say. When someone would ask him how he was doing, he would reply, "If I were any better, I would be twins!"

He was a unique manager because he had several waiters who followed him around from restaurant to restaurant. The reason the waiters followed Jeff was his attitude. He was a natural motivator.

If an employee was having a bad day, Jeff was telling the employee how to look on the positive side of the situation.

Seeing this style really made me curious, so one day I went up to Jeff and said to him, "I don't get it! You can't be a positive person all of the time. How do you do it?"

Jeff replied, "Each morning I wake up and say to myself, 'Jeff, you have two choices today. You can choose to be in a good mood, or you can choose to be in a bad mood.' I choose to be in a good mood. Each time something bad happens, I can choose to be a victim or I can choose to learn from it. I choose to learn from it. Every time someone comes to me complaining, I can choose to accept their complaining or I can point out the positive side of life. I choose the positive side of life."

"Yeah, right, it's not that easy," I protested.

"Yes, it is," Jeff said. "Life is all about choices. When you cut away all the junk, every situation is a choice. You choose how you react to situations. You choose how people will affect your mood. You choose to be in a good mood or a bad mood. The bottom line: It's your choice how you live life."

I reflected on what Jeff said. Soon thereafter, I left the restaurant industry to start my own business. We lost touch, but often I thought about him when I made a choice about life instead of reacting to it.

Several years later, I heard that Jeff did something you are never supposed to do in a restaurant business: he left the back door open one morning and was held up at gun point by three armed robbers. While trying to open the safe, his hand, shaking from nervousness, slipped off the combination. The robbers panicked and shot him.

Luckily, Jeff was found relatively quickly and rushed to the local trauma center. After eighteen hours of surgery and weeks of intensive care, Jeff was released from the hospital with fragments of the bullets still in his body.

I saw Jeff about six months after the accident. When I asked him how he was, he said, "If I were any better, I'd be twins. Wanna see my scars?" I declined to see his wounds but did ask him what had gone through his mind as the robbery took place. "The first thing that went through my mind was that I should have locked the back door," Jeff replied. "Then, as I lay on the floor, I remembered that I had two choices: I could choose to live, or I could choose to die. I chose to live."

"Weren't you scared? Did you lose consciousness?" I asked.

Jeff continued, "The paramedics were great. They kept telling me I was going to be fine. But when they wheeled me into the emergency room and I saw the expressions on the faces of the doctors and nurses, I got really scared. In their eyes, I read, 'He's a dead man.' I knew I needed to take action."

"What did you do?" I asked.

"Well, there was a big, burly nurse shouting questions at me," said Jeff. "She asked if I was allergic to anything. 'Yes,' I replied. The doctors and nurses stopped working as they waited for my reply. I took a deep breath and yelled, 'Bullets!' Over their laughter, I told them, 'I am choosing to live. Operate on me as if I am alive, not dead."

Jeff lived, thanks to the skill of his doctors but also because of his amazing attitude. I learned from him that every day we have the choice to live fully. Attitude, after all, is everything.

This story about Jeff demonstrates that we have the ability to choose our outcomes through our perceptions. Of course, there were several times within this story and certainly within Jeff's life when he could have chosen a different attitude. However, it would not have improved the situation but only made it worse. Consider how you can use Jeff's approach within your own life. Perhaps it will make a difference.

Controlling Worries

One distraction that many individuals experience is getting overwhelmed with daily worries. Unfortunately, this creates unnecessary stress within their lives and *usually* does not improve the situation. Now, it is natural to be concerned about difficulties that you or those you care about are experiencing. However, when has this ever lead to a more favorable outcome?

Think about compartmentalizing your worries into two areas: (1) controllable and (2) noncontrollable. For example, students may be concerned about their grades in particular classes. Understandably, this is important and can be considered a *controllable* concern—controllable because students do possess the power to meet with their instructor and ask for special assistance, meet with a study group, study more, and pursue a myriad of other solutions.

A *non-controllable* concern is one for which the outcome is out of your hands. Imagine someone who is concerned about the direction of the stock market, the weather, or world peace. These concerns clearly are not within an individual's control. Thus, these would be considered noncontrollable situations.

To acquire a clearer understanding of this theory, take out a clean sheet of paper and list a number of situations that you are presently worrying about. Consider such areas as your career, family, finances, friends, health, relationships, school, studies, and others.

Once you have created a list, consider whether these worries are noncontrollable (NC) or controllable (C). Then, simply indicate to the left of each worry whether it is *C* or *NC*. Address the worries that have an *NC* next to them; scratch them out. For those that have a *C* next to them, decide what can be done or needs to be done and take a proactive approach. You might be thinking that it is not that easy. You are right; taking action is not always easy. However, if you are looking to free yourself of unnecessary worries, then it is essential. This activity can help you begin to think of what can be done and prevent your worrying about things that cannot be changed. If this approach does not feel right for you, you may need to consider something else that is more suited for your personality. Remember, within all areas of mental health, there are no *right* or *wrong* ways, just those that are *healthful* for your life.

As discussed in this and previous chapters, it is important to establish a balance in your life. Certainly, you would not be human if you did not worry about difficulties you or those you care about were facing. However, too much worry can immobilize you and keep you from being mentally healthy. Thus, it is advantageous to consider what can be done about a situation rather than to expend energy on things that cannot be controlled.

It seems that the most important theme in mental health is your ability to control yourself, which can occur only if you thoroughly understand what mental health *is* for you. This is not a simple process. It often involves trial and error, as well as experiencing *happy* and *sad, good* and *bad,* and *comfortable* and *uncomfortable.* The following story illustrates this:

One day, a young boy approached a wise old woman who was cradling a cocoon. The boy was quite curious and asked the woman what she was holding. The wise woman responded that she was holding a cocoon that would soon become a beautiful butterfly. The cocoon was vibrating, which captivated the boy's curiosity. After a while, the boy asked if he could hold the cocoon. The wise woman said "yes," but explained that he could not help the butterfly out of the cocoon once the outer wall broke open. She further explained that he could not pull the cocoon apart or in any way assist the butterfly in breaking free. The boy promised, and the wise woman handed the vibrating cocoon to the boy.

The following day, the boy was amazed to see a colorful butterfly attempting to break free from its shelter. The boy watched as the butterfly struggled. He watched the cocoon shake with the effort of the emerging butterfly. However, after watching this for what seemed to be a long time, the boy began to feel sorry for the butterfly and wanted to help. He remembered what the wise woman had said but did not feel a little help would hurt. Besides, he hated to see the butterfly struggle. Thus, the boy slowly pulled the cocoon apart and with amazement watched the butterfly emerge from its shell. The butterfly flapped its wings for a moment and began flying but then slowly fell to the ground and died.

Not knowing what he had done, the young boy visited the wise woman and explained what had happened. The wise woman shook her head and slowly explained. She said, "The reason it takes a while for the butterfly to emerge is that it cannot come out of its cocoon until its wings are strong enough for it to fly. The butterfly flaps its wings against the inner wall of the cocoon until its wings are strong enough for the butterfly to emerge and carry its body. Although our intentions are to help . . . we must allow the butterfly to fly when it is ready. Only he knows. . . ."

Many people struggle from time to time with various issues related to mental health. It is nice to have others help them through their difficulties, and at times it is necessary. However, if people become accustomed to others' help, then they do not struggle and become stronger themselves. Occasionally, it is even necessary to take a step backward in order to take two or three steps forward. In fact, these struggles offered the greatest opportunity for growth. Thomas Jefferson once said, "In order to experience growth, one must undergo dramatic change from time to time."

Understand that, in determining readiness, it is important to focus on the reality of the goals that are being attempted. If the task is too great, it steps away from being a hope for the future and, instead, becomes a frustration of the present. "The optimal state of inner experience is one in which there is *order in consciousness*." This happens when psychic energy, or attention, is invested in realistic goals and when skills match opportunities for action (Csikszentmihalyi, 1990). Worry stems from being overloaded or expecting too much. To make a concern controllable, moderate your level of expectation.

This is not to say that you should water down a dream. Do not lower expectations; just break those big dreams into smaller, more realistic goals. Once these tasks are in a more manageable form, it makes the pursuit of their completion less of a headache and more of a joy. "The pursuit of a goal brings order in awareness because a person must concentrate attention on the task at hand and momentarily forget everything else. These periods of struggling to overcome challenges are what people find to be most enjoyable times in their lives. A person who has achieved control over psychic energy and who has invested it in consciously chosen goals cannot help but grow into a more complex being" (Csikszentmihalyi, 1990).

Summary

This chapter's purpose is to bring the previous chapters together in a way that is useful to you, the reader. The central theme is one that puts the control of your life into your own hands. The aim of this text has been to inform you and educate you regarding the field of mental health and to provide you with solid information regarding the topics in daily life that are most important to everyone. Its purpose has also been to give you the tools to create change in your own life by making choices that affect you in a positive way.

The first associated mental health issue is to realize that *mental health* is multifaceted and the focus and emphasis varies from person to person. The second is to realize the powerful effect your day-to-day choices have on your mental health and emotional well-being. The third is to understand the importance of self-assessment in the mental health field. The value of clear and effective communication, both verbal and nonverbal, cannot be overemphasized. Most importantly, realize that you have the ability to affect your mental attitude, your choices, whether or not you choose to be an optimist or a pessimist, how much your worries and stressors affect your life, and how you feel about yourself.

DISCUSSION QUESTIONS

1. After reading this text, what does mental health mean to *you?* What parts of the definitions presented ring true to you, and what parts seem less important? Why?

2. To help you answer the preceding question, rank the following items from most important to least important for you. Ask yourself where you need to work and where you are satisfied with yourself.
   Emotions
   Self-esteem
   Communication
   Stress management
   Spiritual well-being
   Happiness
   Goals

3. Are you an optimist or a pessimist? How does this characteristic of your personality affect your day-to-day life positively or negatively?

4. How do you feel about mental health treatment? If you thought you needed help, what type of treatment would you seek? Do you feel differently when you apply these questions to other people than when you apply them to yourself?

5. What traits do you possess that you like the most? The least? How could you change these?

6. Are you a clear communicator, both verbally and nonverbally? Identify a situation in your life that was affected in a negative way because of unclear communication. How could you have communicated differently?

7. Complete the activity discussed in the section, *Controlling Worries*. List all the things that worry you, and decide if they are situations you can control. If so, what can you do?

   a. _____
   b. _____
   c. _____
   d. _____
   e. _____
   f. _____
   g. _____
   h. _____
   i. _____
   j. _____

8. Can you identify a situation in your life that is requiring you to "take one step back to take two steps forward?" How do you feel about this? Does it frustrate you, or can you see the need for the setbacks you are experiencing?

9. Carefully consider how the people in your life support you. Do you associate with more people that support you in a positive way than in a negative way? Identifying the way people influence you can help you to make better judgments concerning your relationships.

10. Decide what one thing you can take away from this text, and put it into practice. Make a wholehearted attempt to take control of your life and how you react to situations. Whether this means becoming better at managing stress, developing higher self-esteem, becoming a better communicator, or something else, decide that you will stop thinking about it and take action.

REFERENCES

Csikszentmihalyi, M. (1990). *Flow: The Psychology of Optimal Experience.* New York: Harper & Row.

Helmstetter, S. (1986). *What We Say When We Talk to Ourselves.* New York: Simon and Schuster.

Mental Health: A Report of the Surgeon General [On-line]. (1999). Available: http://www.surgeon-general.gov/library.mentalhealth/toc.html

Seligman M. (1990). *Learned Optimism.* New York: Alfred A. Knopf.

Seligman, M. (1995). *The Optimistic Child.* New York: Houghton Mifflin.

Peale, N. (1952). *The Power of Positive Thinking,* New York: Prentice Hall.

INDEX